SEVENTH EDITION

CONCEPTS IN CLINICAL PHARMACOKINETICS

Robin L. Southwood, PharmD, BC-ADM, CDE
Clinical Associate Professor
College of Pharmacy
University of Georgia
Athens, Georgia

Virginia H. Fleming, PharmD, BCPS
Clinical Assistant Professor
College of Pharmacy
University of Georgia
Athens, Georgia

Gary Huckaby, PharmD
Clinical Director of Pharmacy Services
St. Mary's Health Care System
Athens, Georgia

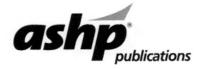

ashp publications

Any correspondence regarding this publication should be sent to the publisher, American Society of Health-System Pharmacists, 4500 East-West Highway, Suite 900, Bethesda, MD 20814, attention: Special Publishing.

The information presented herein reflects the opinions of the contributors and advisors. It should not be interpreted as an official policy of ASHP or as an endorsement of any product.

Because of ongoing research and improvements in technology, the information and its applications contained in this text are constantly evolving and are subject to the professional judgment and interpretation of the practitioner due to the uniqueness of a clinical situation. The editors and ASHP have made reasonable efforts to ensure the accuracy and appropriateness of the information presented in this document. However, any user of this information is advised that the editors and ASHP are not responsible for the continued currency of the information, for any errors or omissions, and/or for any consequences arising from the use of the information in the document in any and all practice settings. Any reader of this document is cautioned that ASHP makes no representation, guarantee, or warranty, express or implied, as to the accuracy and appropriateness of the information contained in this document and specifically disclaims any liability to any party for the accuracy and/or completeness of the material or for any damages arising out of the use or non-use of any of the information contained in this document.

Editorial Project Manager, Books and eLearning Courses: Ruth Bloom

Editorial Project Manager, Publications Production Center: Kristin Eckles

Production Manager: Johnna Hershey

Cover and Page Design: David Wade

Library of Congress Cataloging-in-Publication Data

Names: Southwood, Robin, author. | Fleming, Virginia H., author. | Huckaby, Gary, author. | Preceded by (work): Spruill, William J.

Concepts in clinical pharmacokinetics. | American Society of Health-System Pharmacists, issuing body.

Title: Concepts in clinical pharmacokinetics / Robin Southwood, Virginia H. Fleming, Gary Huckaby.

Description: Seventh edition. | Bethesda, MD : ASHP, [2018] | Preceded by

Concepts in clinical pharmacokinetics / William J. Spruill, William E. Wade, Joseph T. DiPiro, Robert A. Blouin, Jane M. Pruemer. Sixth edition.

2014. | Includes bibliographical references and index.

Identifiers: LCCN 2018006511 | ISBN 9781585285914 (pbk.)

Subjects: | MESH: Pharmacokinetics | Pharmaceutical

Preparations—administration & dosage | Problems and Exercises

Classification: LCC RM301.5 | NLM QV 18.2 | DDC 615/.7—dc23 LC record available at https://lccn.loc.gov/2018006511

ISBN: 978-1-58528-591-4

Printed in Canada

10 9 8 7 6 5 4 3 2 1

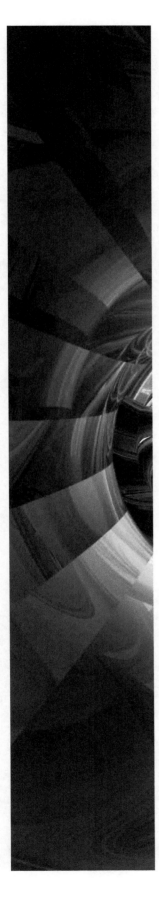

Table of Contents

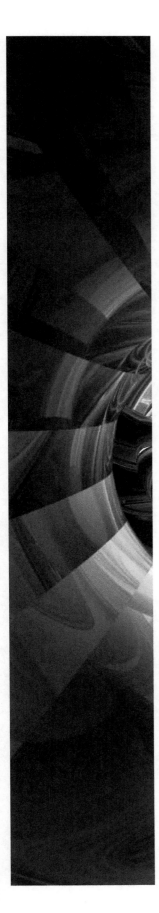

Preface

The term *pharmacokinetics* can evoke a variety of responses. For some, it is the difficult course with complex equations. For others, it is the beautiful science of how the medications move though the human body. And for others, it is an opportunity to enhance patient care through patient-specific dosing. Still others see pharmacokinetics as an area of review for licensure or specialty exam content.

The seventh edition of *Concepts in Clinical Pharmacokinetics* is a combination of new and old. What remains fundamental in this edition is the successful strategy of presenting pharmacokinetic modeling principles in a step-by-step process utilizing defined lessons that explain concepts in straightforward terms and illustrate the concepts through examples within each lesson. Self-assessment opportunities are offered as via in-lesson examples and end-of-lesson practice problems with correct answers provided. The aim of this edition is to provide content in a manner that facilitates learning for students who are introduced to the pharmacokinetic concepts for the first time and/or as a review for practitioners moving from one practice specialty to another. In addition, the review of the concepts is useful for those preparing for board exams or specialty certification exams.

The following have been updated in the seventh edition:

- Assessment of renal function and dosing of aminoglycoside and vancomycin antibiotics

- Content in other chapters with new figures to demonstrate learning points

- All in-lesson and end-of-lesson questions

Pharmacokinetic concepts are further illustrated by application to clinical dosing cases, including aminoglycosides, vancomycin, theophylline, digoxin, and phenytoin. These cases are designed to show the easily understandable, step-by-step approach for performing appropriate clinical dosing calculations. All cases provide the complete mathematical solutions for each calculation, allowing readers to "check their math." Equations are explained in detail, and all similar equations used throughout the text are cross-referenced to the basic concept. There is also a valuable appendix containing basic and drug-specific pharmacokinetic equations.

The goal for this edition, as with the previous six editions, remains the same—to provide the student or practitioner with the concepts and clinical applications needed for a better understanding of this complicated, yet still vital, subject.

Robin L. Southwood
Virginia H. Fleming
Gary Huckaby
August 2018

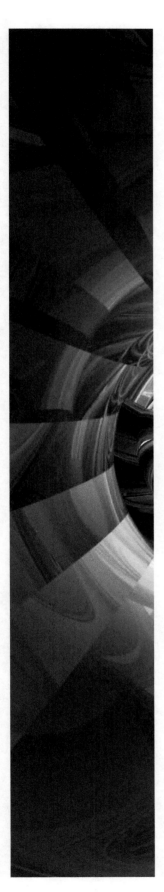

Acknowledgments

We are indebted to our colleagues and mentors Bill Spruill, Joe DiPiro, and the late Bill Wade, for the opportunity to prepare the seventh edition of *Concepts in Clinical Pharmacokinetics.*

A Note from the Authors on Using This Edition

The seventh edition continues the strategy of teaching basic pharmacokinetic concepts, mathematical models, and clinical application principles needed to determine values such as dose, interval, steady-state concentration, half-life, etc. Specific conceptual and mathematical formulas are combined to solve more complex dosing situations. Eleven lessons contain a practice quiz to chart your progress, and there are three separate practice sets of questions with answers. The last four lessons are completely devoted to clinical cases that fully explain, step-by-step, how to dose multiple drugs that generally require serum drug concentration monitoring. This edition has all new problems in each lesson. Content in the aminoglycoside and vancomycin lessons have been updated.

We strongly encourage you to attempt to solve these cases without looking at the step-by-step explanations, and then when finished, check your answers against the key. We wish you much success in your endeavors and hope you enjoy the book!

Robin L. Southwood
Virginia H. Fleming
Gary Huckaby

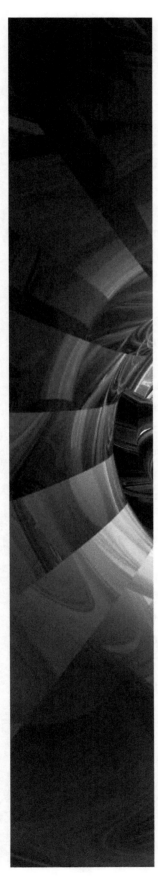

$\boldsymbol{\alpha}$:   distribution rate constant for two-compartment model

AUC :   area under plasma drug concentration versus time curve

AUMC :   area under the (drug concentration × time) versus time (moment) curve

$\boldsymbol{\beta}$:   terminal elimination rate constant

C :   concentration

$\overline{C}$	average steady-state concentration
C_0, C_1, C_2	initial (just after infusion), first, second concentrations
C_{in}	concentration in blood on entering organ
C_{last}	last measured concentration
C_{max}	maximum concentration
C_{max1}, C_{max2}	first, second maximum concentrations
$C_{ss\,max}$	steady-state maximum concentration
$C_{ss\,min}$	steady-state minimum concentration
C_{min}	minimum concentration
C_{out}	concentration in blood on leaving organ
C_{peak}	peak concentration
C_{ss}	steady-state concentration
C_t	concentration at time t
C_{trough}	trough concentration

Cl :   clearance

Cl_b	biliary clearance
Cl_h	hepatic (liver) clearance
Cl_i	intrinsic clearance
Cl_m	clearance by metabolism (mainly liver)
$Cl_{other\ organs}$	clearance by other organs
$Cl_{P \rightarrow mX}$	formation clearance for a given metabolite X
$Cl_{P \rightarrow m\,1}$	fractional clearance of parent drug (P) to form metabolite 1 (m_1)
Cl_r	renal clearance
Cl_t	total body clearance

conc :   concentration

$\boldsymbol{\Delta}$:   change in

$\boldsymbol{E}$:   extraction ratio

continued on next page

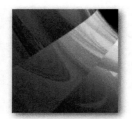

e : base of natural logarithm

F : fraction of drug absorbed that reaches systemic circulation (bioavailability)

    F_{m1} fraction of m_1 formed from a single dose of the parent drug

    F_p fraction of unbound drug in plasma

    F_t fraction of unbound drug in tissue

GFR : glomerular filtration rate

GI : gastrointestinal

K : elimination rate constant

    K_0 rate of drug infusion

    K_{12} rate constant for transfer of drug from compartment 1 to compartment 2

    K_{21} rate constant for transfer of drug from compartment 2 to compartment 1

    K_a absorption rate constant

    K_m Michaelis–Menten constant (drug concentration at which elimination rate = ½ Vmax)

λ : terminal elimination rate constant

m_1, m_2, m_3 : metabolites 1, 2, and 3

$m_{1,u}, m_{2,u}, m_{3,u}$: amount of m_1, m_2, or m_3 excreted in the urine

MRT : mean residence time

n : number of doses

Q : bloodflow

    Q_h hepatic bloodflow

S : salt form of drug

SST : serum separator tube

τ : dosing interval

t : time (after dose)

    t' time after end of infusion ($t' = \tau - t$ for trough concentration)

    t'' time (duration) of loading infusion

    t_0 time zero

    $T½$ half-life

    $t_{90\%}$ time required to reach 90% of steady-state concentration

V : volume; volume of distribution

    V_{area} volume of distribution by area

    V_c volume of central compartment

    V_{extrap} extrapolated volume of distribution

    V_p plasma volume

    V_{ss} steady-state volume of distribution

    V_t tissue volume

    V_{max} maximum rate of the elimination process

X : amount of drug

    X_0 dose (or initial dose) of drug

    X_1, X_2 amount of drug at different times

    X_c amount of drug in central compartment

    X_d daily dose of drug

    X_p amount of drug in peripheral compartment

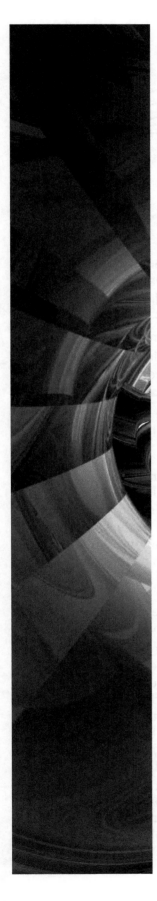

Introduction to Pharmacokinetics and Pharmacodynamics

OBJECTIVES

After completing Lesson 1, you should be able to:

1. Define and differentiate between *pharmacokinetics* and *clinical pharmacokinetics*.

2. Define *pharmacodynamics* and relate it to pharmacokinetics.

3. Describe the concept of the *therapeutic concentration range*.

4. Identify factors that cause interpatient variability in drug disposition and drug response.

5. Describe situations in which routine clinical pharmacokinetic monitoring would be advantageous.

6. List the assumptions made about drug distribution patterns in both one- and two-compartment models.

7. Represent graphically the typical natural log of plasma drug concentration versus time curve for a one-compartment model after an intravenous (IV) dose.

Pharmacokinetics is currently defined as the study of the time course of drug absorption, distribution, metabolism, and excretion. *Clinical pharmacokinetics* is the application of pharmacokinetic principles to the safe and effective therapeutic management of drugs in an individual patient.

Primary goals of clinical pharmacokinetics include enhancing efficacy and decreasing toxicity of a patient's drug therapy. Other uses include assessment of adherence and indirect assessment of organ function. The development of strong correlations between drug concentrations and their pharmacologic responses has enabled clinicians to apply pharmacokinetic principles to actual patient situations.

A drug's effect is often related to its concentration at the site of action, so it would be useful to monitor this concentration. Receptor sites of drugs are generally inaccessible to our observations or are widely distributed in the body; therefore, direct measurement of drug concentrations at these sites is not practical. For example, the receptor sites for digoxin are thought to be within the myocardium. Obviously we cannot directly sample drug concentration in this tissue. However, we can measure drug concentration in the blood or plasma, urine, saliva, and other easily sampled fluids (**Figure 1-1**). *Kinetic homogeneity* describes the predictable relationship between plasma drug concentration and concentration at the receptor site where a given drug produces its therapeutic effect (**Figure 1-2**). Changes in the plasma drug concentration reflect changes in drug concentrations

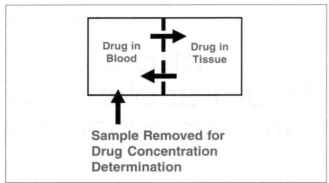

FIGURE 1-1.
Blood is the fluid most often sampled for drug concentration determination.

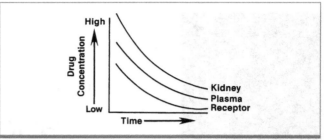

FIGURE 1-3.
Drug concentration versus time.

at the receptor site, as well as in other tissues. As the concentration of drug in plasma increases, the concentration of drug in most tissues will increase proportionally.

Similarly, if the plasma concentration of a drug is decreasing, the concentration in tissues will also decrease. **Figure 1-3** is a simplified plot of the drug concentration versus time profile after an IV drug dose and illustrates this concept.

The property of kinetic homogeneity is important for the assumptions made in clinical pharmacokinetics. It is the foundation on which all therapeutic and toxic plasma drug concentrations are established. That is, when studying concentrations of a drug in plasma, we assume that these plasma concentrations directly relate to concentrations in tissues where the disease process is to be modified by the drug (e.g., the central nervous system in Parkinson's disease or bone in osteomyelitis). This assumption, however, may not be true for all drugs.

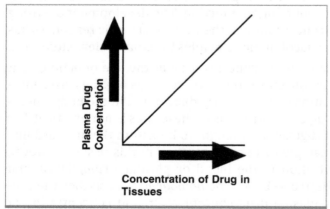

FIGURE 1-2.
Relationship of plasma to tissue drug concentrations.

Clinical Correlate

Drugs concentrate in some tissues because of physical (such as molecular size or weight) or chemical (such as lipophilicity/hydrophilicity or ionization) properties. Examples include digoxin, which concentrates in the myocardium, and lipid-soluble drugs, such as benzodiazepines, which concentrate in fat.

Basic Pharmacodynamic Concepts

Pharmacodynamics refers to the relationship between drug concentration at the site of action and the resulting effect, including the time course and intensity of therapeutic and adverse effects. The effect of a drug present at the site of action is determined by that drug's binding with a receptor. Receptors may be present on neurons in the central nervous system (i.e., opiate receptors) to depress pain sensation, on cardiac muscle to affect the intensity of contraction, or even within bacteria to disrupt maintenance of the bacterial cell wall.

For most drugs, the concentration at the site of the receptor determines the intensity of a drug's effect (**Figure 1-4**). However, other factors affect drug response as well. The density of receptors on the cell surface, the mechanism by which a signal is transmitted into the cell by second messengers (substances within the cell), or the regulatory factors that control gene translation and protein production may influence drug effect. This multilevel regulation results in variation of sensitivity to drug effect from one individual to another and also determines enhancement of, or tolerance to, drug effects that can result in intrapatient variation.

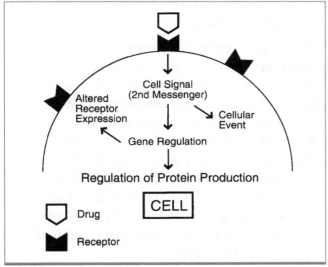

FIGURE 1-4.
Relationship of drug concentration to drug effect at the receptor site.

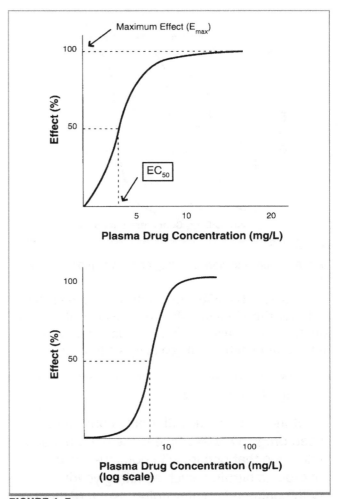

FIGURE 1-5.
Relationship of drug concentration at the receptor site to effect (as a percentage of maximal effect).

In the simplest examples of drug effect, there is a relationship between the concentration of drug at the receptor site and the pharmacologic effect. If enough concentrations are tested, a maximum effect (E_{max}) can be determined (**Figure 1-5**). When the logarithm of concentration is plotted versus effect (Figure 1-5), one can see that there is a concentration below which no effect is observed and a concentration above which no greater effect is achieved.

One way of comparing *drug potency* is by the concentration at which 50% of the maximum effect is achieved. This is referred to as the *50% effective concentration* or *EC_{50}*. When two drugs are tested in the same individual, the drug with a lower EC_{50} would be considered more potent. This means that a lesser amount of a more potent drug is needed to achieve the same effect as a less potent drug.

The EC_{50} does not, however, indicate other important determinants of drug response, such as the duration of effect. Duration of effect is determined by a complex set of factors, including the time that a drug is engaged on the receptor as well as intracellular signaling and gene regulation.

For some drugs, the effectiveness can decrease with continued use. This is referred to as *tolerance*. Tolerance may be caused by pharmacokinetic factors, such as increased drug metabolism, that decrease the concentrations achieved with a given dose. There can also be pharmacodynamic tolerance, which occurs when the same concentration at the receptor site results in a reduced effect with repeated exposure. An example of drug tolerance is the use of opiates in the management of chronic pain. It is not uncommon to find these patients requiring increased doses of the opiate over time. Tolerance can be described in terms of the dose-response curve, as shown in **Figure 1-6**. When tolerance occurs, efficacy may be regained by increasing drug dose. Drug-free intervals do not usually restore efficacy. Tachyphylaxis is a form of tolerance that occurs rapidly and is unique because loss of efficacy does not respond to dose increases but does return with drug-free intervals.

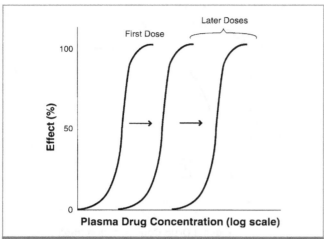

FIGURE 1-6.
Demonstration of tolerance to drug effect with repeated dosing.

To assess the effect that a drug regimen is likely to have, the clinician should consider pharmacokinetic and pharmacodynamic factors. Both are important in determining a drug's effect.

Clinical Correlate

Tolerance can occur with many commonly used drugs. One example is the hemodynamic tolerance that occurs with continued use of organic nitrates, such as nitroglycerin. With continued uninterrupted use, the effect of this drug is reduced. Nitrates exhibit tachyphylaxis, a tolerance that can be reversed by interspersing drug-free intervals during chronic drug use. Another example of tolerance occurs with narcotic analgesics. With chronic continual use, receptors are downgraded so that higher doses of the drugs are required to achieve the same level of analgesia. Tolerance may also occur with side effects of certain drugs so that when titrated slowly over time, the patient is able to tolerate higher doses of the drug without being limited by unpleasant or burdensome side effects. These types of tolerance are referred to as *physiologic tolerance,* which should be differentiated from *psychological dependence* in which the patient believes strongly that they need a drug and feel anxiety when separated from the drug.

Clinical Correlate

One way to compare potency between two drugs that are in the same pharmacologic class is to compare EC_{50}. The drug with a lower EC_{50} is considered more potent. The potency of a drug, however, does not necessarily determine which drug is "better" than another. It correlates to the amount of drug (dose) needed to achieve a desired effect, which may be larger than one drug than for another, but as long as equipotent doses of the two agents are given, a similar effect should be seen.

Therapeutic Drug Monitoring

Therapeutic drug monitoring is defined as the use of assay procedures for determination of drug concentrations in plasma, and the interpretation and application of the resulting concentration data to develop safe and effective drug regimens. If performed properly, this process allows for the achievement of therapeutic concentrations of a drug more rapidly and safely than can be attained with empiric dose changes. Together with observations of the drug's clinical effects, it should provide the safest approach to optimal drug therapy.

The usefulness of plasma drug concentration data is based on the concept that pharmacologic response is closely related to drug concentration at the site of action. For certain drugs, studies in patients have provided information on the plasma concentration range that is safe and effective in treating specific diseases: the therapeutic range (**Figure 1-7**). Within this therapeutic range, the desired effects of the drug are observed. Below it, there is greater probability that the therapeutic benefits are not realized; above it, toxic effects may occur.

No absolute boundaries divide subtherapeutic, therapeutic, and toxic drug concentrations. A gray area usually exists for most drugs in which these concentrations overlap due to variability in individual patient response. Numerous pharmacokinetic characteristics of a drug may result in variability in the plasma concentration achieved with a given dose when administered to various patients

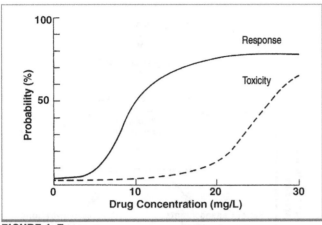

FIGURE 1-7.

Relationship between drug concentration and drug effects for a hypothetical drug.

Source: Adapted with permission from Evans WE, ed. General principles of applied pharmacokinetics. In: *Applied Pharmacokinetics.* 3rd ed. Vancouver, WA: Applied Therapeutics; 1992:1–3.

(**Figure 1-8**). This interpatient variability is primarily attributed to one or more of the following:

- Variations in drug absorption
- Variations in drug distribution
  - Including variation in protein binding
- Differences in an individual's ability to metabolize and eliminate the drug (e.g., genetics)
- Disease states (renal or hepatic insufficiency) or physiologic states (e.g., extremes of age, obesity, sepsis/distributive shock of critical illness) that alter drug absorption, distribution, or elimination
- Drug interactions

Therapeutic monitoring using drug concentration data is valuable when the following occurs:

- A good correlation exists between the pharmacologic response and plasma concentration. Over at least a limited concentration range, the intensity of pharmacologic effects should increase with plasma concentration. This relationship allows us to predict pharmacologic effects with changing plasma drug concentrations (**Figure 1-9**).
- Wide intersubject variation in plasma drug concentrations results from a given dose.
- The drug has a narrow therapeutic index (i.e., the therapeutic concentration is close to the toxic concentration).
- The drug's desired pharmacologic effects cannot be assessed readily by other simple means (e.g., blood pressure measurement for antihypertensives).

The value of therapeutic drug monitoring is limited in situations as follows:

- There is no well-defined therapeutic plasma concentration range.
- The formation of pharmacologically active metabolites of a drug complicates the application of plasma drug concentration data to clinical effect unless metabolite concentrations are also considered.
- Toxic effects may occur at unexpectedly low drug concentrations as well as at high concentrations (i.e., side effects of concern are *not* dose related).
- There are no significant consequences associated with too high or too low levels.

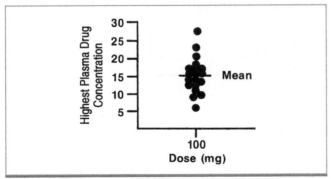

FIGURE 1-8.

Example of variability in plasma drug concentration among subjects given the same drug dose.

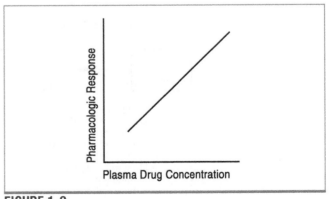

FIGURE 1-9.

When pharmacologic effects relate to plasma drug concentrations, the latter can be used to predict the former.

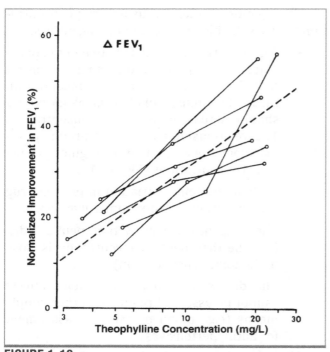

FIGURE 1-10.
Relationship between plasma theophylline concentration and change in forced expiratory volume (FEV) in asthmatic patients.

Source: Reproduced with permission from Mitenko PA, Ogilvie RI. Rational intravenous doses of theophylline. *N Engl J Med.* 1973;289:600–3. Copyright ©1973, Massachusetts Medical Society.

Theophylline is an excellent example of a drug in which significant interpatient variability in pharmacokinetic properties exists. This is important from a clinical standpoint as subtle changes in serum concentrations may result in marked changes in drug response. **Figure 1-10** shows the relationship between theophylline concentration (*x*-axis,

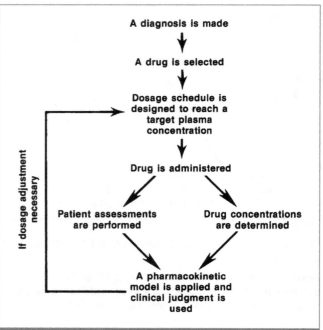

FIGURE 1-11.
Process for reaching dosage decisions with therapeutic drug monitoring.

on a logarithmic scale) and its pharmacologic effect (changes in pulmonary function [*y*-axis]). This figure illustrates that as the concentration of theophylline increases, so does the intensity of the response for some patients. Wide interpatient variability is also shown.

Figure 1-11 outlines the process clinicians may choose to follow in making drug dosing decisions by using therapeutic drug monitoring. **Figure 1-12** shows the relationship of pharmacokinetic and pharmacodynamic factors.

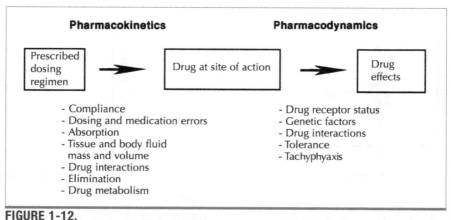

FIGURE 1-12.
Relationship of pharmacokinetics and pharmacodynamics and factors that affect each.

TABLE 1-1. Therapeutic Ranges for Commonly Used Drugs

Drug	Range
Digoxin	0.5–2 ng/mL
Lidocaine	1.5–5 mg/L
Lithium	0.6–1.4 mEq/L
Phenobarbital	15–40 mg/L
Phenytoin (total)	10–20 mg/L
Quinidine	2–5 mg/L
Cyclosporine	150–400 ng/mL
Valproic acid	50–100 mg/L
Carbamazepine	4–12 mcg/L
Ethosuximide	40–100 mg/L
Primidone	5–12 mg/L

Source: Adapted with permission from Bauer LA. Clinical pharmacokinetics and pharmacodynamics. In: DiPiro JT, Talbert RL, Yee GC, et al., eds. *Pharmacotherapy: a Pathophysiologic Approach.* 8th ed. New York, NY: McGraw-Hill. http://Accesspharmacy.com.

Examples of therapeutic ranges for commonly used drugs are shown in **Table 1-1**. As can be seen in this table, most drug concentrations are expressed as a unit of mass per volume.

Clinical Correlate

A drug's effect may also be determined by the amount of time that the drug is present at the site of action. An example is with beta-lactam antimicrobials. The rate of bacterial killing by beta-lactams is usually determined by the length of time that the drug concentration remains above the minimal concentration that inhibits bacterial growth (MIC) at the site of action (the bacterial cell wall). This is because for beta-lactams to inhibit cell wall synthesis, drug must be present for periods of time when the cell is actively dividing and growing—so time at the site of action is the most important determinant of efficacy (assuming the concentration is above the MIC). The pharmacokinetic term for this is *T>MIC* (or *time over the MIC*) and it is the parameter used to determine the best dosing strategy for beta-lactams to achieve appropriate bacterial killing.

Pharmacokinetic Models

The handling of a drug by the body can be very complex, as several processes (such as absorption, distribution, metabolism, and elimination) work to alter drug concentrations in tissues and fluids. Simplifications of body processes are necessary to predict a drug's behavior in the body. One way to make these simplifications is to apply mathematical principles to the various processes.

To apply mathematical principles, a model of the body must be selected. A basic type of model used in pharmacokinetics is the *compartmental model,* which is categorized by the number of compartments needed to describe the drug's behavior in the body. There are one-compartment, two-compartment, and multicompartment models. The compartments do not represent a specific tissue or fluid but may represent a group of similar tissues or fluids. These models can be used to predict the time course of drug concentrations in the body (**Figure 1-13**).

Compartmental models are termed *deterministic* because the observed drug concentrations determine the type of compartmental model required to describe the pharmacokinetics of the drug. This concept will become evident when we examine one- and two-compartment models.

To construct a compartmental model as a representation of the body, simplifications of body structures are made. Organs and tissues in which drug distribution is similar are grouped into one compartment. For example, distribution into adipose tissue differs from distribution into renal tissue for most drugs. Therefore, these tissues may be in different compartments. The highly perfused organs (e.g., heart, liver, and kidneys) often have similar drug distribution patterns, so these areas may be considered as one compartment. The compartment that includes blood (plasma), heart, lungs,

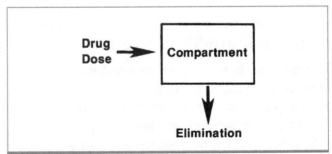

FIGURE 1-13.
Simple compartmental model.

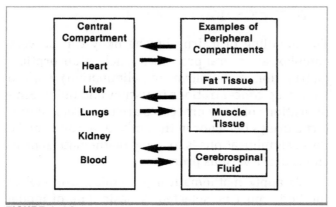

FIGURE 1-14.
Typical organ groups for central and peripheral compartments.

liver, and kidneys is usually referred to as the *central compartment* or the *highly blood-perfused compartment* (**Figure 1-14**). The other compartment that includes fat tissue, muscle tissue, and cerebrospinal fluid is the peripheral compartment, which is less well perfused than the central compartment.

Another simplification of body processes concerns the expression of changes in the amount of drug in the body over time. These changes with time are known as *rates*. The *elimination rate* describes the change in the amount of drug in the body due to drug elimination over time. Most pharmacokinetic models assume that elimination does not change over time.

The value of any model is determined by how well it predicts drug concentrations in fluids and tissues. Generally, it is best to use the simplest model that accurately predicts changes in drug concentrations over time. If a one-compartment model is sufficient to predict plasma drug concentrations (and those concentrations are of most interest to us), then a more complex (two-compartment or more) model is not needed. However, more complex models are often required to predict tissue drug concentrations.

Clinical Correlate

Drugs that do not extensively distribute into extravascular tissues, such as aminoglycosides, are generally well described by one-compartment models. Extent of distribution is partly determined by the chemistry of the agents. Aminoglycosides

are polar molecules, so their distribution is limited primarily to extracellular water. Drugs extensively distributed in tissue (such as lipophilic drugs like the benzodiazepines) or that have extensive intracellular uptake may be better described by the more complex models.

Compartmental Models

The one-compartment model is the most frequently used model in clinical practice. In structuring the model, a visual representation is helpful. The compartment is represented by an enclosed square or rectangle, and rates of drug transfer are represented by straight arrows (**Figure 1-15**). The arrow pointing into the box simply indicates that drug is put into that compartment; the arrow pointing out of the box indicates that drug is leaving the compartment.

This model is the simplest because there is only one compartment. All body tissues and fluids are considered a part of this compartment. Furthermore, it is assumed that after a dose of drug is administered, it distributes instantaneously to all body areas. Common abbreviations are shown in Figure 1-15.

Some drugs do not distribute instantaneously to all parts of the body even after IV bolus administration; therefore, consideration must be given to optimal time for sampling serum drug concentrations. *IV bolus dosing* means administering a dose of drug over a very short time period. A common distribution pattern is for the drug to distribute rapidly in the bloodstream and to the highly perfused organs, such as the liver and kidneys. Then, at a slower rate, the drug distributes to other body tissues. This pattern of drug distribution may be represented by a two-compartment model. Drug

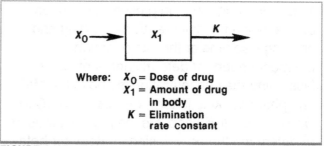

Where: X_0 = Dose of drug
X_1 = Amount of drug in body
K = Elimination rate constant

FIGURE 1-15.
One-compartment model.

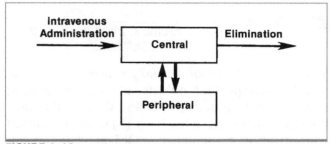

FIGURE 1-16.
Compartmental model representing transfer of drug to and from central and peripheral compartments.

moves back and forth between these compartments to maintain equilibrium (**Figure 1-16**).

Figure 1-17 simplifies the difference between one- and two-compartment models. Again, the one-compartment model assumes that the drug

is distributed to tissues very rapidly after IV administration.

The two-compartment model can be represented as in **Figure 1-18**, where

X_0 = dose of drug

X_1 = amount of drug in central compartment

X_2 = amount of drug in peripheral compartment

K = elimination rate constant of drug from central compartment to outside the body

K_{12} = elimination rate constant of drug from central compartment to peripheral compartment

K_{21} = elimination rate constant of drug from peripheral compartment to central compartment

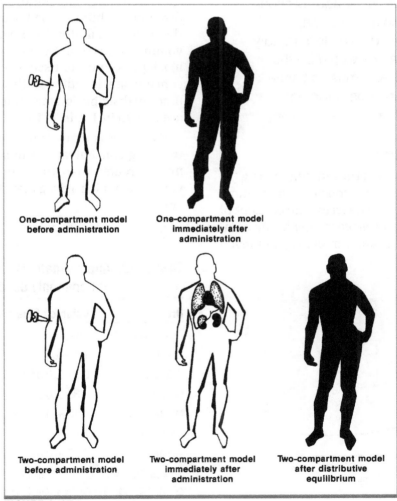

One-compartment model before administration

One-compartment model immediately after administration

Two-compartment model before administration

Two-compartment model immediately after administration

Two-compartment model after distributive equilibrium

FIGURE 1-17.
Drug distribution in one- and two-compartment models.

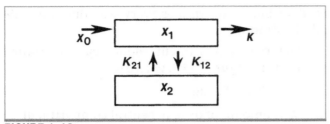

FIGURE 1-18.
Two-compartment model.

Clinical Correlate

Digoxin, particularly when given intravenously, is an example of a drug that is well described by two-compartment pharmacokinetics. After an IV dose is administered, plasma concentrations rise and then rapidly decline as drug distributes out of plasma and into muscle tissue. After equilibration between drug in tissue and plasma, plasma concentrations decline less rapidly (**Figure 1-19**). The plasma would be the central compartment, and muscle tissue would be the peripheral compartment.

Volume of Distribution

Until now, we have spoken of the amount of drug (X) in a compartment. If we also consider the volume of the compartment, we can describe the concept of drug concentration. *Drug concentration* in the compartment is defined as the amount of drug in a given volume, such as mg/L:

$$\boxed{\text{1-1}} \quad \text{concentration} = \frac{\text{amount of drug in body}}{\substack{\text{volume in which drug} \\ \text{is distributed}}} = \frac{X}{V}$$

Volume of distribution (usually expressed as V, Vd, or V_D) is an important indicator of the extent of drug distribution into body fluids and tissues. V relates the amount of drug in the body (X) to the measured concentration in the plasma (C). Thus, V is the volume required to account for all of the drug in the body if the concentrations in all tissues are the same as the plasma concentration:

$$\text{volume of distribution} = \frac{\text{amount of drug}}{\text{concentration}}$$

A large volume of distribution usually indicates that the drug distributes extensively into body tissues and fluids. Conversely, a small volume of distribution often indicates limited drug distribution.

Volume of distribution indicates the extent of distribution but not the tissues or fluids into which the drug distributes. Two drugs can have the same volume of distribution, but one may distribute primarily into muscle tissues, whereas the other may concentrate in adipose tissues. Approximate volumes of distribution for some commonly used drugs are shown in **Table 1-2**.

When V is many times the volume of the body, the drug concentrations in some tissues should be much greater than those in plasma. The smallest volume in which a drug may distribute is the plasma volume.

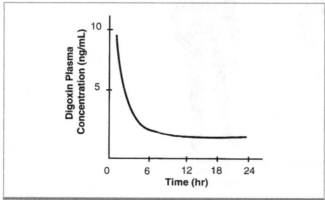

FIGURE 1-19.
Plasma concentrations of digoxin after an IV dose.

TABLE 1-2. Approximate Volumes of Distribution of Commonly Used Drugs

Drug	Volume of Distribution (L/kg)
Amlodipine	16 ± 4
Ganciclovir	1.1 ± 0.2
Ketorolac	0.21 ± 0.04
Lansoprazole	0.35 ± 0.05
Montelukast	0.15 ± 0.02
Sildenafil	1.2 ± 0.3
Valsartan	0.23 ± 0.09

Source: Brunton LL, Lazo JS, Parker KL, eds. *The Pharmacologic Basis of Therapeutics.* 11th ed. New York, NY: McGraw-Hill; 2006:1798, 1829, 1839, 1840, 1851, 1872, and 1883.

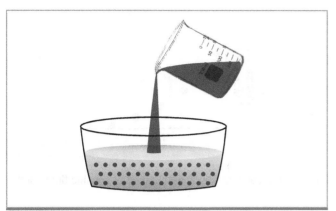

FIGURE 1-20.
The volume of a tank can be determined from the amount of substance added and the resulting concentration.

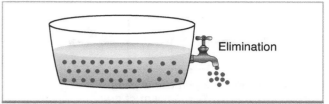

FIGURE 1-21.
Drug elimination complicates the determination of the volume of the body from drug concentrations.

To illustrate the concept of volume of distribution, let us first imagine the body as a tank filled with fluid as the body is primarily composed of water. To calculate the volume of the tank, we can place a known quantity of substance into it and then measure its concentration in the fluid (**Figure 1-20**). If the amount of substance (X) and the resulting concentration (C) is known, then the volume of distribution (V) can be calculated using the simplified equations:

$$X = VC \text{ or } C = \frac{X}{V} \text{ or } V = \frac{X}{C}$$

X = amount of drug in body

V = volume of distribution

C = concentration in the plasma

As with other pharmacokinetic parameters, volume of distribution can vary considerably from one person to another because of differences in physiology or disease states. ***Note:*** The dose of a drug (X_0) and the amount of drug in the body (X) are essentially the same thing because all of the dose goes into the body (for drugs administered intravenously or that are 100% orally bioavailable).

In this example, important assumptions have been made, such as that instantaneous distribution occurs, and it occurs equally throughout the tank. In the closed tank, there is no elimination. This example is analogous to a one-compartment model of the body after IV bolus administration. However, there is one complicating factor—during the entire time that the drug is in the body, elimination is taking place. So, if we consider the body as a tank with an open outlet valve, the concentration used to calculate the volume of the tank would be constantly changing (**Figure 1-21**).

We can use the relationship given in **Equation 1-1** for volume, amount of drug administered, and resulting concentration to estimate a drug's volume of distribution in a patient. If we give a known dose of a drug and determine the concentration of that drug achieved in the plasma, we can calculate a volume of distribution. However, the concentration used for this estimation must take into account changes resulting from drug elimination, as discussed in Lessons 3 and 9.

If 100 mg of drug X is administered intravenously and the plasma concentration is determined to be 5 mg/L just after the dose is given, then

$$\text{volume of distribution} \atop (V) = \frac{\text{dose}}{\text{resulting concentration}} = \frac{X_0}{C} = \frac{100 \text{ mg}}{5 \text{ mg/L}} = 20 \text{ L}$$

Clinical Correlate

The volume of distribution is easily approximated for many drugs. For example, if the first 80-mg dose of gentamicin is administered intravenously and results in a peak plasma concentration of 8 mg/L, volume of distribution would be calculated as follows:

$$\text{volume of distribution} \atop (V) = \frac{\text{dose}}{\text{resulting concentration}} = \frac{X_0}{C} = \frac{80 \text{ mg}}{8 \text{ mg/L}} = 10 \text{ L}$$

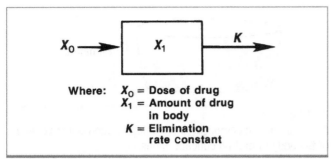

FIGURE 1-22.
One-compartment model.

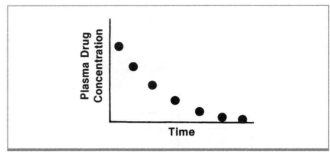

FIGURE 1-24.
Plasma drug concentrations determined at specific time points.

Clinical Correlate

Drugs that have extensive distribution outside of plasma appear to have a large volume of distribution. Examples include digoxin, diltiazem, imipramine, labetalol, metoprolol, meperidine, and nortriptyline.

Plasma Drug Concentration Versus Time Curves

With the one-compartment model (**Figure 1-22**), if we continuously measure the concentration of a drug in the plasma after an IV bolus dose and then plot these plasma drug concentrations against the times they are obtained, the curve shown in **Figure 1-23** would result. Note that this plot is a curve and that the plasma concentration is highest just after the dose is administered at time zero (t_0).

Because of cost limitations and patient convenience in clinical situations, only a small number of plasma samples are usually obtained for measuring drug concentrations (**Figure 1-24**). From these

known values, one is able to predict plasma drug concentrations at times when no samples are available (**Figure 1-25**). In clinical situations, it is rare to collect more than two samples after a dose.

The prediction of drug concentrations based on known concentrations can be subject to multiple sources of error. However, if we realize the assumptions used to make the predictions, some errors can be avoided. These assumptions are pointed out as we review the one-compartment system.

From a mathematical standpoint, the prediction of plasma concentrations is easier if we know that the concentrations are all on a straight line rather than a curve. This conversion can be accomplished for most drugs by plotting the natural logarithm (ln) of the plasma drug concentration versus time. The plot of a curve (Figure 1-25) is, in effect, converted to a straight line by using the natural log of the plasma drug concentration (**Figure 1-26**).

A straight line is obtained from the natural log of plasma drug concentration versus time plot only for drugs that follow first-order elimination processes and exhibit one-compartment distribution. *First-order elimination* occurs when the amount of

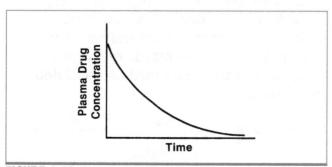

FIGURE 1-23.
Typical plasma drug concentration versus time curve for a one-compartment model.

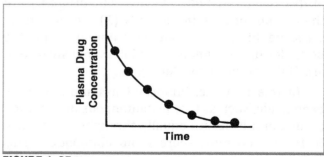

FIGURE 1-25.
Plasma drug concentrations can be predicted for times when they were not determined. Concentrations on the line drawn through the measured concentrations are predicted concentrations.

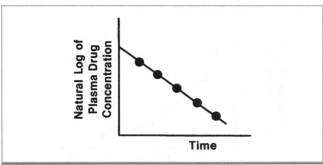

FIGURE 1-26.
With a simple one-compartment IV bolus model, a plot of the natural log of plasma concentration versus time results in a straight line.

drug eliminated from the body in a specific time is dependent on the amount of drug in the body at that time. This concept is explained further in Lesson 2.

An alternative to calculating the natural log values is to plot the actual concentration and time values on semilogarithmic (or semilog) paper (**Figure 1-27**), a special graph paper that automatically adjusts for the logarithmic relationship by altering the distance between lines on the *y*-axis. The lines on the *y*-axis are not evenly spaced but rather are logarithmically related within each log cycle (or multiple of 10). So when the actual values of plasma drug concentrations are plotted against the time values, a straight line results. The *x*-axis has evenly spaced lines; there is no logarithmic conversion of those values. (The term *semilogarithmic* indicates that only one axis is converted.) The numbers on the *y*-axis may be used to represent 0.1 through 1, 1 through 10, 10 through 100, or any series with a 10-fold difference in the range of values.

Clinical Correlate

Semilog graph paper can be found via google.com or other sites (e.g., printfreegraphpaper.com).

If a series of plasma concentration versus time points are known and plotted on semilog paper, a straight line can be drawn through the points by visual inspection or, more accurately, by linear regression techniques. *Linear regression* is a mathematical method used to determine the line that best represents a set of plotted points. From this line, we can predict plasma drug concentrations at times for which no measurements are available (**Figure 1-28**).

Clinical Correlate

For a typical patient, plasma concentrations resulting from an 80-mg dose of gentamicin may be as shown in **Table 1-3**. The plasma concentrations plotted on linear and semilogarithmic graph paper are shown in **Figure 1-29**. With the semilog paper, it is easier to predict what the gentamicin plasma concentration would be 10 hours after the dose is administered.

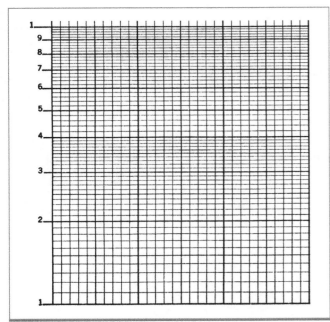

FIGURE 1-27.
Paper with one log-scale axis is called semilog paper.

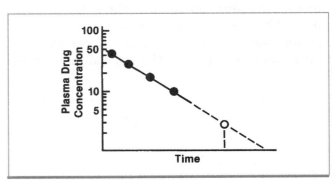

FIGURE 1-28.
When plasma concentration versus time points fall on a straight line, concentrations at various times can be predicted simply by picking a time point and matching concentration on the line at that time.

TABLE 1-3. Time Course of Plasma Gentamicin Concentration

Concentration (mg/L)	Time after Dose (hr)
6	1
4.4	2
2.4	4
0.7	8

Math Principle

The *log of a number* is the power to which a given base number must be raised to equal that number. With natural logarithms, the base is 2.718. For example, the natural logarithm of 8.0 is x, where $2.718^x = 8.0$ and $x = 2.08$. Natural logarithms are used because they relate to natural processes such as drug elimination, radioactive decay, and bacterial growth. Instead of 2.718 to indicate the base of the natural log function, the abbreviation e is used. Also, instead of writing natural logarithm of 8.0, we shall use the abbreviation *ln 8.0*.

Natural logarithms can be related to common logarithms (base 10 logarithms) as follows:

$$\log \text{base } 10 = \frac{\log \text{base } e}{2.303}$$

Using the Calculator with Natural Log and Exponential Keys

There are two major keys that will be used to calculate pharmacokinetic values from either known or estimated data. These are the *ln* key and the e^x key. Certain calculators do not have the e^x key. Instead, they will have an *ln* key and an *INV* key or a *2nd* key. Pressing the *INV* key or the *2nd* key and then the *ln* key will give e^x values. The calculators included

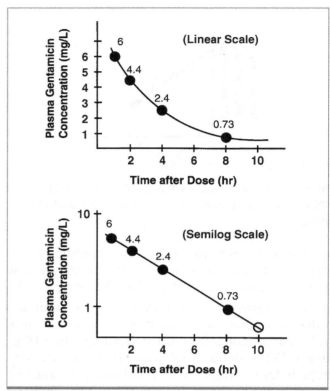

FIGURE 1-29.
Predicting plasma drug concentrations with semilog scale.

on mobile devices may not offer these functions; however, device application stores generally offer scientific calculator applications for download (may require purchase).

Clinically Important Equations Identified in This Chapter

1. $C = X/V$

2. $V = X/C$

REVIEW QUESTIONS

1-1. The predictable relationship between plasma drug concentration and concentration at the receptor site where a given drug produces its therapeutic effect is called _____.

A. Pharmacodynamics

B. Drug concentration

C. Pharmacokinetics

D. Kinetic homogeneity

1-2. The application of pharmacokinetic principles to the safe and effective therapeutic management of drugs in an individual patient is known as _____.

A. Pharmacodynamics

B. Clinical pharmacokinetics

1-3. The most accurate way to measure drug concentrations at a specific tissue would be to measure a sample of the tissue or fluid.

A. True

B. False

1-4. Pharmacodynamics refers to the relationship of drug _____.

A. Dose to drug concentration in plasma

B. Dose to drug concentration at the receptor site

C. Concentrations to drug effect

D. Dose to drug effect

1-5. Which of the following affects drug pharmacodynamics?

A. Drug concentration at the receptor site

B. Density of receptors on the target cell surface

C. Mechanism by which a signal is transmitted into the cell by secondary messengers

D. Regulatory factors that control gene translation and protein degradation

E. All the above influence drug pharmacodynamics.

1-6. The EC_{50} refers to the drug concentration at which _____.

A. One half of the maximum response is achieved

B. One half of the recipients experience toxicity

B. The maximal effect is achieved

C. One half of the recipients experience tolerance

1-7. The therapeutic range is the range of plasma drug concentrations that will _____.

A. Most likely result in desired drug effect and minimal risk of drug toxicity

B. Most likely result in minimal risk of drug toxicity

C. Most likely result in drug toxicity

D. None of the above

1-8. The most important concept in therapeutic drug monitoring is _____.

A. The medication is well absorbed

B. The medication is efficacious

C. The pharmacologic response is related to the drug concentration in plasma

D. The pharmacologic response is related to the rate of renal elimination

1-9. One factor that may result in variability in plasma drug concentrations after the same drug dose is given to different patients includes variations in _____.

A. Drug absorption

B. The EC_{50} of the drug

C. Genetic differences in metabolism

D. Body weight

E. All but B

1-10. An example of a situation that would not support therapeutic drug monitoring with plasma drug concentrations would be one in which _____.

A. A wide variation in plasma drug concentrations is achieved in different patients given a standard drug dose

B. The toxic plasma concentration is many times the therapeutic concentration range

C. Correlation between a drug's plasma concentration and therapeutic response is positive

D. Unwanted side effects frequently occur above the therapeutic range

1-11. For a drug with a narrow therapeutic index, the plasma concentration required for therapeutic effects is near the concentration that produces toxic effects.

A. True

B. False

1-12. Therapeutic drug monitoring would be beneficial in which of the following scenarios associated with use of a drug?

A. Seizures can occur for a drug when levels exceed a known therapeutic range.

B. Osteonecrosis can occur when a patient receives a drug chronically over many years at the established maintenance dose.

C. Side effects of a drug occur at any drug level whether in or above target range.

D. A drug needs to penetrate the blood–brain barrier.

1-13. Because of tolerance, patients may have different levels of effect from the same dose of a certain drug.

A. True

B. False

1-14. The central compartment includes fat tissue, muscle tissue, and cerebrospinal fluid.

A. True

B. False

1-15. The most commonly used model in clinical pharmacokinetic situations is the _____.

A. One-compartment model

B. Two-compartment model

C. Multicompartment model

D. Zero order elimination

1-16. Instantaneous distribution to most body tissues and fluids is assumed in which of the following models?

A. One-compartment model

B. Two-compartment model

C. Multicompartment model

1-17. The amount of drug per unit of volume is defined as the _____:

A. Volume of distribution

B. Concentration

C. Rate

1-18. The theoretical volume required to account for all of the drug in the body, if the concentration in all tissues is the same as the plasma concentration, is defined as the _____:

A. Volume of distribution

B. Concentration

C. Rate

D. Order

1-19. If 3 g of a drug are added and distributed throughout a tank and the resulting concentration is 0.15 g/L, calculate the volume of the tank.

A. 10 L

B. 20 L

C. 30 L

D. 200 L

1-20. For a drug that has first-order elimination and follows a one-compartment model, which of the following plots would result in a curved line?

A. Plasma concentration versus time

B. Natural log of plasma concentration versus time

1-21. A drug that follows a one-compartment model is given as an IV injection, and the following plasma concentrations are determined at the times indicated:

Plasma Concentration (mg/L)	Time after Dose (hr)
95	1
81	2
70	3

Using semilog graph paper, determine the approximate concentration in plasma at 6 hours after the dose.

A. 58 mg/L

B. 44 mg/L

C. 30 mg/L

ANSWERS

1-1. A. *Incorrect answer.* Pharmacodynamics deals with the relationship between the drug concentration at the site of action and the resulting effect.

B. *Incorrect answer.* Drug concentrations in plasma and tissues result from pharmacokinetic processes.

C. *Incorrect answer.* Pharmacokinetics describes drug absorption, distribution, metabolism and excretion.

D. CORRECT ANSWER

1-2. A. *Incorrect answer.* Pharmacodynamics alone is not sufficient for effective therapeutic management, as it does not account for absorption, distribution, metabolism, and excretion.

B. CORRECT ANSWER

1-3. A. CORRECT ANSWER. The plasma drug concentration is not the same as that in the tissue but rather is related to the tissue concentration by the volume of distribution (*V*). Plasma drug concentrations are commonly used because

blood, being readily accessible via venipuncture, is the body fluid most often collected for drug measurement.

B. *Incorrect answer*

1-4. A, B. *Incorrect answers.* These statements are definitions of pharmacokinetics.

C. CORRECT ANSWER

D. *Incorrect answer.* This statement refers to the effect of pharmacokinetic and pharmacodynamic processes.

1-5. E. CORRECT ANSWER (A through D describe components of Pharmacodynamics.)

1-6. A. CORRECT ANSWER

B, C. *Incorrect answers.* The "50" in EC_{50} refers to 50% of the maximal effect.

D. *Incorrect answer.* The term EC_{50} refers to pharmacologic effect and not to tolerance.

1-7. A. CORRECT ANSWER. The therapeutic drug range is the range within which most patients will experience desired outcomes.

B, C, D. *Incorrect answers.* The therapeutic range of a drug describes a range of plasma drug concentrations generally considered safe and effective in a patient population; no absolute boundaries divide subtherapeutic, therapeutic, and toxic drug concentrations for an individual patient. Both pharmacodynamic and pharmacokinetic factors influence a patient's response.

1-8. A. *Incorrect answer.* Absorption is a drug specific factor that might influence outcome but is not the critical factor.

B. *Incorrect answer.* A medication should not be utilized if a there is no expectation of efficacy.

C. CORRECT ANSWER. Therapeutic monitoring depends on the correlation of drug concentration to expected outcome.

D. *Incorrect answer.* Elimination might influence dosing, but only if a relationship between plasma concentration and therapeutic (or toxic) outcome exists.

1-9. A, C, D. *Incorrect answers.* These responses are factors that may influence plasma concentrations.

     B. *Incorrect answer.* The EC_{50} is a way of comparing drug potency. The EC_{50} is the concentration at which 50% of the maximum effect of the drug is achieved.

     E. CORRECT ANSWER

1-10. A. *Incorrect answer.* A wide variation in plasma drug concentrations would be a good justification for therapeutic drug level monitoring.

     B. CORRECT ANSWER. When the toxic plasma concentration is much greater than the therapeutic concentration range, there is less need for drug level monitoring.

     C. *Incorrect answer.* A positive correlation between concentration and response makes therapeutic drug level monitoring more useful.

     D. *Incorrect answer.* Because it would be helpful to measure serum drug concentrations because the target range does predict risk of toxicity.

1-11. A. CORRECT ANSWER. For a drug with a narrow therapeutic index, the plasma concentration required for therapeutic effects is near the concentration that produces toxic effects. The dosage of such a drug must be chosen carefully.

     B. *Incorrect answer.*

1-12. A. CORRECT ANSWER. There is a correlation between plasma drug level and the occurrence of an adverse event, indicating that monitoring of level and reduce risk.

     B. *Incorrect answer.* Not needed for side effects that are not dose-related.

C. *Incorrect answer.* The risk of side effect is not directly related to serum drug concentration, and therapeutic monitoring would not predict risk of side effect.

D. *Incorrect answer.* Need to anticipate challenges of crossing the blood–brain barrier (BBB), but again not always required to do therapeutic drug monitoring to achieve that except with certain drugs that also have narrow therapeutic indices (although dose recommendations in that case may be higher to achieve penetration) (For example, serotonin reuptake inhibitors for treatment of depression). More dependent on chemical properties to cross BBB than just on dose (although that is also considered in these cases).

1-13. A. CORRECT ANSWER. For some drugs, the effectiveness can decrease with continued use. Every patient has tried the drug for different periods of time affecting the effectiveness of the drug differently per patient.

     B. *Incorrect answer*

1-14. A. *Incorrect answer.* The peripheral compartment is generally made up of less well-perfused tissues, such as muscle and fat.

     B. CORRECT ANSWER

1-15. A. CORRECT ANSWER

     B. *Incorrect answer.* Although a two-compartment model is often used, it is not used as commonly as a one-compartment model.

     C. *Incorrect answer.* Multicompartment models are used occasionally for research purposes but are not normally used in clinical pharmacokinetics.

     D. *Incorrect answer.* Zero order elimination is not a pharmacokinetic model of drug distribution.

1-16.   A.   CORRECT ANSWER

   B.   *Incorrect answer.* In a two-compartment model, it is assumed that drug distribution to some tissues proceeds at a lower rate than for other tissues.

   C.   *Incorrect answer.* In a multicompartment model, it is also assumed that drug distribution to some tissues proceeds at a lower rate than for other tissues.

1-17.   A.   *Incorrect answer.* The volume of distribution refers to the dose over the resulting concentration.

   B.   CORRECT ANSWER

   C.   *Incorrect answer.* The amount per unit of volume is a static value and would not change over time; therefore, it would not be considered a rate.

1-18.   A.   CORRECT ANSWER. This is the fundamental definition of the estimated volume of distribution.

   B, C, D.   *Incorrect answers.*

1-19.   A, C, D. *Incorrect answers.* A math error must have been made. The answer can be found by dividing 3 g by 0.15 g/L.

   B.   CORRECT ANSWER

1-20.   A.   CORRECT ANSWER

   B.   *Incorrect answer.* This plot would be a straight line (see Figure 1-29).

1-21.   A, C. *Incorrect answers.* These results might vary slightly if determined using linear graph paper due to minor variance during the plotting process. Larger variances likely reflect incorrect plotting of data points.

   B.   CORRECT ANSWER

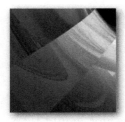

Discussion Points

D1. An proton pump inhibitor is given to control gastric pH and prevent stress ulcer related bleeding. The following gastric pHs were observed when steady-state concentrations of the drug were achieved. What are the E_{max} and EC_{50} of this drug?

Plasma Concentration (mg/L)	Resulting pH
0.25	1
0.5	1
1	1.4
2	2.6
3	3.8
4	4.8
5	4.8

D2. The relationship shown in **Figure 1-30** is observed from a clinical study. What are some of the likely reasons for this result?

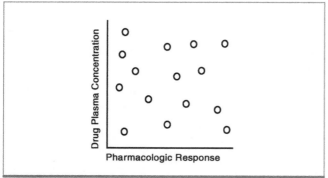

FIGURE 1-30.
Pharmacologic response versus drug plasma concentration.

D3. The models shown in **Figure 1-31** both well represent actual plasma concentrations of a drug after a dose. Which one should be preferred to predict plasma levels? Provide a justification for your answer.

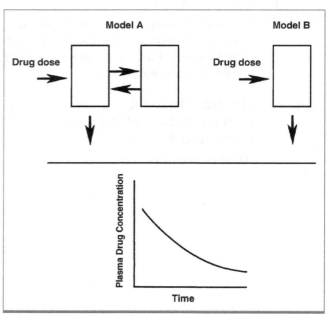

FIGURE 1-31.
Models for predicting plasma drug concentrations over time.

D4. Would you expect a small drug molecule that does not cross physiologic membranes very well and is not lipid soluble to have a relatively high or low volume of distribution? Explain your answer.

D5. When plotting plasma drug concentration (*y*-axis) versus time (*x*-axis), what are the advantages of using a natural log scale for the y-axis rather than a linear scale?

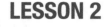
Basic Pharmacokinetics

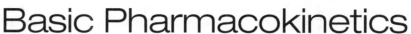

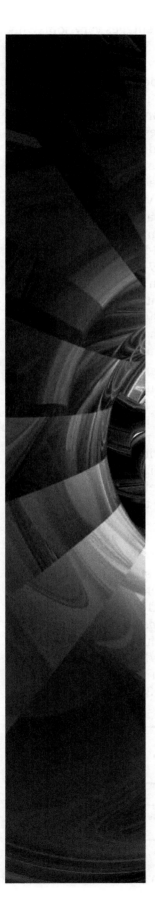

OBJECTIVES

After completing Lesson 2, you should be able to:

1. Define the concept of apparent volume of distribution and use an appropriate mathematical equation to calculate this parameter.

2. Identify the components of body fluids that make up extracellular and intracellular fluids and know the percentage of each component.

3. Describe the difference between whole blood, plasma, and serum.

4. Define drug clearance.

5. Describe the difference between first- and zero-order elimination and how each appears graphically.

To examine the concept of volume of distribution further, let's return to our example of the body as a tank described in Lesson 1. We assumed that no drug was being removed from the tank while we were determining volume. In reality, drug concentration in the body is constantly changing, primarily due to elimination. This flux makes it more difficult to calculate the volume in which a drug distributes.

One way to calculate the apparent volume of drug distribution in the body is to measure the plasma concentration immediately after intravenous administration before elimination has had a significant effect. The concentration just after intravenous administration (at time zero, t_0) is abbreviated as C_0 (**Figure 2-1**). The volume of distribution can be calculated using the equation:

$$\text{volume of distribution} = \frac{\substack{\text{amount of drug} \\ \text{administered (dose)}}}{\substack{\text{initial drug} \\ \text{concentration}}} \text{ or } V(\text{L}) = \frac{X_0(\text{mg / L})}{C_0(\text{mg / L})}$$

(See **Equation 1-1**.)

C_0 can be determined from a direct measurement or estimated by back-extrapolation from concentrations determined at any time after the dose. If two concentrations have been determined, a line containing the two values and extending through the y-axis can be drawn on semilog paper. The point where that line crosses the y-axis gives an estimate of C_0. Both the direct measurement and back-extrapolation approaches assume that the drug distributes instantaneously into a single homogeneous compartment.

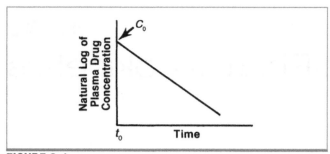

FIGURE 2-1.
Concentration resulting immediately after an intravenous injection of a drug is referred to as C_0.

The volume of distribution is an important parameter for determining proper drug dosing regimens. Often referred to as the *apparent* volume of distribution, it does not have an exact physiologic significance, but it can indicate the extent of drug distribution and aid in determination of dosage requirements. Generally, dosing is proportional to the volume of distribution. For example, the larger the volume of distribution, the larger a dose must be to achieve a desired target concentration. This would be true for a single dose of an intravenous medication or a single dose of an oral medication that is 100% bioavailable. For multiple drug dosing, clearance would also affect dosing requirements. Bioavailability would also be accounted for with drugs that are not 100%.

To understand how distribution occurs, you must have a basic understanding of body fluids and tissues (**Figure 2-2**). The fluid portion (water) in an adult makes up approximately 60% of total body weight and is composed of intracellular fluid (35%) and extracellular fluid (25%). Extracellular fluid is made up of plasma (4%) and interstitial fluid (21%). Interstitial fluid surrounds cells outside the vascular system. These percentages vary somewhat in a child.

Volume of distribution can vary greatly when comparing medications depending on the medication's ability to distribute into peripheral tissue. There is no specific definition for classifying volume of distribution into categories such as large or small. If a drug has a volume of distribution of approximately 15–18 L in a 70-kg person, we might assume that its distribution is limited to extracellular fluid, as that is the approximate volume of extracellular fluid in the body. If a drug has a volume of distribution of about 40 L, the drug may be distributing into all body water because a 70-kg person has approximately 40 L of body water (70 kg × 60%). If the volume of distribution is much greater than 40–50 L, the drug probably is concentrated in tissue outside the plasma and interstitial fluid. For this reason, volume of distribution is often expressed in terms of units of volume per kilogram in dosing references.

If a drug distributes extensively into tissues, the volume of distribution calculated from plasma concentrations could be much higher than the actual physiologic plasma volume in which it distributes. For example, by measuring plasma concentrations, it appears that digoxin distributes in approximately 440 L in an adult. Because digoxin binds extensively to muscle tissue, plasma levels are fairly low relative to concentrations in muscle tissue. For other drugs, tissue concentrations may not be as high as the plasma concentration, so it may appear that these drugs distribute into a relatively small volume.

It is also important to distinguish among blood, plasma, and serum. *Blood* refers to the fluid portion in combination with formed elements (white cells, red cells, and platelets). *Plasma* refers only to the fluid portion of blood (including soluble proteins but not formed elements). When the soluble protein fibrinogen is removed from plasma, the remaining product is *serum* (**Figure 2-3**).

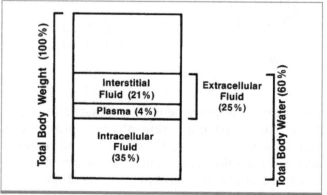

FIGURE 2-2.
Fluid distribution in an adult.

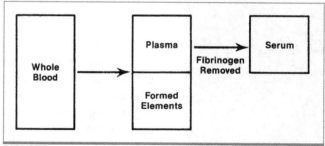

FIGURE 2-3.
Relationship of whole blood, plasma, and serum.

These differences in biologic fluids must be recognized when considering reported drug concentrations. The plasma concentration of a drug may be much less than the whole blood concentration if the drug is preferentially sequestered by red blood cells.

Clinical Correlate

Most drug concentrations are measured using plasma or serum that usually generates similar values. It is more relevant to use plasma or serum than whole blood measurements to estimate drug concentrations at the site of effect. However, some drugs, such as antimalarials, are extensively taken up by red blood cells. In these situations, whole blood concentrations would be more relevant, although they are not commonly used in clinical practice.

Clearance

Another important parameter in pharmacokinetics is clearance. *Clearance* is a measure of the removal of drug from the body. Plasma drug concentrations are affected by the rate at which drug is administered, the volume in which it distributes, and its clearance. A drug's clearance and the volume of distribution determine its half-life. The concept of half-life and its relevant equations are discussed in Lesson 3.

Clearance (expressed as volume/time) describes the removal of drug from a volume of plasma in a given unit of time. Clearance does not indicate the amount of drug removed from the body. It indicates the volume of plasma (or blood) from which the drug is completely removed, or cleared, in a given time period (hence is expressed as volume/time). **Figures 2-4** and **2-5** represent two ways of

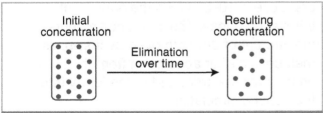

FIGURE 2-4.
Decrease in drug concentration due to drug clearance.

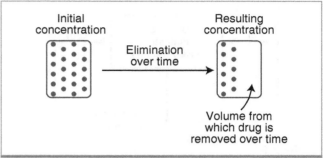

FIGURE 2-5.
Clearance may be viewed as the volume of plasma from which drug is totally removed over a specified period.

thinking about drug clearance. In Figure 2-4, the amount of drug (the number of dots) decreases but fills the same volume, resulting in a lower concentration. Another way of viewing the same decrease would be to calculate the volume that would be drug-free if the concentration were held constant.

Drugs can be cleared from the body by many different mechanisms, pathways, or organs, including hepatic biotransformation and renal and biliary excretion. *Total body clearance* of a drug is the sum of all the clearances by various mechanisms.

2-1
$$Cl_t = Cl_r + Cl_m + Cl_b + Cl_{other}$$

where

Cl_t = total body clearance (from all mechanisms, where t refers to total)

Cl_r = renal clearance (through renal excretion)

Cl_m = clearance by liver metabolism or biotransformation

Cl_b = biliary clearance (through biliary excretion)

Cl_{other} = clearance by all other routes (gastrointestinal tract, pulmonary, etc.)

For an agent removed primarily by the kidneys, renal clearance (Cl_r) makes up most of the total body clearance. For a drug primarily metabolized by the liver, hepatic clearance (Cl_m) is most important.

A good way to understand clearance is to consider a single well-perfused organ that eliminates drug. Blood flow through the organ is referred to as Q (mL/min) as seen in **Figure 2-6**, where C_{in} is the drug concentration in the blood entering the

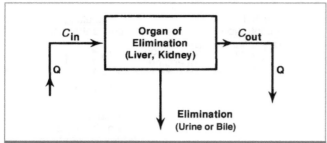

FIGURE 2-6.
Model for organ clearance of a drug.

TABLE 2-2. Effect on Clearance

Extraction Ratio (E)	Blood Flow (Q) (L/hr)	Clearance (Cl) (L/hr)
High (0.7–1.0)	Low	Low
Low (<0.3)	High	Low
High (0.7–1.0)	High	High
Low (<0.3)	Low	Low

organ, and C_{out} is the drug concentration in the exiting blood. If the organ eliminates some of the drug, C_{in} is greater than C_{out}.

We can measure an organ's ability to remove a drug by relating C_{in} and C_{out}. This extraction ratio (E) is:

$$E = \frac{C_{in} - C_{out}}{C_{in}}$$

This ratio must be a fraction between zero and one. Organs that are very efficient at eliminating a drug will have an extraction ratio approaching one (i.e., 100% extraction). **Table 2-1** is used as a general guide. The drug clearance of any organ is determined by blood flow and the extraction ratio:

organ clearance = blood flow × extraction ratio

or:

2-2 $Cl_{organ} = Q \times \dfrac{C_{in} - C_{out}}{C_{in}}$ or $Cl_{organ} = QE$

If an organ is very efficient in removing drug (i.e., extraction ratio near one) but blood flow is low, clearance will also be low. Also, if an organ is inefficient in removing drug (i.e., extraction ratio close to zero) even if blood flow is high, clearance would again be low. See **Table 2-2**.

TABLE 2-1. Rating of Extraction Ratios

Extraction Ratio (E)	Rating
>0.7	High
0.3–0.7	Intermediate
<0.3	Low

The equations noted previously are not used routinely in clinical drug monitoring, but they describe the concept of drug clearance. Examination of a single well-perfused organ to understand clearance is a noncompartmental approach; no assumptions about the number of compartments have to be made. Therefore, *clearance* is said to be a model-independent parameter. Clearance also can be related to the model-dependent parameters volume of distribution and elimination rate (discussed in Lesson 3).

Clearance may also be a useful parameter for constructing dosage recommendations in clinical situations. It is an index of the capacity for drug removal by the body's organs.

Clinical Correlate

Blood flow and the extraction ratio will determine a drug's clearance. Propranolol is a drug that is eliminated exclusively by hepatic metabolism. The extraction ratio for propranolol is greater than 0.9, so most of the drug presented to the liver is removed by one pass through the liver. Therefore, clearance is approximately equal to liver blood flow (Cl = Q × E: when E ~ 1.0, Cl ~ Q). One indication of the high extraction ratio is the relatively high oral dose of propranolol compared with the intravenous dose; an oral dose is 10–20 times the equivalent intravenous dose. The difference reflects the amount of drug removed by first-pass metabolism after absorption from the gastrointestinal tract and before entry into the general circulation.

TABLE 2-3. Average Clearances of Common Drugs

Amlodipine	5.9 ± 1.5 mL/min/kg
Ganciclovir	3.4 ± 0.5 mL/min/kg
Ketorolac	0.50 ± 0.15 mL/min/kg
Lansoprazole	6.23 ± 1.60 mL/min/kg
Montelukast	0.70 ± 0.17 mL/min/kg
Sildenafil	6.0 ± 1.1 mL/min/kg
Valsartan	0.49 ± 0.09 mL/min/kg

Sources: Brunton LL, Lazo JS, Parker KL, eds. *The Pharmacologic Basis of Therapeutics*, 11th ed. New York, NY: McGraw-Hill; 2006:1798, 1829, 1839, 1840, 1851, 1872, and 1883.

The average clearances of some commonly used drugs are shown in **Table 2-3**. These values can vary considerably between individuals and may be altered by disease.

First-Order and Zero-Order Elimination

The simplest example of drug elimination in a one-compartment model is a single intravenous bolus dose of a drug. The following are first assumed:

1. Distribution and equilibration to all tissues and fluids occur instantaneously so a one-compartment model applies.

2. Elimination is first order.

Most drugs are eliminated by a first-order process, and the concept of first-order elimination must be understood. With *first-order elimination*, the amount of drug eliminated in a set amount of time is directly proportional to the amount of drug in the body. The result is that the literal amount of drug eliminated (e.g., mg) over a certain time period increases as the amount of drug in the body increases; likewise, the amount of drug eliminated per unit of time decreases as the amount of drug in the body decreases; however, the percentage of drug eliminated per unit of time remains constant.

With the first-order elimination process, although the amount of drug eliminated may change with the amount of drug in the body, the fraction of a drug in the body eliminated over a given time remains constant. In practical terms, the fraction or percentage of drug removed is the same with either high or low drug concentrations. For example, if 1000 mg of a drug is administered and the drug follows first-order elimination, we might observe the patterns in **Table 2-4**.

The actual amount of drug eliminated is different for each fixed time period depending on the initial amount in the body, but the fraction removed is the same, so this elimination is first order. Because the elimination of this drug (like most drugs) occurs by a first-order process, the amount of drug eliminated decreases as the concentration in plasma decreases. The actual fraction of drug eliminated over any given time (in this case 12%) depends on the drug itself and the individual patient's capacity to eliminate the drug.

With *zero-order elimination*, the amount of drug eliminated per unit of time does not change with the amount or concentration of drug in the body, but the

TABLE 2-4. Comparison of Zero-Order and First-Order Elimination

	First Order							
Time after Drug Administration (hr)	0	1	2	3	0	5	6	7
Amount of Drug in Body	1000	880	774	681	599	527	464	408
Amount of Drug Eliminated over Preceding Hour (mg)	—	120	106	93	82	72	63	
Fraction of Drug Eliminated over Preceding Hour (mg)	—	0.12	0.12	0.12	0.12	0.12	0.12	0.12

	Zero Order							
Time after Drug Administration (hr)	0	1	2	3	4	5	6	7
Amount of Drug in Body	1000	850	700	550	400	250	100	—
Amount of Drug Eliminated over Preceding Hour (mg)	—	150	150	150	150	150	150	100*
Fraction of Drug Eliminated over Preceding Hour (mg)	—	0.15	0.18	0.21	0.27	0.38	0.6	1

*Because at this moment less than 150 mg of drug remains in the body, only the remaining amount of drug can be eliminated.

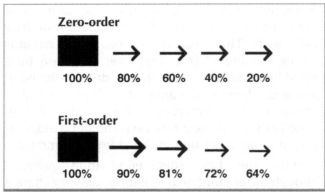

FIGURE 2-7.
Zero- versus first-order elimination. The size of the arrow represents the amount of drug eliminated over a unit of time. Percentages are the fraction of the initial drug amount remaining in the body.

fraction removed varies (**Figure 2-7**). For example, if 1000 mg of a drug is administered and the drug follows zero-order elimination, we might observe the patterns in Table 2-4.

Now that we have examined zero- and first-order elimination, let's return to our simple one-compartment, intravenous bolus situation. If the plasma drug concentration is continuously measured and plotted against time after administration of an intravenous dose of a drug with first-order elimination, the plasma concentration curve shown in **Figure 2-8** would result. To predict

concentrations at times when we did not collect samples, we must linearize the plot by using semi-log paper (**Figure 2-9**).

Clinical Correlate

Most antimicrobial agents (e.g., aminoglycosides, cephalosporins, and vancomycin) display first-order elimination when administered in usual doses. The pharmacokinetic parameters for these drugs are not affected by the size of the dose given. As the dose and drug concentrations increase, the amount of drug eliminated per hour increases while the fraction of drug removed remains the same. Some drugs (e.g., phenytoin), when given in high doses, display zero-order elimination. *Zero-order elimination* occurs when the body's ability to eliminate a drug has reached its maximum capability (i.e., all transporters are being used). As the dose and drug concentrations increase, the amount of drug eliminated per hour does not increase, and the fraction of drug removed declines.

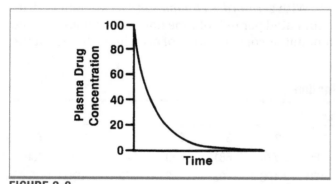

FIGURE 2-8.
Plasma drug concentration versus time after an intravenous (bolus) drug dose, assuming a one-compartment model with first-order elimination (linear *y*-scale).

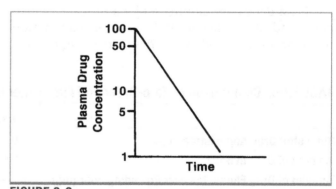

FIGURE 2-9.
As in Figure 2-8, but with a log scale *y*-axis.

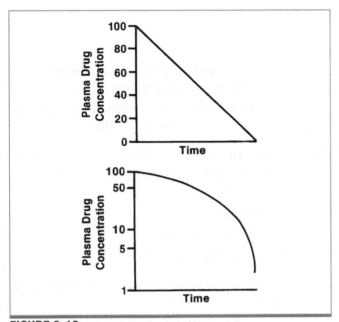

FIGURE 2-10.
Plasma drug concentrations versus time after an intravenous (bolus) drug dose, assuming a one-compartment model with zero-order elimination (**A**, linear plot; **B**, log plot).

For a drug with first-order elimination, the natural log of plasma concentration versus time plot is a straight line. Conversely, plots with zero-order elimination would be as shown in **Figure 2-10**. Note that for a drug with zero-order elimination, the plot of the plasma concentration versus time is linear (plot A in Figure 2-10), whereas on semilog paper (representing the natural log of plasma concentration versus time), it is a curve (bottom plot in Figure 2-10). If the natural log of a plasma drug concentration versus time plot is linear, it generally can be assumed that the drug follows first-order elimination.

REVIEW QUESTIONS

2-1. After an intravenous bolus dose drawn immediately after administration, drug concentration equals _____ divided by the apparent volume of distribution.

A. Clearance

B. Amount of drug administered

C. Half-life

D. Absorption rate constant

2-2. A dose of 500 mg of a drug is administered to a patient, and the following concentrations result at the indicated times below. Assume a one-compartment model.

Plasma Concentration (mg/L)	Time after Dose (hr)
127	0
100	2
55	4
30	6

An estimate of the volume of distribution would be _____.

A. 9.1 L

B. 16.6 L

C. 2.75 L

D. 3.9 L

2-3. If a drug is well distributed to tissues, its apparent volume of distribution is probably _____.

A. Large

B. Small

2-4. The volume of distribution can be helpful in determining drug dosing requirements.

A. True

B. False

2-5. For the body fluid compartments below, rank them from the lowest volume to the highest, in a typical 70-kg person.

A. Plasma < extracellular fluid < intracellular fluid < total body water

B. Extracellular fluid < intracellular fluid < plasma < total body water

C. Intracellular fluid < extracellular fluid < plasma < total body water

D. Total body water < plasma < intracellular fluid < extracellular fluid

2-6. Select the site from which drug concentrations are most commonly measured:

A. Serum

B. Whole blood

C. Formed elements

D. Interstitial fluid

2-7. Clearance is expressed using the following units:

A. Concentration/half-life

B. Dose/volume

C. Half-life/dose

D. Volume/time

2-8. Total body clearance is the sum of clearance via all possible routes of elimination (the kidneys, liver, and other routes of elimination).

A. True

B. False

2-9. Clearance describes the amount of drug removed from the body per unit time.

A. True

B. False

2-10. Drug clearance can only be calculated for drugs that fit a one-compartment model.

A. True

B. False

2-11. With a drug that follows first-order elimination, the amount of drug eliminated per unit time _____.

A. Is directly proportional to the amount of drug in the body

B. Decreases as the amount of drug in the body increases

C. Increases as the amount of drug in the body decreases

D. All of the above are correct.

ANSWERS

2-1.   A, C, D. *Incorrect answers*

   B.   CORRECT ANSWER. You can determine the correct answer from the units in the numerator and denominator. They should cancel to yield a volume unit. *Grams* divided by *grams per liter* would leave you with *liter* as the unit. The volume is therefore determined from the dose, or amount of drug given, and the resulting initial concentration.

2-2.   A.   *Incorrect answer.* You may have used 100 mg/L as the initial concentration.

   B.   *Incorrect answer.* You may have used an incorrect initial concentration.

   C.   CORRECT ANSWER. To find the initial concentration, plot the given plasma concentration and time values on semilog paper, connect the points, and read the value of the *y*-axis (concentration) when *x* (time) = 0. This should be approximately 182 mg/L. You can then determine the volume of distribution using the equation volume of distribution = dose/initial concentration.

   D.   *Incorrect answer.* You may have used an incorrect initial concentration, or you may have used linear graph paper instead of semilog paper.

2-3.   A.   CORRECT ANSWER

   B.   *Incorrect answer.* Drug concentrations are generally measured in plasma. When drug distributes well into tissues, the plasma level will be decreased. Examining the equation volume of distribution = dose/initial concentration, as the initial concentration increases, the volume will increase.

2-4.   A.   CORRECT ANSWER. The apparent volume of distribution affects the "change" in serum drug concentration (from trough to peak) achieved with each dose of medication. It influences both the loading and maintenance dose.

   B.   *Incorrect answer*

2-5.   A.   CORRECT ANSWER. See Figure 2-2. Plasma would be 2.8 L, extracellular fluid would be 18 L, intracellular fluid would be 25 L, and total body water would be 42 L.

   B, C, D. *Incorrect answers.* Plasma is the most readily available site for measurement. Whole blood would represent on a portion of plasma concentration. Formed elements would not be expected to be a site of distribution for medications. Interstitial fluid would be difficult to assess.

2-6.   A.   CORRECT ANSWER

   B, C, D. *Incorrect answers*

2-7.   A, B, C. *Incorrect answers.* The units for clearance are volume/time.

   D.   CORRECT ANSWER

2-8.   A.   CORRECT ANSWER. Total body clearance can be determined as the sum of individual clearances from all organs or routes of elimination.

   B.   *Incorrect answer*

2-9.   A.   CORRECT ANSWER. As described in questions 2-6 and 2-7, clearance is a rate—expressed as units of drug eliminated per unit of time.

   B.   *Incorrect answer*

2-10.   A.   *Incorrect answer*

   B.   CORRECT ANSWER. It is not necessary to specify a model to determine drug clearance.

2-11.   A.   CORRECT ANSWER

   B, C, D. *Incorrect answers.* With first-order elimination, the amount of drug eliminated in any time period is determined by the amount of drug present at the start. Although the amount of drug eliminated in successive time periods may decrease, the fraction of the initial drug that is eliminated remains constant.

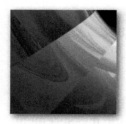

Discussion Points

D1. Drug Y is given by an intravenous injection, and plasma concentrations are then determined as follows:

Time after Injection (hr)	Concentration (mg/L)
0	18
1	16.2
2	14.6
3	13.1
4	11.8
5	10.6
6	9.6
7	8.6
8	7.7

Is this drug eliminated by a first-order or zero-order process? Justify your answer.

D2. Which of the following patient scenarios is associated with a smaller volume of distribution (if the initial serum concentration is drawn immediately after injection)?

A. Dose = 500 mg and initial serum concentration is 30 mg/L

B. Dose = 30 mg and initial serum concentration is 10 mg/L

D3. Explain how a person who weighs 70 kg can have a volume of distribution for a drug of 700 L.

D4. For drug X, individual organ clearances have been determined as follows:

Renal clearance	200 mL/min
Hepatic clearance	25 mL/min
Pulmonary clearance	6.5 mL/min

How would you describe the clearance of drug X?

Which organ system failure would most likely result in increased serum drug concentrations?

D5. Volume of distribution is often referred to as "apparent" volume of distribution. Why is this concept employed, and what is the significance of the volume of distribution concept to thinking about drug dosing recommendations?

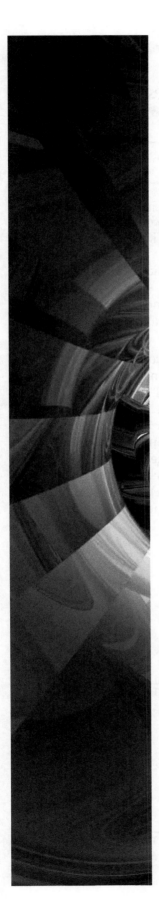

Half-Life, Elimination Rate, and AUC

OBJECTIVES

After completing Lesson 3, you should be able to:

1. Calculate the elimination rate constant given a natural log (ln) of plasma drug concentration versus time curve.

2. Define *half-life*.

3. Calculate a drug's half-life given a natural log of plasma drug concentration versus time curve.

4. Define the relationship between half-life and elimination rate constant.

5. Calculate a drug's half-life given its elimination rate constant.

6. Define *drug clearance*, and relate it to the area under the plasma drug concentration curve and drug dose.

7. Calculate a drug's concentration at time zero and area under the plasma concentration versus time curve (AUC), given plasma concentration data after an intravenous bolus drug dose.

In Lesson 2, we learned that for most drugs (those following first-order elimination), a straight line can describe the change in natural log of plasma concentration over time. Recognizing this relationship, we can now develop mathematical methods to predict drug concentrations. Whenever you have a straight line such as that in **Figure 3-1**, the line is defined by the equation:

$$Y = mX + b$$

where m is the slope of the line, and b is the intercept of the y-axis. If you know the slope and the y-intercept, you can find the value of Y for any given X value.

As the value for the y-intercept may be obtained easily by visual inspection, the only part of the equation that must be calculated is the slope of the line. A slope is calculated from the change in the y-axis (the vertical change) divided by the change in the x-axis (the horizontal change), as in **Figure 3-2**:

$$\text{slope} = \frac{\Delta Y}{\Delta X} \text{ or slope} = \frac{Y_2 - Y_1}{X_2 - X_1}$$

where Δ means "change in."

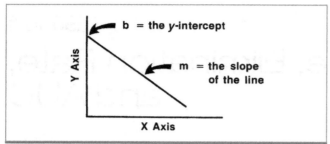

FIGURE 3-1.
Straight-line plot showing slope and *y*-intercept.

The slope is obtained by selecting two different points on the line and calculating the difference between their values. We can apply these same mathematical principles to the natural log of plasma concentration versus time plot (**Figure 3-3**).

The slope is the change in the natural log of plasma concentrations divided by the change in time between the concentrations:

$$slope = \frac{\Delta \ln conc}{\Delta \ time} \ or \ slope = \frac{\ln C_1 - \ln C_0}{t_1 - t_0}$$

If, for example, 10 mg/L is the first concentration (C_0) drawn immediately after administration ($t_0 = 0$ hour) and 1 mg/L is the second concentration (C_1) drawn 2.5 hours after administration ($t_1 = 2.5$ hours):

$$slope = \frac{\ln C_1 - \ln C_0}{t_1 - t_0}$$

$$= \frac{\ln 1 - \ln 10}{2.5 \ hr - 0 \ hr} = \frac{0 - 2.303}{2.5 \ hr}$$

$$= -0.92 \ hr^{-1}$$

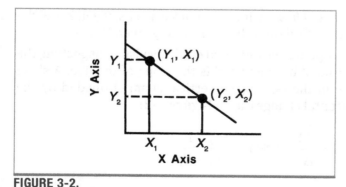

FIGURE 3-2.
The slope of a straight line can be determined from any two points on the line.

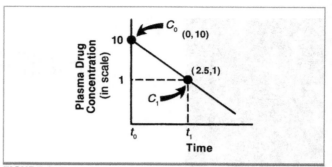

FIGURE 3-3.
The slope of the natural log of plasma concentration versus time curve can be determined if two plasma concentrations and their corresponding times are known.

Note that the slope is calculated using $\ln C_1 - \ln C_0$ or $\ln (C_1/C_0)$ and not $\ln (C_1 - C_0)$. The latter would give an incorrect result. A negative slope indicates that the log of concentration declines with increasing time.

When the log of drug concentration is plotted versus time and a straight line results, as in the previous example, the slope of that line indicates the rate of drug elimination. A steeper slope (**Figure 3-4**, top graph) indicates a faster rate of elimination than does a flatter slope (Figure 3-4, bottom graph). For first-order processes, the rate of elimination (expressed as the fraction of drug in the body removed over a unit of time) is the same at high or low concentrations and is therefore called an *elimination rate constant* (K).

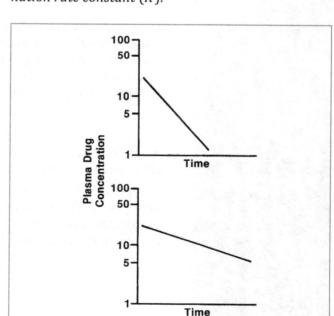

FIGURE 3-4.
A steeper slope (top) indicates a faster rate of elimination.

Therefore, when drug elimination is first order, the negative slope of the natural log of drug concentration versus time plot equals the drug's elimination rate constant (K):

slope = − elimination rate constant

or:

− slope = elimination rate constant

One must carefully examine the mathematical differences in positive and negative slope and elimination rate constant (K) values as they apply to various dosing equations. The slope value from two plasma drug concentrations is always a negative number since the concentration is decreasing (and is negative in the mathematical calculation because the second number is less than the first). However, the K can be used in either its positive or negative form by simple application of one of the rules of logarithms: Log [A/B] = Log A − Log B.

Remember that the elimination rate constant is the fraction of drug removed over a unit of time. If the elimination rate constant is 0.25 hr^{-1}, then 25% of the drug remaining in the body is removed each hour.

Because we know that a plot of the natural log of drug concentration over time is a straight line for a drug following first-order elimination, we can predict drug concentrations for any time after the dose if we know the equation for this line. Remember that all straight lines can be defined by:

$$Y = mX + b$$

As shown in Figure 3-3:

Y axis = natural log of drug concentration in plasma

X axis = time after dose

m = slope of line, or negative elimination rate constant

b = intercept on natural log of plasma drug concentration axis (y-intercept)

Now, when we convert to our new terms:

ln drug concentration = (− elimination rate constant × time after dose) + ln concentration at y-intercept

If we know the slope of the line and the intercept of the y-axis, we can predict the natural log of drug concentration at any time after a dose.

Drug concentrations can be predicted using these mathematical methods instead of the previously described graphical methods. With mathematical methods, our predictions of drug concentrations over time are more accurate. So, if the negative slope of the natural log of drug concentration versus time plot equals the elimination rate constant, our equation for the line:

$$Y = mX + b$$

becomes:

ln (drug concentration) = (− elimination rate constant × time after dose) + ln y-intercept

To simplify our terminology here, let:

ln C = natural log of drug concentration

K = elimination rate constant

t = time after dose

Also, we call the y-intercept "ln C_0," the drug concentration immediately after a dose is administered (at time zero, or t_0). Therefore, our equation becomes:

$$\ln C = (-K \times t) + \ln C_0 \quad \text{or} \quad -K = \frac{\ln C - \ln C_0}{t}$$

This last equation is valuable in therapeutic drug monitoring. If two plasma drug concentrations and the time between them are known, then the elimination rate can be calculated. If one plasma drug concentration and the elimination rate are known, then the plasma concentration at any later time can be calculated. Note that the previous equation can also be expressed to solve for K as a positive value as follows:

$$K = \frac{\ln C_0 - \ln C}{t}$$

Note: C_0 and C have changed locations. Last, either version of this equation can now be rewritten in a calculator-friendly version by applying the log rule, Log [A/B] = Log A − Log B, yielding:

$$K = \frac{\ln \dfrac{C_0}{C}}{t} \quad \text{or} \quad K = \frac{\ln \dfrac{C_1}{C_2}}{t}$$

Clinical Correlate

The concepts presented in this lesson can be used to predict plasma concentrations in some situations. For example, if a patient with renal dysfunction received a dose of vancomycin, and plasma concentrations of 40 mg/L and 20 mg/L were determined 24 and 48 hours after the dose, then the two plasma concentrations could be plotted on semilog paper to determine when the concentration would reach 10 mg/L (**Figure 3-5**). This would be approximately 88 hours after the infusion. This information can be used to determine when the next dose should be given.

Elimination Rate Constant

As stated in the previous section, the elimination rate constant (K) represents the fraction of drug removed per unit of time and has units of reciprocal time (e.g., minute^{-1}, hour^{-1}, and day^{-1}). These units are evident from examination of the calculation of K. For example, in **Figure 3-6**, C_0 is the first plasma drug concentration measured just after the dose is given, and C_1 is the second plasma drug concentration measured at a later time (t_1). From our previous discussion, we know that the equation for this line ($y = mX + b$) is:

$$\ln C_1 = -Kt + \ln C_0$$

Furthermore, we can rearrange this equation to create a more useful version of this equation.

3-1
$$-K = \frac{\ln C_1 - \ln C_0}{t_1 - t_0}$$

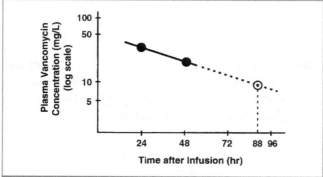

FIGURE 3-5.
Predicting plasma drug concentrations.

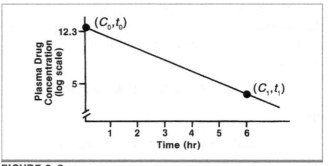

FIGURE 3-6.
Determination of a line (log scale) from two known plasma drug concentrations.

It is a property of logarithms that:

$$\ln C_1 - \ln C_0 = \ln \frac{C_1}{C_0}$$

Then, using numbers from Figure 3-6:

$$-K = \frac{\ln \dfrac{C_1}{C_0}}{t_1 - t_0} = \frac{\ln\left(\dfrac{5\ \text{mg/L}}{12.3\ \text{mg/L}}\right)}{6\ \text{hr} - 0\ \text{hr}}$$

So, $-K = -0.15$ hr^{-1}, or $K = 0.15$ hr^{-1}.

In this case, the elimination rate constant is 0.15 hr^{-1}. Note that the elimination rate is a positive number since we are solving for $-K$. This means that 15% of the drug remaining in the body is removed each hour, so an initial plasma concentration of 10 mg/L will decrease 15% (0.15 × 10 mg/L = 1.5 mg/L) to 8.5 mg/L by the end of the first hour. By the end of the second hour, the concentration will be 7.2 mg/L, a 15% reduction from 8.5 mg/L (0.15 × 8.5 mg/L = 1.3).

The equation $\ln C = -Kt + \ln C_0$ is important, because it allows the estimation of the concentration at any given time. Remember that it is in the form of an equation for a line, $Y = mX + b$. Remembering the rule of logarithms that $\ln X^p = P \ln X$, if we take the antilog of each part of this equation, we get:

3-2
$$C = C_0 e^{-Kt}$$

where:

C = plasma drug concentration at time = t

C_0 = plasma drug concentration at time = 0

K = elimination rate constant (fraction removed per unit of time)

t = time after dose

e = base of the natural log (approximately 2.718)

e^{-Kt} = percent or fraction remaining after time (t)

In "plain English," this equation is saying that a concentration at some time (C) is equal to some previous concentration (C_0) "multiplied by" e^{-Kt}, the fraction of C_0 remaining after t hours. To determine the e^{-Kt} portion on a calculator, enter the value for $-Kt$ and then the function for e^x, or inverse natural log, or raise 2.718 to the power of the value of $-Kt$. The antilog of a number is equal to e (or 2.718) raised to a power equal to that number. The preceding equation can also be used to predict the concentration at any time, given an initial concentration of C_0 and an elimination rate of K.

In addition, C_0 and C are used to represent any two serum drug concentrations where C_0 is the first (and in the case of elimination rate constant the larger), and C is the second serum drug concentration. We could just as easily use C_1 and C_2 in our equation. This is only true for medications with first-order elimination, which fortunately is most commonly utilized medications. We will review prediction of elimination rate and serum drug concentrations for agents with nonlinear elimination in Lessons 10 and 15.

Clinical Correlate

If we know that the plasma drug concentration just after a gentamicin dose is 8 mg/L and the patient's elimination rate constant is 0.25 hr^{-1}, we can predict what the concentration will be 8 hours later:

$$C = C_0 e^{-Kt}$$

where:

C_0 = 8 mg/L,

K = 0.25 hr^{-1}, and

t = 8 hours.

$$C_{at\ 8\ hr} = 8\ mg/L \times e^{-0.25\ hr^{-1}\ (8\ hr)}$$

$$= 8\ mg/L\ (0.135)$$

$$= 1.1\ mg/L$$

Note: The term e^{-Kt} indicates the fraction of the initial dose of drug that remains in the body at time t; 0.135 (or 13.5%) remains in the body 8 hours after the initial dose in this example. Conversely, the term $1 - e^{-Kt}$ would indicate the percent or fraction excreted in the time between drug dosing (t_0) and time (t).

Half-Life

Another important parameter that relates to the rate of drug elimination is half-life ($T\frac{1}{2}$). The *half-life* is the time necessary for the concentration of drug in the plasma to decrease by one-half. A drug's half-life is often related to its duration of action and also may indicate when another dose should be given.

One way to estimate the half-life is to visually examine the natural log of plasma drug concentration versus time plot and note the time required for the plasma concentration to decrease by one-half. For example, in **Figure 3-7**, the decrease from 10 to 5 mg/L takes approximately 1.5 hours. It also takes 1.5 hours for the concentration to decrease from 5.0 to 2.5 mg/L, from 7.0 to 3.5 mg/L, etc. At any point, the decrease in concentration by one-half takes approximately 1.5 hours, even when the decrease is from a concentration as low as 0.05 to 0.025 mg/L. Thus, the half-life can be estimated to be 1.5 hours.

There is another way to estimate the half-life from two known concentrations. Because the half-life is the time for a concentration to decrease by one-half, $T\frac{1}{2}$ can be estimated by halving the initial concentration, then taking one-half of that concentration to get a second concentration, and so on until the final concentration is reached. The number of halves required to reach the final desired concentration, divided into the time between the two concentrations, is the *estimated half-life*. For example, the following two concentrations were determined at the times stated after a dose was administered:

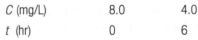

C (mg/L)	8.0	4.0
t (hr)	0	6

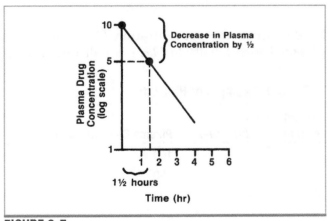

FIGURE 3-7.
Half-life can be determined from the natural log of plasma concentration versus time plot.

Because the concentration drops from 8.0 to 4.0 mg/L in 6 hours, the half-life is 6 hours. Consider a case in which concentrations and times were as follows:

C (mg/L)	12.0	3.0
t (hr)	8	12

The concentration drops from 12 to 3 mg/L in 4 hours. To get from 12 to 3 requires a halving of 12 to 6 and a halving of 6 to 3, representing two half-lives in 4 hours, or one half-life of 2 hours.

The half-life and the elimination rate constant express the same idea. They indicate how quickly a drug is removed from the plasma and, therefore, how often a dose has to be administered. As with the elimination rate constant, calculation of drug half-life using this method is only accurate if the medication has first-order elimination.

If the half-life and peak plasma concentration of a drug are known, then the plasma drug concentration at any time can be estimated. For example, if the peak plasma concentration is 100 mg/L after an intravenous dose of a drug with a 2-hour half-life, then the concentration will be 50 mg/L 2 hours after the peak concentration (a decrease by half). At 4 hours after the peak concentration, it will have decreased by half again, to 25 mg/L, and so on, as shown in **Table 3-1**. Half-life may be mathematically calculated with the following equation:

3-3
$$T\tfrac{1}{2} = \frac{0.693}{K}$$

The equation represents the important relationship between the half-life and the elimination rate constant shown by mathematical manipulation. We already know that:

$$\ln C = C_0 - Kt$$

By definition, the concentration (C) at the time (t) equal to the half-life ($T\tfrac{1}{2}$) is half the original

TABLE 3-1. Example of Half-Life

Time after Peak Concentration (half-life)	Plasma Concentration (mg/L)
0	100
2	50
4	25
6	12.5
8	6.25
10	3.125

concentration (C_0). Therefore, at one half-life, the concentration is half of what it was initially. So, we can say that at $t = T\tfrac{1}{2}$, $C = \tfrac{1}{2}C_0$. For simplicity, let's assume that $C_0 = 1$. Therefore:

$$\ln 0.5 C_0 = \ln C_0 - K(T\tfrac{1}{2})$$

$$\ln 0.5 = \ln 1 - K(T\tfrac{1}{2})$$

Transforming this equation algebraically gives:

$$K(T\tfrac{1}{2}) = \ln(1) - \ln(0.5)$$

$$T\tfrac{1}{2} = \frac{0 - (-0.693)}{K}$$

$$T\tfrac{1}{2} = \frac{0.693}{K}$$

and

$$K = \frac{0.693}{T\tfrac{1}{2}}$$

Therefore, the half-life can be determined if we know the elimination rate constant, and conversely, the elimination rate constant can be determined if we know the half-life. This relationship between the half-life and elimination rate constant is important in determining drug dosages and dosing intervals.

Clinical Correlate

For medications with first-order elimination, half-life can be calculated from two plasma concentrations after a dose is given. First, the elimination rate constant (K) is calculated as shown previously. For example, if a dose of gentamicin is administered and a peak plasma concentration is 6 mg/L after the infusion is completed and is 1.5 mg/L 4 hours later, the elimination rate constant is calculated as follows:

$$-K = \frac{\ln C_1 - \ln C_0}{t_1 - t_0}$$

$$= \frac{\ln 1.5 - \ln 6}{4\ \text{hr} - 0\ \text{hr}}$$

$$= \frac{-1.39}{4\ \text{hr}}$$

$$= -0.348\ \text{hr}^{-1}$$

Therefore:

$$K = 0.348 \text{ hr}^{-1}$$

Then:

$$T\,\tfrac{1}{2} = \frac{0.693}{0.348 \text{ hr}^{-1}}$$
$$= 2 \text{ hr}$$

Clinical Correlate

The average plasma half-lives of some commonly used drugs are shown in **Table 3-2**. These may vary considerably between individuals and may be altered by disease. Note that drug effects may persist for a period of time longer than would be predicted by a drug's half-life. The greater the value of the half-life, the longer the drug stays in the body. As an example from Table 3-2, half of a dose of vancomycin takes approximately 5.6 hours to be eliminated from the body (no matter the size of the dose). Also, half of a dose of cefazolin is eliminated in approximately 2.2 hours after administration, and so on.

Relationships among Pharmacokinetic Parameters

In previous lessons, we discussed elimination rate, volume of distribution, and clearance. These

TABLE 3-2. Half-Lives of Common Drugs

Drug	Half-Life (hr)
Amlodipine	39
Amoxicillin	1.7
Morphine	1.9
Moxifloxacin	15.4
Sertraline	23
Simvastatin	2–3
Valsartan	9.4
Vancomycin	5.6

Sources: Brunton LL, Lazo JS, Parker KL, eds. *The Pharmacologic Basis of Therapeutics.* 11th edition. New York, NY: McGraw-Hill; 2006:1800, 1806, 1817, 1821, 1830, 1842, 1843, and 1883.

important parameters aid in calculating a drug dosage regimen. All three relate to how fast a drug effect will terminate. There are significant relationships among these parameters, the drug dose, and plasma drug concentrations. In this lesson, we begin to explore these relationships so that we can better predict plasma drug concentrations achieved with drug doses.

Although clearance is a model-independent pharmacokinetic parameter and is not physiologically dependent only on elimination rate, it is sometimes useful to relate it to such parameters as the elimination rate constant (K) and the volume of distribution (V). Mathematically, systemic clearance (Cl_t) is related to V and K by:

$$\text{Cl}_t / V = K$$

or:

$$\text{Cl}_t = V \times K$$

3-4

Clearance and volume are independent factors that together determine K (and $T\tfrac{1}{2}$). Because V has units of volume (milliliters or liters) and clearance has units of volume/time (usually milliliters per minute), K has units of reciprocal time (minute^{-1}, hour^{-1}, or day^{-1}). It is important to understand that the elimination rate constant and plasma drug concentration versus time curve are determined by drug clearance and volume of distribution.

Clearance can be related to drug dose by first evaluating the plasma drug concentration versus time curve after a dose. In examining this curve (**Figure 3-8**), we see that there is a definite area under the curve, referred to as the *area under the plasma drug concentration versus time curve* or *AUC*.

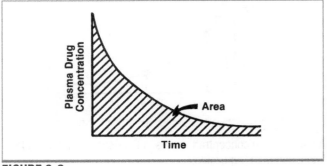

FIGURE 3-8.
Area under the plasma drug concentration versus time curve.

For intravenously administered drugs or those with 100% BA, the AUC is determined by drug clearance and the dose given:

3-5
$$AUC = \frac{\text{dose administered}}{\text{drug clearance}}$$

When clearance remains constant, the AUC is directly proportional to the dose administered. If the dose doubled, the AUC would also double. Another way to think about this concept is that clearance is the parameter relating the AUC to the drug dose.

We usually know the dose of drug being administered and can determine plasma drug concentrations over time. From the plasma concentrations, the AUC can be estimated and drug clearance can be determined easily by rearranging the previous equation to:

$$\text{drug clearance} = \frac{\text{dose administered}}{AUC}$$

With a one-compartment model, first-order elimination, and intravenous drug administration, the AUC can be calculated easily:

$$AUC = \frac{\text{initial concentration } (C_0)}{\text{elimination rate constant } (K)}$$

C_0 has units of concentration, usually milligrams per liter (mg/L), and K is expressed as reciprocal time (usually hour^{-1}), so the AUC is expressed as milligrams per liter times hours (mg × hr)/L. These units make sense graphically as well because when we multiply length times width to measure area, the product of the axes (concentration in milligrams per liter and time in hours) would be expressed as milligrams per liter times hours.

AUC can be calculated by computer modeling of the above AUC equation, or by applying the *trapezoidal rule*. The trapezoidal rule method is rarely used but provides visual means to understand AUC. If a line is drawn vertically to the *x*-axis from each measured concentration, a number of smaller areas are described (**Figure 3-9**). Because we are using the determined concentrations rather than their natural logs, the plasma drug concentration versus time plot is curved. The tops of the resulting shapes are curved as well, which makes their areas difficult to calculate. The area of each shape can be estimated, however, by drawing a straight line between adjacent concentrations and calculating the area of the resulting trapezoid (**Figure 3-10**).

If the time between measurements (and hence the width of the trapezoid) is small, only a slight error results. These smaller areas can be summed to estimate the AUC, as shown in the following equation:

$$AUC = \left[\left(\frac{C_2 + C_1}{2}\right)(t_2 - t_1)\right] + \left[\left(\frac{C_3 - C_2}{2}\right)(t_3 - t_2)\right] \cdots \text{etc.}$$

To calculate drug clearance, however, we need the AUC from time zero to infinity, and the preceding

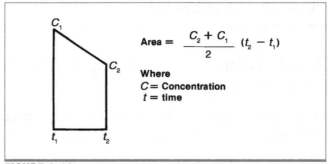

FIGURE 3-10.
Calculation of the area of a trapezoid.

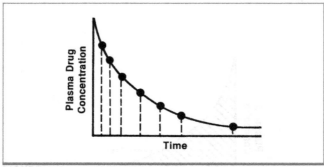

FIGURE 3-9.
A plasma drug concentration versus time curve can be divided into a series of trapezoids.

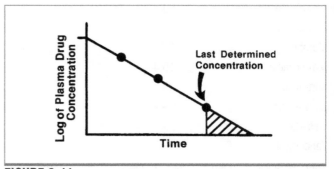

FIGURE 3-11.
Terminal area.

method only estimates the AUC to the final measured drug concentration.

The terminal part of the AUC is estimated by dividing the last measured plasma concentration by the elimination rate constant (**Figure 3-11**):

$$\text{terminal area} = \frac{C_{last}}{K}$$

Add the terminal area to the value of AUC from the preceding equation to find the value of AUC from zero to infinity.

Clinical Correlate

The AUC can be used to determine a drug's clearance. For an individual patient, when the same drug dose is given over a period of time and the volume of distribution remains constant, changes in clearance can be assessed by changes in the AUC. For example, a doubling of the AUC would result if clearance decreased by half. For orally administered drugs, this would only be true if the fraction of drug absorbed from the gastrointestinal tract remained constant. AUC is only rarely used in clinical situations to determine clearance. It is used more frequently in clinical research.

To calculate drug clearance, divide drug dose by AUC. By knowing how to calculate clearance by the area method, it is not necessary to decide first which model (i.e., one, two, or more compartments) best fits the observed plasma levels.

Clinically Important Equations Identified in This Chapter

1. $-K = \dfrac{\ln C_1 - \ln C_0}{t_1 - t_0}$ **Equation 3-1**

2. $C = C_0 e^{-Kt}$ **Equation 3-2**

3. $T\frac{1}{2} = \dfrac{0.693}{K}$ **Equation 3-3**

4. $Cl_t = V \times K$ **Equation 3-4**

REVIEW QUESTIONS

3-1. Which of the following is the equation for a straight line?

   A. $X = mY + b$

   B. $b = mY + X$

   C. $Y = mX + b$

   D. $mX + Y = b$

3-2. Which letter in the equation from question 3-1 represents a parameter that can be identified by visual inspection of a time-concentration graph?

   A. X

   B. m

   C. Y

   D. b

3-3. Slope of a line can be calculated by which of the following methods?

   A. $\Delta Y / \Delta X$

   B. $\Delta X / \Delta Y$

   C. $(Y_2 - Y_1)/(X_2 - X_1)$

   D. $(X2 - X1)/(Y2 - Y1)$

   E. A and C

   F. B and D

3-4. Which of the following would be the slope (and hence the negative elimination rate constant) of the straight line in **Figure 3-12**?

   A. $\ln (C_0 - C_1)$

   B. $t_0 - t_1$

   C. $C_0 - t_0$

   D. $(\ln C_1 - \ln C_0)/(t_1 - t_0)$

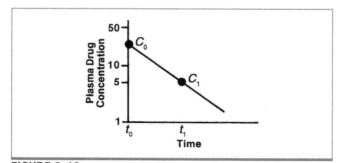

FIGURE 3-12.
Plasma drug concentration versus time.

3-5. Which of the following is the elimination rate constant for **Figure 3-13**?

   A. −0.173

   B. 0.52

   C. 0.231

   D. 0.173

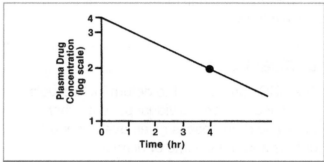

FIGURE 3-13.
Plasma drug concentration versus time.

3-6. If two patients receive the same drug and the plots in **Figure 3-14** result, which patient has the larger elimination rate constant (faster elimination)?

   A. Patient A

   B. Patient B

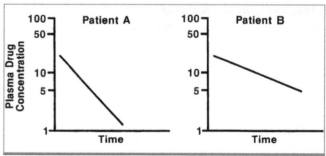

FIGURE 3-14.
Plasma drug concentration versus time.

3-7. A patient with renal dysfunction received a dose of vancomycin. Plasma concentrations were 25 and 18 mg/L at 24 and 48 hours after infusion, respectively. Plot these two plasma concentrations on semilog paper, and determine how many additional hours will be required for the concentration to fall from 18 mg/L to 10 mg/L.

   A. 42 hours

   B. 56 hours

C. 72 hours

D. 84 hours

3-8. Using the equation $C = C_0 e^{-Kt}$, determine the plasma concentration of a drug 18 hours after a peak level of 15 mg/L is observed if the elimination rate constant is 0.03 hr^{-1}.

A. 8.74 mg/L

B. 25.74 mg/L

C. 18.1 mg/L

3-9. Which of the following is a proper unit for the elimination rate constant?

A. minutes

B. mg/min

C. hr^{-1}

D. mg/L

3-10. If the elimination rate constant is 0.15 hr^{-1}, the percent of drug removed per hour is _____.

A. 15%

B. 1.5%

C. 0.15%

D. 85%

3-11. If the plasma concentration just after a gentamicin dose is 20 mg/L and the patient's elimination rate constant is 0.17 hr^{-1}, predict what the plasma concentration will be 8 hours later.

A. 6.73 mg/L

B. 3.42 mg/L

C. 5.13 mg/L

D. 4.97 mg/L

3-12. For a drug that has an initial plasma concentration of 80 mg/L and a half-life of 4 hours, what would the plasma concentration be 12 hours after the initial concentration?

A. 5 mg/L

B. 10 mg/L

C. 15 mg/L

D. 20 mg/L

3-13. From **Figure 3-15**, the approximate *T½* is _____.

A. 5 hours

B. 10 hours

C. 20 hours

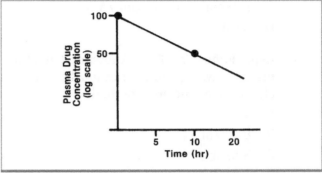

FIGURE 3-15.
Plasma drug concentration versus time.

3-14. If a drug has an elimination rate constant of 0.087 hr^{-1}, what is the half-life?

A. 7.97 hours

B. 11.5 hours

C. 12.6 hours

3-15. To calculate drug clearance by the area method, it is necessary to first determine whether the drug best fits a one- or two-compartment model.

A. True

B. False

3-16. In the trapezoid shown in **Figure 3-16**, what is the area?

A. 150 (mg/L) × hour

B. 300 (mg/L) × hour

C. 100 (mg/L) × hour

D. 25 (mg/L) × hour

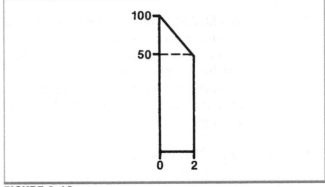

FIGURE 3-16.
Trapezoid.

3-17. If the dose of an intravenously administered drug (X_0) and AUC are known, the clearance (area method) is calculated by _____.

    A. AUC/dose

    B. Dose/AUC

    C. Plasma concentration/AUC

    D. K/AUC.

3-18. Using **Figure 3-17** and knowing that a 500-mg dose was given intravenously, calculate clearance by the area method.

    A. 42 L/hr

    B. 8.4 L/hr

    C. 3 L/hr

    D. 4.2 L/hr

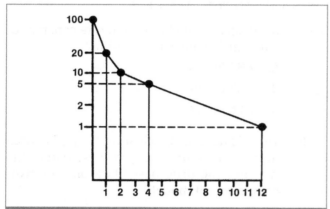

FIGURE 3-17.
Plasma drug concentration versus time.

ANSWERS

3-1. A, B, D. *Incorrect answers*

    C. CORRECT ANSWER. The slope is m, and b is the y-intercept.

3-2. D. CORRECT ANSWER. b can be determined by visual inspection since it represents the y- axis intercept of the graph; slope must be calculated from the change in the y-axis (the vertical change) divided by the change in the x-axis (the horizontal change).

3-3. E. CORRECT ANSWER

3-4. A. *Incorrect answer.* This value should be ($\ln C_1 - \ln C_0$) and should be divided by the change in time ($t_1 - t_0$).

    B. *Incorrect answer.* The numerator [($\ln C_1 - \ln C_0$)] hasn't been included.

    C. *Incorrect answer*

    D. CORRECT ANSWER. The slope is the natural log of change in concentration divided by the change in time: ($\ln C_1 - \ln C_0$)/($t_1 - t_0$).

3-5. A. *Incorrect answer.* The elimination rate constant would not have a negative value; this is merely the slope of the line.

    B. *Incorrect answer.* You may have added ln 2 and ln 4 rather than subtracted ln 4 from ln 2.

    C. *Incorrect answer.* You may have used 3 hours in the denominator rather than 4 hours for change in time.

    D. CORRECT ANSWER. The K itself is a positive number. As stated in response A, the negative sign would represent the slope of the line (–slope = –K).

3-6. A. CORRECT ANSWER. The larger the slope of the line is (i.e., the steeper the line is), the larger the elimination rate constant will be.

    B. *Incorrect answer.* Note that the slope of the line is smaller (i.e., the line is less steep).

3.7. B, C, D. *Incorrect answers.* Be sure your points are plotted on paper that has a log scale for y (concentration) values. Double-check the placement of your points.

    A. CORRECT ANSWER

3-8. A. CORRECT ANSWER

    B. *Incorrect answer.* You may have used Kt and not –Kt.

    C. *Incorrect answer.* Check the –Kt term, which should be –0.03 hr^{-1} × 18 hours (or –0.54, thus e-0.54 would be 0.58 × 15 = 8.74).

3-9. A. *Incorrect answer.* A rate constant is a unit change per time expressed as reciprocal time units (e.g., minute^{-1}).

   B. *Incorrect answer.* The elimination rate constant does not include mass units.

   C. CORRECT ANSWER

   D. *Incorrect answer.* These are the proper units for concentration.

3-10. A. CORRECT ANSWER

   B, C, D. *Incorrect answers.* The elimination rate constant is 0.15 hr^{-1}, meaning 15% of the drug remaining in the body is eliminated per hour.

3-11. A, B, D. *Incorrect answers*

   C. CORRECT ANSWER. $C_{8\,hr} = C_0 e{-}Kt$, where $C_0 = 20$ mg/L, $K = 0.017$ hr^{-1}, and $t = 8$ hours.

3-12. A, C, D. *Incorrect answers*

   B. CORRECT ANSWER. $C_{12\,hr} = C_0 e^- Kt$, where $C_0 = 80$ mg/L, $K = 0.173$ hr^{-1}, and $t = 12$ hours. K is calculated from half-life ($K = 0.693/T\frac{1}{2}$). Also, 12 hours represents three half-lives. We would expect the concentration to decrease from 80 to 40 mg/L, then to 20 mg/L, and finally, to 10 mg/L.

3-13. A, C. *Incorrect answers*

   B. CORRECT ANSWER. To find the $T\frac{1}{2}$ of 10 hours, find the interval of time necessary for the concentration to decrease from 100 to 50.

3-14. A. CORRECT ANSWER

   B. *Incorrect answer. You may have used $T\frac{1}{2}$ = 1/0.087 rather than $T\frac{1}{2}$ = 0.693/K.*

   C. *Incorrect answer.* You may have used $T\frac{1}{2}$ = K/0.693 (and moved the decimal place) rather than $T\frac{1}{2}$ = 0.693/K.

3-15. A. *Incorrect answer*

   B. CORRECT ANSWER. When using the area method, it does not matter if the drug best fits any particular model.

3-16. A. CORRECT ANSWER

   B. *Incorrect answer.* You may have neglected to divide the sum of 100 plus 50 by 2 before then multiplying by the width of 2.

   C, D. *Incorrect answers.* Be sure you calculated the height correctly as the average of 50 and 100.

3-17. A, C, D. *Incorrect answers*

   B. CORRECT ANSWER. Remember, clearance has units of volume/time, so the units in the equation must result in volume/time. Dose/AUC has units of mg/(mg/L) × hour, which reduces to L/hr.

3-18. A, B, C. *Incorrect answers*

   D. CORRECT ANSWER. To calculate clearance, the AUC from time zero to infinity must be used. The AUC from time zero to 12 hours can be calculated, and to this area is added the estimated area from 12 hours to infinity. This area is estimated by dividing the drug concentration at 12 hours, 1 mg/L, by the elimination rate constant, 0.20 hr^{-1} (estimated by the slope of the line between the last two points), thereby obtaining an area of 5 (mg/L) × hour from 12 hours to infinity. Clearance = dose/AUC. Dose is 500 mg. AUC is 119 mg/L, which is the sum of 114 mg/L (from 0 to 12 hours) and 5 mg/L (from 12 hours to infinity).

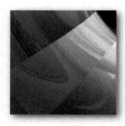

Discussion Points

D-1. Drug X is given by intravenous administration to two patients. Two plasma concentrations are then determined, and the slope of the plasma concentration versus time curve is calculated. Determine which patient (A or B) has the greater elimination rate constant.

	Patient A	Patient B
Slope of plasma concentration versus time curve	−0.55	−0.23

D-2. Drug X is given to two patients, and two plasma drug concentrations are then determined for each patient. Determine which patient has the greater elimination rate constant.

Time after Dose (hr)	Plasma Concentration (mg/L)	
	Patient A	Patient B
8	22	30
16	5	8

D-3. Why is the half-life of most drugs the same at high and low plasma concentrations?

D-4. The plasma concentration versus time curves for two different drugs are exactly parallel; however, one of the drugs has much higher plasma concentrations. What can you say about the two drugs' half-lives?

D-5. For drug X, the AUC determines the intensity of drug effect. Explain why a reduction of drug clearance by 50% would result in the same intensity of effect as doubling the dose.

D-6. Discuss the mathematical consequences of using a negative versus a positive value for elimination rate constant (k). How do the rules of logarithms affect the arrangements of the equations used to calculate elimination rate constant and desired dosing interval (τ)?

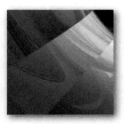

The following problems are for your review. Definitions of symbols and key equations are provided here:

X_0 = dose administered

K = elimination rate constant

V = volume of distribution

$T\frac{1}{2}$ = half-life

t_0 = time immediately after drug administration

C_0 = concentration of drug in plasma at t_0

$C_t = C_0 e^{-Kt}$ = concentration of drug in plasma at any time (t) after drug administration

AUC = area under plasma concentration versus time curve

Cl_t = total drug clearance from body = dose/AUC

$$K = \frac{\ln C_0 - \ln C_1}{t_1 - t_0}$$

QUESTIONS

The following applies to **Questions PS1-1 to PS1-3**. A 1.5-g dose of drug X is administered by intravenous injection, and the following plasma concentrations result (a one-compartment model is assumed):

Time after Dose (hr)	Plasma Concentration (mg/L)
2	28
4	22
6	17.2

PS1-1. The plasma concentration at 9 hours after the dose estimated from a plot of the points on semilog graph paper* is _____.

    A. 10.5 mg/L

    B. 12 mg/L

    C. 13.9 mg/L

    D. 14.8 mg/L

    *Hint: 3-cycle semilog graph paper can often be found free via an Internet search.

PS1-2. An estimate for the volume of distribution would be approximately _____.

    A. 67 L

    B. 42 L

    C. 53 L

PS1-3. For this same example, the half-life would be _____.

    A. 2.2 hours

    B. 4.5 hours

    C. 3.1 hours

    D. 5.8 hours

The following applies to **Questions PS1-4 to PS1-6**. An 100-mg dose of drug Y is administered as an intravenous bolus, and the following plasma concentrations result:

Time after Dose (hr)	Plasma Concentration (mg/L)
0	19.2
0.5	18.1
1	16.5
2	13.5
4	8.5
8	2.2

PS1-4. Using the plasma concentrations at 4 and 8 hours, K is _____.

    A. 0.118 hr^{-1}

    B. 0.338 hr^{-1}

    C. 0.478 hr^{-1}

    D. 0.675 hr^{-1}

PS1-5. Using the trapezoidal rule, calculate the area under the curve from 0 to infinity (∞).

Remember: $AUC_{0 \to \infty}$ equals AUC_{0-8} plus the area under the curve after 8 hours. This terminal area is calculated by taking the final concentration (at 8 hours) and dividing by *K* above.

    A. 6.51 (mg/L) × hr

    B. 76.38 (mg/L) × hr

    C. 82.89 (mg/L) × hr

    D. 47.35 (mg/L) × hr

PS1-6. For this same example, the clearance calculated by the area method would be _____.

    A. 0.82 L/hr

    B. 0.974 L/hr

    C. 1.52 L/hr

    D. 1.21 L/hr

ANSWERS

PS1-1. A, C. *Incorrect answers*. You may have used linear graph paper rather than semilog paper.

    B   CORRECT ANSWER

    D. *Incorrect answer.* Be sure your *x*-scale for time is correct and that you extrapolated the concentration for 9 hours.

PS1-2. A, C. *Incorrect answers*

    B. CORRECT ANSWER. First, estimate C_0 by drawing a line back to time = 0 (t_0) using the three plotted points. This should equal 36 mg/L.

    Then, $V = dose/C_0 = 1500 \text{ mg}/36 \text{ mg/L} = 41.6$ or 42 L.

PS1-3. A. *Incorrect answer.* You may have calculated the numerator incorrectly.

    B, C. *Incorrect answers*. You may have used the wrong time interval.

    D. CORRECT ANSWER. Half life = 0.693/*K*, where: $K = (\ln 22 - \ln 28)/(4 \text{ hr} - 2 \text{ hr}) = 0.12 \text{ hr}^{-1}$. So, half-life = 0.693/0.12 = 5.78 hr.

PS1-4. A, C, D. *Incorrect answers*

    B. CORRECT ANSWER

$$K = \frac{\ln 2.2 - \ln 8.5}{8 \text{ hr} - 4 \text{ hr}} = \frac{0.79 - 2.14}{4 \text{ hr}}$$

$$= 0.338 \text{ hr}^{-1}$$

PS1-5. A. *Incorrect answer.* You may have included just the area from 8 hours to infinity.

    B. *Incorrect answer.* You may not have included the area from 8 hours to infinity.

    C. CORRECT ANSWER.

For AUC from 0 to 8 hours:

$$\frac{18.1 \text{ mg/L} + 19.2 \text{ mg/L}}{2}(0.5 \text{ hr}) = 9.325 \text{ mg*hr/L}$$

$$\frac{16.5 \text{ mg/L} + 18.1 \text{ mg/L}}{2}(0.5 \text{ hr}) = 8.65 \text{ mg*hr/L}$$

$$\frac{13.5 \text{ mg/L} + 16.5 \text{ mg/L}}{2}(1 \text{ hr}) = 15 \text{ mg*hr/L}$$

$$\frac{8.5 \text{ mg/L} + 13.5 \text{ mg/L}}{2}(2 \text{ hr}) = 22 \text{ mg*hr/L}$$

$$\frac{2.2 \text{ mg/L} + 8.5 \text{ mg/L}}{2}(4 \text{ hr}) = 21.4 \text{ mg*hr/L}$$

$$9.325 + 8.65 + 15 + 22 + 21.4$$
$$= 76.38 \text{ (mg} \times \text{hr)/L}$$

For AUC from 8 hours to infinity:

$$AUC = \frac{2.2 \text{ mg/L}}{0.338 \text{ hr}^{-1}} = 6.51 \text{ (mg} \times \text{hr)/L}$$

Therefore, the AUC from time zero to infinity equals:

$$76.375 \, \text{(mg/L)} \times \text{hr} + 6.51 \, \text{(mg/L)} \times \text{hr}$$
$$= 82.89 \, \text{(mg/L)} \times \text{hr}$$

D. *Incorrect answer.* You may not have multiplied by ½ when calculating the area from 8 hours to infinity.

PS1-6. A. *Incorrect answer.* You may have inverted the formula.

B, C. *Incorrect answers*

D. CORRECT ANSWER

$$\text{Clearance} = \frac{\text{dose}}{\text{AUC}} = \frac{100 \, \text{mg}}{82.89 \, \text{(mg/L)} \times \text{hr}}$$
$$= 1.21 \, \text{L/hr}$$

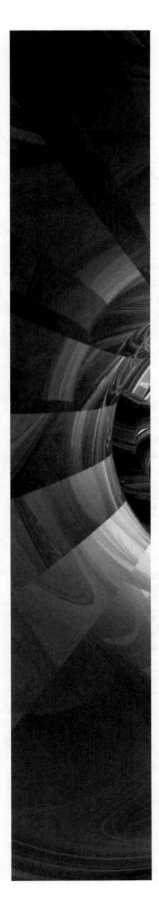

Intravenous Bolus Administration, Multiple Drug Administration, and Steady-State Average Concentrations

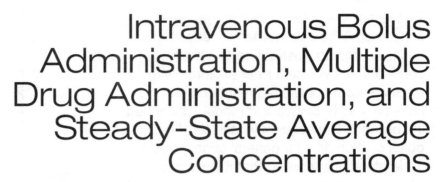

OBJECTIVES

After completing Lesson 4, you should be able to:

1. Describe the principle of superposition and how it applies to multiple drug dosing.

2. Define *steady state*, and describe how it relates to a drug's half-life.

3. Calculate the estimated peak plasma concentration after multiple drug dosing (at steady state).

4. Calculate the estimated trough plasma concentration after multiple drug dosing (at steady state).

5. Understand the equation for accumulation factor at steady state.

In clinical practice, most pharmacokinetic dosing is performed with one-compartment, intermittent infusion models at steady state. Using these models, we can obtain, from population estimates or patient-specific calculation, an elimination rate constant (K) and a dosing interval (τ) based on this K value. Volume of distribution (V) can likewise be either estimated or calculated from patient-specific values. So far, our discussion has been limited to a single intravenous (IV) bolus dose of drug; however, most clinical situations require a therapeutic effect for time periods extending beyond the effect of one dose. In these situations, multiple doses of drug are given. The goal is to maintain a therapeutic effect by keeping the amount of drug in the body, as well as the concentration of drug in the plasma, within a fairly constant range (the therapeutic range). In this lesson, we construct equations for predicting drug concentrations after multiple IV bolus (i.e., IV push) doses. Intermediate equations are used simply to illustrate the derivation of the final equations that can be applied clinically. Full understanding of this simpler IV bolus model will aid in the understanding of the slightly more complicated yet more clinically relevant IV intermittent infusion equations used later in this book.

Clinical Correlate

This lesson describes a one-compartment, first-order, IV bolus pharmacokinetic model. It is used only to illustrate certain math concepts that will be further explored with the more commonly used IV intermittent infusion (i.e., IV piggyback) models described in Lesson 5. Consequently, read this IV bolus section only for general conceptual understanding, knowing that it is seldom applied clinically.

Intravenous Bolus Dose Model

Although not used often clinically, the simplest example of multiple dosing is the administration of rapid IV doses (IV boluses) of drug at constant time intervals, in which the drug is represented by a one-compartment model with first-order elimination (i.e., one-compartment, first-order model).

The first dose produces a plasma drug concentration versus time curve like the one in **Figure 4-1**. C_0 is now referred to as C_{max}, meaning maximum concentration, to group it with the other peak concentrations that occur with multiple dosing.

If a second bolus dose is administered before the first dose is completely eliminated, the maximum concentration after the second dose ($C_{max\ 2}$) will be higher than that after the first dose ($C_{max\ 1}$) (**Figure 4-2**). The second part of the curve will be similar to the first curve but will be higher (have a greater concentration), because some drug remains from the first dose when the second dose is administered.

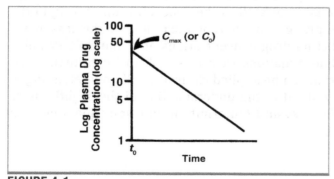

FIGURE 4-1.
Plasma drug concentrations after a first dose.

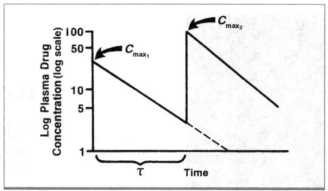

FIGURE 4-2.
Plasma drug concentrations resulting from a second dose.

The *dosing interval* is the time between administrations of doses. The dosing interval, symbolized by the Greek letter tau (τ), is commonly determined by a drug's half-life. Rapidly eliminated drugs (i.e., those having a short half-life [$T\frac{1}{2}$]) generally have to be given more frequently (shorter τ) than drugs with a longer half-life.

If a drug follows first-order elimination (i.e., the fraction of drug eliminated per unit of time is constant), then plasma drug concentrations after multiple dosing can be predicted from concentrations after a single dose. This method uses the principle of superposition, a simple overlay technique.

If the early doses of drug do not affect the pharmacokinetics (e.g., absorption and clearance) of subsequent doses, then plasma drug concentration versus time curves after each dose will look the same; they will be superimposable. The only difference is that the actual concentrations are higher until steady state is achieved because drug has accumulated.

Recall that the y-intercept is called C_0, and the slope of the line is $-K$. Furthermore, the drug concentration at any time (C_t) after the first IV bolus dose is given by:

$$\ln C_t = \ln C_0 - Kt \quad \text{(See \textbf{Equation 3-2}.)}$$

or:

$$C_t = C_0 e^{-Kt}$$

A second IV bolus dose is administered after the dosing interval (τ) but before the first dose is completely eliminated. Because $C_t = C_0 e^{-Kt}$ at any time (t) after the first dose, it follows that:

$$C_{min1} = C_{max1}\ e^{-K\tau}$$

where $C_{\min 1}$ is the concentration just before the next dose is given, and τ, the dosing interval, is the time from $C_{\max}$ to $C_{\min}$.

$C_{\max 2}$ is the sum of $C_{\min 1}$ and $C_{\max 1}$ (**Figure 4-3**), as the same dose is given again:

$$C_{\max 2} = C_{\max 1} + C_{\min 1}$$

We showed that:

$$C_{\min 1} = C_{\max 1} e^{-K\tau}$$

so:

$$C_{\max 2} = C_{\max 1} + C_{\max 1} e^{-K\tau}$$

By rearranging, we get:

$$C_{\max 2} = C_{\max 1}\left(1 + e^{-K\tau}\right)$$

A third IV bolus dose can be administered after the same dosing interval (τ). The plasma drug concentration versus time profile reveals a further increase in the maximum concentration immediately after the third dose, as shown in **Figure 4-4**. Just as after the first dose:

$$C_{\min 2} = C_{\max 2} e^{-K\tau}$$

which, by substitution for $C_{\max 2} = C_{\max 1}(1 + e^{-K\tau})e^{-K\tau}$. Moreover:

$$C_{\max 3} = C_{\max 2} + C_{\max 1}$$

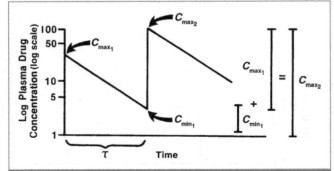

FIGURE 4-3.
$C_{\max 2}$ calculation.

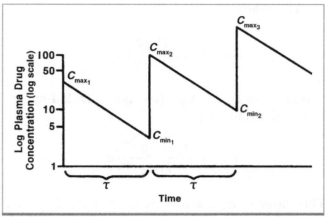

FIGURE 4-4.
Increase in $C_{\max}$ with repeated doses.

which, substituting for $C_{\min 2} = C_{\max 1}(1 + e^{-K\tau})e^{-K\tau} + C_{\max 1}$. This simplifies as follows:

$$C_{\max 3} = C_{\max 1}[(1 + e^{-K\tau})(e^{-K\tau}) + 1]$$

$$= C_{\max 1}[e^{-K\tau} + e^{-2K\tau} + 1]$$

$$= C_{\max 1}[1 + e^{-K\tau} + e^{-2K\tau}]$$

As we can see, a pattern emerges—after any number of dosing intervals, the maximum concentration will be:

$$C_{\min n} = C_{\max 1}[1 + e^{-K\tau} + e^{-2K\tau} + \ldots + e^{-(n-1)K\tau}]$$

where n is the number of doses given. This equation can be simplified by mathematical procedures to a more useful form:

$$C_{\max n} = C_{\max 1}\frac{(1 - e^{-nK\tau})}{(1 - e^{-K\tau})}$$

where $C_{\max n}$ is the concentration just after n number of doses are given. So, if we know $C_{\max 1}$, the elimination rate, and the dosing interval, we can predict the maximum plasma concentration after any number (n) of doses.

We also know that $C_{\min n}$ (concentration just before a dose is given) equals $C_{\max n} e^{-K\tau}$.

Therefore:

$$C_{\max n} = C_{\max 1} \frac{(1 - e^{-nK\tau})}{(1 - e^{-K\tau})} e^{-K\tau}$$

and because $C_{\max 1} = X_0/V$ (i.e., dose divided by volume of distribution):

$$C_{\min n} = \frac{X_0}{V} \frac{(1 - e^{-nK\tau})}{(1 - e^{-K\tau})} e^{-K\tau}$$

This latter change allows us to calculate $C_{\min}$ if we know the dose and volume of distribution, a likely situation in clinical practice.

In each of the preceding equations, the term $(1 - e^{-nK\tau})/(1 - e^{-K\tau})$ appears. It is called the *accumulation factor*, because it relates drug concentration after a single dose to drug concentration after n doses with multiple dosing. This factor is a number greater than 1, which indicates how much higher the concentration will be after n doses compared with the first dose. For example, if 100 doses of a certain drug are given to a patient, where $K = 0.05$ hr^{-1} and $\tau = 8$ hours, the accumulation factor is calculated as follows:

$$\frac{(1 - e^{-nK\tau})}{(1 - e^{-K\tau})} = \frac{(1 - e^{-100(0.05\ hr^{-1})8\ hr})}{(1 - e^{-(0.05\ hr^{-1})8\ hr})} = 3.03$$

This means that the peak (or trough) concentration after 100 doses will be 3.03 times the peak (or trough) concentration after the first dose.

The accumulation factor for two or three doses can also be calculated to predict concentrations before achievement of steady state.

Remember:

4-1   accumulation factor $= \dfrac{(1 - e^{-nK\tau})}{(1 - e^{-K\tau})}$

So for the second IV bolus dose:

$$\text{accumulation factor (two doses)} = \frac{(1 - e^{-2(0.05\ hr^{-1})8\ hr})}{(1 - e^{-(0.05\ hr^{-1})8\ hr})}$$

$$= \frac{(1 - 0.449)}{(1 - 0.670)}$$

$$= 1.67$$

For the third IV bolus dose:

$$\text{accumulation factor (three doses)} = \frac{(1 - e^{-3(0.05\ hr^{-1})8\ hr})}{(1 - e^{-(0.05\ hr^{-1})8\ hr})}$$

$$= \frac{(1 - 0.301)}{(1 - 0.670)}$$

$$= 2.12$$

Therefore, after two or three doses, the observed peak drug concentration will be 1.67 or 2.12 times the peak concentration after the first dose, respectively. The concept of accumulation factor is discussed in more detail in the Accumulation Factor section later in this lesson.

These equations are used later to predict drug concentrations for given dosage regimens. For certain drugs (e.g., aminoglycosides), it is important to predict peak ($C_{\max}$) and trough ($C_{\min}$) concentrations in various clinical situations.

Clinical Correlate

If a drug has a very short half-life (much less than the dosing interval), then the plasma concentrations resulting from each dose will be the same, and accumulation of drug will not occur because the fraction remaining after the previous dose approaches zero and does not contribute to $C_{\max}$ (as shown in **Figure 4-5**). An example would be a drug such as gentamicin given every 8 hours intravenously to a patient whose excellent renal function results in a drug half-life of 1.0–1.5 hours.

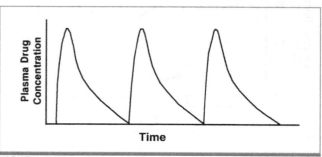

FIGURE 4-5.
Plasma drug concentration versus time.

Intravenous Bolus Equations at Steady State

As successive doses of a drug are administered, the drug begins to accumulate in the body. With first-order elimination, the amount of drug eliminated per unit of time is proportional to the amount of drug in the body. Accumulation continues until the rate of elimination approaches the rate of administration:

Rate of drug going in = rate of drug going out

As the rate of drug elimination increases and then approaches that of drug administration, the maximum (peak) and minimum (trough) concentrations increase until equilibrium is reached. After that point, there will be no additional accumulation; the maximum and minimum concentrations will remain constant with each subsequent dose of drug (**Figure 4-6**).

When this equilibrium occurs, the maximum (and minimum) drug concentrations are the same for each additional dose given (assuming the same dose and dosing interval are used). When the maximum (and minimum) drug concentrations for successive doses are the same, the amount of drug eliminated over the dosing interval (rate out) equals the dose administered (rate in), and the condition of *steady state* is reached.

Steady state will always be reached after repeated drug administration at the same dosing interval if the drug follows first-order elimination. However, the time required to reach steady state varies from drug to drug, depending on the elimination rate constant. With a higher elimination rate constant (more rapid elimination and shorter half-life), steady state is reached sooner than with a lower one (more less rapid elimination and longer half-life) (**Figure 4-7**).

Steady state is the point at which the amount of drug administered over a dosing interval equals the amount of drug being eliminated over that same period, and it is totally dependent on the elimination rate constant. Therefore, when the elimination rate is higher, a greater amount of drug is eliminated over a given time interval; it then takes a shorter time for the amount of drug eliminated and the amount of drug administered to become equivalent (and, therefore, achieve steady state). If the half-life of a drug is known, the time to reach steady state can be determined. If repeated doses of drug are given at a fixed interval, then in one half-life, the plasma concentrations will reach 50% of those at steady state. By the end of the second half-life, the concentrations will be 75% of steady state, and so on, as shown in **Table 4-1**. The plasma concentrations will increase by progressively smaller increments. For all practical purposes, steady state will be reached after approximately four or five half-lives; the concentrations at steady state may be abbreviated as C_{ss}.

For a drug such as gentamicin, with a 1- to 4-hour half-life in patients with normal renal function, steady-state concentration is achieved within 10–20 hours. For agents with longer half-lives, such as digoxin and phenobarbital, however, a week or longer may be needed to reach steady state.

With multiple drug doses (**Figure 4-8**), steady state is reached when the drug from the first dose is almost entirely eliminated from the body. At this

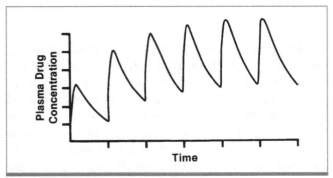

FIGURE 4-6.
Multiple-dose drug administration.

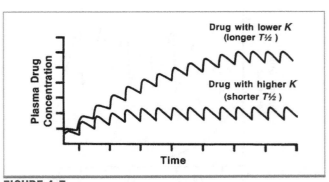

FIGURE 4-7.
Steady state is reached sooner with a drug having a shorter half-life.

TABLE 4-1. Percentage of Steady-State Concentration Reached

Duration of Drug Administration (half-lives)	Steady-State Concentration Reached (%)
1	50
2	75
3	87.5
4	93.75
5	96.875
6	98.4735
7	99.25

TABLE 4-2. Time to Reach Steady State for Commonly Used Drugs[a]

Drug	Time (hr)
Amlodipine	195
Amoxicillin	8.5
Morphine	9.5
Moxifloxacin	77
Sertraline	115
Simvastatin	10–15
Valsartan	47
Vancomycin	28

[a]Calculated from average drug half-lives, Table 3-2.

point, the amount of drug remaining from the first dose does not contribute significantly to the total amount of drug in the body. After a single dose, approximately four or five half-lives are required for the body to eliminate the amount of drug equivalent to one dose. However, at steady state, the amount of drug equivalent to one dose is eliminated over one dosing interval. This apparently faster elimination is a result of accumulation of drug in the body. Although the same proportion (usually expressed as percentage) of drug is eliminated per hour, the greater amount of drug in the body at steady state causes a greater amount to be eliminated over the same time period.

The average times to reach steady state for some commonly used drugs are shown in **Table 4-2**. These values may vary considerably between individuals and may be altered by disease. For some

drugs (e.g., aspirin, ranitidine, and gentamicin), the therapeutic effects will begin before steady-state plasma concentrations are reached. For others (e.g., zidovudine or lovastatin), a much longer time period than that needed to reach steady state is necessary for full therapeutic benefits.

Clinical Correlate

Time to achieve steady state is a physiologic function based solely on the drug's K or half-life, and the amount of time it takes to achieve steady state cannot be increased or decreased. However, administration of a loading dose for drugs that take many hours to reach steady state is commonly used to achieve a concentration within the therapeutic range from the outset of therapy.

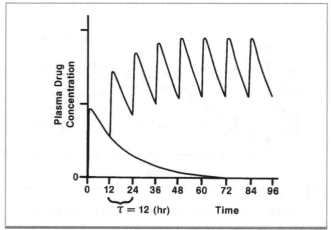

FIGURE 4-8.
At steady state, the time required to eliminate one dose of drug is one dosing interval.

The time to reach steady state is determined by the drug's elimination rate constant (K), but what determines the actual plasma drug concentrations achieved? At steady state, the levels achieved depend on the drug's clearance, volume of distribution, dose, and dosing interval (τ). When equivalent doses are given, a drug with a low elimination rate constant and small volume of distribution should achieve higher steady-state plasma concentrations than an otherwise similar agent with a high elimination rate constant and large volume of distribution. In the remainder of this lesson, we examine some aspects of multiple drug dosing.

Steady-state concentrations are commonly increased in two ways:

- Method 1—Increase the drug dose but maintain the same dosing interval (τ), as shown in **Figure 4-9**, which results in wider fluctuations between the maximum (peak) and minimum (trough) concentrations after each dose.

- Method 2—Keep the same dose but give it more frequently, as shown in **Figure 4-10**, which reduces the differences between the peak and trough concentrations.

Note that the time to achieve steady state is the same in both figures.

Clinical Correlate

You may wish to change a patient's steady-state drug concentrations. For example, the patient is not receiving maximal benefits, because the steady-state concentrations are relatively low or the steady-state levels are high, causing the patient to experience toxic effects. Remember from earlier in this lesson that repeated doses of drug require approximately four or five half-lives to reach steady state. Clinically, this means that each time a dose or dosing interval is changed, four or five half-lives are needed to reach a new steady state. Of course, a drug with a long half-life will require a longer time to achieve the new steady state than a drug with a relatively short half-life. For example, Drug A has a half-life of 6 hours; if the dose or dosing interval is changed, steady state will not be reached for 24–30 hours after the change. If Drug B has a half-life of 3 hours, steady state will be reached in 12–15 hours after a change in the dose or dosing interval.

In deciding on a specific dosing regimen for a patient, the goal is to achieve a certain plasma concentration of drug at steady state. Ideally, peak and trough concentrations will both be within the therapeutic range (**Figure 4-11**).

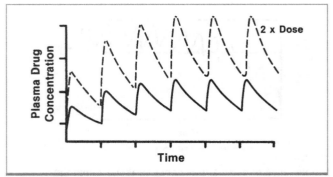

FIGURE 4-9.
Dose increase with no change in dosing interval to achieve higher concentrations.

Accumulation Factor

Equations can describe the plasma concentrations and pharmacokinetics of a drug at steady state. Remember, steady state will be reached only after four or five half-lives.

Recall that with an IV bolus injection of a drug fitting a one-compartment model and first-order elimination, the drug concentration at any time (t) after any number of doses (n), not necessarily at steady state, can be described by:

$$C_{n(t)} = \frac{X_0}{V} \left(\frac{1 - e^{-nKt}}{1 - e^{-Kt}} \right) e^{-Kt}$$

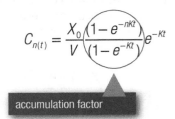

accumulation factor

Note the inclusion of the accumulation factor from Equation 4-1 as part of this equation.

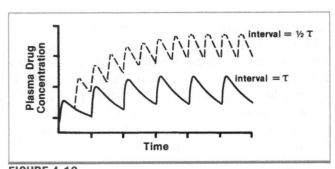

FIGURE 4-10.
Dosing interval decrease with no change in dose to achieve higher concentrations.

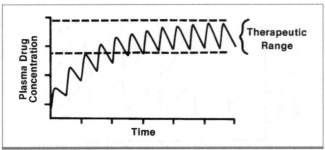

FIGURE 4-11.
Maintenance of plasma drug concentrations within the therapeutic range.

To predict the plasma concentration of a drug at any time t after n number of doses, we therefore need to know four values:

- drug dose (X_0),
- volume of distribution (V),
- elimination rate constant (K), and
- dosing interval (τ).

If we wish to predict the steady-state peak concentration immediately after an IV bolus dose, where $t = 0$ and $e^{-0} = 1$, the previous equation for $C_{n(t)}$ becomes:

$$C_{peak\,(n)} = \frac{X_0}{V}\frac{(1-e^{-nK\tau})}{(1-e^{-K\tau})}$$

because time after the dose equals zero ($t = 0$, and $e^{-0} = 1$).

As multiple drug doses are administered and n becomes sufficiently large (more than four or five doses), n increases and approaches infinity (abbreviated as $n\rightarrow\infty$). The preceding equation can then be simplified. As n becomes a large number, $e^{-nK\tau}$ approaches $e-\infty$, which approaches zero, so $1 - e^{-nK\tau}$ approaches 1. As $1 - e^{-nK\tau}$ approaches 1, the value of this numerator becomes 1, and the resultant numerator/denominator combination is termed the *accumulation factor at steady state*:

4-2
$$\frac{1}{(1-e^{-K\tau})}$$

The equation for $C_{peak(n)}$ now becomes the equation for $C_{ss\,peak}$ and can be written as:

$$C_{ss\,peak} = \frac{X_0}{V}\left[\frac{1}{(1-e^{-K\tau})}\right]$$

We can estimate the minimum or trough concentration at steady state. The trough concentration occurs just before the administration of the next dose (at $t = \tau$). In this situation, the general equation for $C_{n(t)}$ becomes:

$$C_{ss\,trough} = \frac{X_0}{V}\left[\frac{1}{(1-e^{-K\tau})}\right]e^{-K\tau}$$

Clinical Correlate

In most clinical situations, it is preferable to wait until a drug concentration is at steady state before obtaining serum drug concentrations. Use of steady-state concentrations is more accurate and makes the numerous required calculations easier.

Note the similarity between the equations for $C_{ss\,peak}$ and $C_{ss\,trough}$. The expression for $C_{ss\,trough}$ simplifies to $C_{ss\,peak}$ times e^{-Kt}. An almost identical equation (following) can be used to calculate the concentration at any time after the peak. The only difference is that t is replaced by the time elapsed since the peak level.

Therefore:

$$C_{(t)} = C_{ss\,peak}e^{-Kt}$$

where t is the time after the peak.

This last relationship is very useful in clinical pharmacokinetics. It is really the same as an equation presented earlier. (See **Equation 3-2**.)

$$C_t = C_0 e^{-Kt}$$

The preceding equation, stated in words, means a concentration at any time (C_t) is equal to some previous concentration (C_0) multiplied by the fraction (or percent) of that previous concentration (i.e., e^{-Kt}) remaining after it has been allowed to be eliminated from the body for a number of hours represented by t.

If two drug concentrations and the time between them are known, K can be calculated. If one concentration after a dose (e.g., a peak concentration) and K are known, then other concentrations at any time after a dose (but before the next dose) can be estimated.

$$-K = \frac{\ln C_1 - \ln C_2}{t_1 - t_2}$$

Average Steady-State Concentration with Intravenous Bolus Dosing

We now have examined both the maximum and minimum concentrations that occur at steady state. Another useful parameter in multiple IV dosing situations is the average concentration of drug in the plasma at steady state (C_{ss}) (**Figure 4-12**). Because C_{ss} is independent of any pharmacokinetic model, it is helpful to the practicing clinician (model assumptions do not have to be made). C_{ss} is not an arithmetic or geometric mean.

Several mathematical methods may be used to calculate the average drug concentration, but only one is presented here. A plasma drug concentration versus time curve, after steady state has been achieved with IV dosing, is illustrated in **Figure 4-13**. By knowing the dose given (X_0) and the dosing interval (τ), we can determine the average concentration if we also know the area under the plasma drug concentration versus time curve (AUC) over τ. Therefore:

$$C_{ss} = \frac{AUC}{\tau}$$

$$AUC = C_{ss} \times \tau$$

and since:

$$AUC = \frac{dose}{drug\ clearance}$$

$$C_{ss} = \frac{dose}{drug\ clearance \times \tau}$$

therefore:

$$\frac{D}{C} = \frac{C_{ss}}{Cl \times \tau}$$

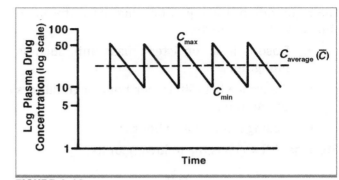

FIGURE 4-12.
Average plasma drug concentration at steady state.

Finally we get the equation:

4-3
$$C_{ss} = \frac{dose}{Cl_t \times \tau}$$

is very useful, particularly with drugs having a long half-life, in which the difference between peak and trough steady-state levels may not be large.

It is important to recognize from the equations that C_{ss} at steady state is determined by the clearance and drug dose (dose/τ). If the dose remains the same (n = a time period such as a day [e.g., 80 mg every 8 hours {80×3} or 120 mg every 12 hours {120×2}]), while τ is changed, C_{ss} would remain the same. Also, changes in V or K that are not related to a change in clearance would not alter C_{ss}. With multiple drug dosing at steady state, changes in τ, K, or V (with no change in clearance) would alter the observed peak and trough drug concentrations but not C_{ss}.

In dealing with such equations, it is helpful to remember that the units of measure on both sides must be the same. For example, in Equation 4.3, C_{ss} should be in micrograms per milliliter, milligrams per liter, or similar concentration units. Therefore,

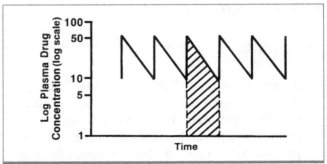

FIGURE 4-13.
AUC for one dosing interval.

the right side of the equation must have the same units, as in the following:

- Dose is in a consistent mass unit, such as milligrams.
- Clearance is in liters per hour or milliliters per minute.
- Dosing interval is in hours.

So, dose/(Cl × τ) has the following units:

$$\frac{\text{amount}}{(\text{volume} / \text{time}) \times \text{time}}$$

Then, as both hour terms cancel out, we see that amount per volume (concentration) is left.

Predicting Steady-State Concentration

The equation for $C_{ss\,peak}$ derived previously (and shown following) is valuable because it allows us to predict the peak plasma concentration achieved when a drug is given in a specified dose (X_0) at a consistent and repeated interval (τ). To predict peak concentration at steady state, however, we also must have an estimate of the elimination rate (K) and the volume of distribution (V); therefore, the following equation is used only for IV bolus dosing:

$$C_{ss\,peak} = \frac{X_0}{V}\left[\frac{1}{(1-e^{-K\tau})}\right]$$

It is possible to estimate a patient's K and V from published reports of similar patients. For example, most patients with normal renal function will have a gentamicin V of 0.20–0.30 L/kg and a K of 0.035–0.2 hr^{-1}. In a clinical setting in which a drug is administered and plasma concentrations are then determined, it is possible to calculate a patient's actual K and V using plasma concentrations. Such calculations can be performed as follows.

EXAMPLE 1

A patient receives 500 mg of drug X intravenously every 6 hours until steady state is reached. Just after the dose is administered, a blood sample is drawn to determine a peak plasma concentration. Then, 5 hours later, a second plasma concentration is determined. Using the two plasma concentrations, we first calculate K, as described previously:

$$K = \frac{\ln C_{peak} - \ln C_{5\,hr}}{5\ hr}$$

Then we insert the known C_{peak}, K, X_0, and τ values in the equation for C_{peak}. By rearranging the equation to isolate the only remaining unknown variable, we can then use it to calculate V:

$$V = \frac{X_0}{C_{ss\,peak}}\left[\frac{1}{(1-e^{-K\tau})}\right]$$

Now we know the values of all the variables in the equation (V, K, C_{peak}, X_0, and τ) and can use this information to calculate a new C_{peak} if we change the dose (e.g., if the previous C_{peak} is too high or too low). For example, if we want the peak level to be higher and wish to calculate the required dose to reach this new peak level, we can rearrange our equation:

$$X_0 = V \times C_{ss\,peak}(1-e^{-Kt})$$

and substitute our calculated V and K and the desired C_{peak}. Or we can choose a new dose (X_0) and calculate the resulting C_{peak} by inserting the calculated K and V with τ into the original equation:

$$C_{ss\,peak} = \frac{X_0}{V}\left[\frac{1}{(1-e^{-K\tau})}\right]$$

Remember that each time we calculate a peak plasma level (C_{peak}), the trough plasma level also can be calculated if we know K and τ:

$$C_{trough} = C_{peak}e^{-K\tau}$$

If the dosing interval is not changed, new doses and concentrations are directly proportional if nothing else changes (i.e., K or V). So,

$$X_{0\,(new)} = \frac{C_{ss\,peak\,(new)}}{C_{ss\,peak\,(old)}} \times X_{0\,(old)}$$

and,

$$C_{ss\,peak\,(new)} = \frac{X_{0\,(new)}}{X_{0\,(old)}} \times C_{ss\,(old)}$$

Clinically Important Equations Identified in This Chapter

1. $C_{ss\,peak} = \dfrac{X_0}{V}\left[\dfrac{1}{(1-e^{-K\tau})}\right]$

    This equation is developed from the equation in Lesson 1:

    $$C = X/V$$

    by attaching the steady-state accumulation factor.

2. $C_{trough} = C_{peak}e^{-Kt}$

    This equation is similar to Equation 3-2 in Lesson 3.

3. $\overline{C} = \dfrac{dose}{Cl_t \times \tau}$ Equation 4-3

REVIEW QUESTIONS

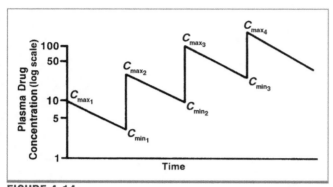

FIGURE 4-14.
Plasma drug concentration versus time.

Note: Refer to **Figure 4-14** when answering questions 4-1 through 4-2.

4-1. If $C_{max\,1}$, K, and τ are 200 mg/L, 0.60 hr^{-1}, and 6 hours, respectively, what is the value of $C_{max\,2}$?
   A. 200 mg/L
   B. 5.4 mg/L
   C. 205.4 mg/L
   D. 223 mg/L

4-2. For the example given in the previous question, what is the value of $C_{min\,2}$?
   A. 5.4 mg/L
   B. 5.5 mg/L
   C. 211 mg/L
   D. 6.2 mg/L

4-3. What is the maximum concentration after 15 doses of a drug if the dose (X_0) is 600 mg and the volume of distribution (V) is 30 L? Assume that τ equals 8 hours and K equals 0.50 hr^{-1}.
   A. 20.4 mg/L
   B. 26.7 mg/L
   C. 39 mg/L

   D. 76 mg/L

4-4. When multiple drug doses are given and steady state is reached, the amount of drug eliminated during one dosing interval (τ) is equal to the drug dose.
   A. True
   B. False

4-5. A drug with a relatively large K (short $T\frac{1}{2}$) takes a longer time to reach steady state than a drug with a small K.
   A. True
   B. False

4-6. If a drug with a $T\frac{1}{2}$ of 8 hours is given every 12 hours and a peak concentration at steady state is 20 mg/L, what will be the approximate peak concentration just after the third dose is administered?
   A. 10 mg/L
   B. 12 mg/L
   C. 15 mg/L
   D. 19 mg/L

4-7. A 100-mg dose of drug X is given to two different patients every 8 hours. Which patient (A or B) is likely to achieve higher steady-state plasma concentrations?

Patient	Elimination Rate (hr^{-1})	Volume of Distribution (L)
A	0.2	10
B	0.4	20

   A. Patient A
   B. Patient B

4-8. Increasing the dosing interval while keeping the dose constant will result in lower steady-state concentrations.
   A. True
   B. False

4-9. Which of the following dosage techniques results in the greatest difference between maximum (peak) and minimum (trough) concentrations after a dose?

  A. Large doses given at a long dosing interval

  B. Small doses given at a short dosing interval

4-10. What is the peak drug X concentration attained at steady state if 50 mg is given by IV injection every 6 hours, the patient's $K = 0.35$ hr^{-1}, and $V = 10$ L? (Assume a one-compartment distribution.)

  A. 1.5 mg/L

  B. 4.4 mg/L

  C. 5.7 mg/L

  D. 35 mg/L

4-11. What would be the trough level for the example in question 4-10?

  A. 0.41 mg/L

  B. 0.7 mg/L

  C. 2 mg/L

  D. 5 mg/L

4-12. A 1000-mg dose of drug X is given every 8 hours until steady-state levels are reached. At steady state, the AUC for one dosing interval is 84 (mg/L) × hour. What is the average concentration over that dosing interval?

  A. 6.1 mg/L

  B. 10.5 mg/L

  C. 12.5 mg/L

  D. 22 mg/L

4-13. A patient receives an antimicrobial dose of 500 mg IV every 8 hours. After steady state is reached, a peak level of 14 mg/L is determined; the level 5 hours after the peak is 5 mg/L. What dose is required to attain a peak plasma level of 40 mg/L? (Assume IV bolus drug administration.)

  A. 500 mg

  B. 1000 mg

  C. 1430 mg

  D. 2000 mg

4-14. For the example given in Question 4-13, when the peak plasma level is 40 mg/L, what will the trough plasma level be?

  A. 2.3 mg/L

  B. 3.2 mg/L

  C. 4.8 mg/L

  D. 6.7 mg/L

ANSWERS

4-1. A. *Incorrect answer.* This is the value of $C_{\text{max 1}}$. $C_{\text{max 2}}$ is calculated as the sum of $C_{\text{max 1}}$ and $C_{\text{min 1}}$.

  B. *Incorrect answer.* This value is the minimum concentration after the first dose. Remember to add the value of $C_{\text{max 1}}$, which was 200 mg/L.

  C. **CORRECT ANSWER**

  D. *Incorrect answer.* This is close to the $C_{\text{max 2}}$ but is actually the steady-state C_{max}. $C_{\text{max 2}}$ is calculated as the sum of $C_{\text{max 1}}$ and $C_{\text{min 1}}$.

4-2. A. *Incorrect answer.* This is $C_{\text{min 1}}$.

  B. **CORRECT ANSWER.** $C_{\text{min 2}}$ can be found from $C_{\text{max 2}}$ as follows: $C_{\text{min 2}} = C_{\text{max 2}} (e^{-Kt})$, so $C_{\text{min 2}} = 205.4$ mg/L$(e^{-0.6/\text{hr}} \times 6$ hr$) = 205.4 \times 0.027 = 5.5$ mg/L.

  C, D. *Incorrect answers*

4-3. A. **CORRECT ANSWER**

$$C_{\text{max}\,n} = C_{\text{max}1} \frac{(1 - e^{-nK\tau})}{1 - e^{-K\tau}}$$

$$C_{\text{max}1} = \frac{X_0}{V} = \frac{600 \text{ mg}}{30 \text{ L}}$$

Then

$$C_{\text{max}15} = \left(\frac{600 \text{ mg}}{30 \text{ L}}\right)\left[\frac{(1 - e^{-15(0.5 \text{ hr}^{-1})8 \text{ hr}})}{(1 - e^{-(0.5 \text{ hr}^{-1})8 \text{ hr}})}\right]$$

$$C_{\text{max}15} = 20.4 \text{ mg/L}$$

  B, C, D. *Incorrect answers*

4-4.   A.   CORRECT ANSWER. When steady state is reached, the amount of drug eliminated over one dosing interval is equal to the dose.

      B.   *Incorrect answer*

4-5.   A.   *Incorrect answer*

      B.   CORRECT ANSWER. The half-life directly relates to the time required to reach steady state. Approximately five half-lives are required to reach steady state. A longer half-life (lower K) will mean that more time is required to reach steady state.

4-6.   A, C, D. *Incorrect answers*

      D.   CORRECT ANSWER. Administration of three doses would take 36 hours, which is four and one-half drug half-lives. Using Table 4-1 as a reference, this would be 95.3% of steady state. Therefore, the peak after the third dose = 95.3% of 20 mg/L = 19 mg/L.

4-7.   A.   CORRECT ANSWER. Higher concentrations would result with a lower clearance ($K \times V$).

$Cl = K \times V$, therefore

$Cl_A = (0.2 \ hr^{-1})(10 \ L) = 2 \ L/hr$

$Cl_B = (0.4 \ hr^{-1})(20 \ L) = 8 \ L/hr$

      B.   *Incorrect answer*

4-8.   A.   CORRECT ANSWER. By increasing the dosing interval, the amount of drug administered per unit of time will decrease, and steady-state concentrations will decrease, since more time for clearance to occur is allowed.

      B.   *Incorrect answer*

4-9.   A.   CORRECT ANSWER

      B.   *Incorrect answer.* A small dose given very frequently results in a smaller change from peak to trough concentrations.

4-10.   A, B, D. *Incorrect answers*

      C.   CORRECT ANSWER. The peak concentration is calculated as follows:

$$C_{peak} = (X_0/V)(1/[1-e^{-K\tau}])$$

$$= (50 \ mg/10 \ L)(1/[1-e^{-0.35 \ hr^{-1} \times 6 \ hr}])$$

$$= 5.7 \ mg/L$$

4-11.   A, C, D. *Incorrect answers*

      B.   CORRECT ANSWER. The trough concentration is calculated as follows:

$$C_{trough} = C_{peak} \times e^{-K\tau}$$

$$= 5.7 \ mg/L \times e^{-0.35 \ hr^{-1} \times 6 \ hr}$$

$$= 0.7 \ mg/L$$

In this case, the elapsed time t is equal to τ.

4-12.   A, C, D. *Incorrect answers*

      B.   CORRECT ANSWER. The average plasma concentration is determined as follows:

$$C = AUC/\tau$$

$$= 84 \ (mg/L) \times hr / 8hr$$

$$= 10.5 \ mg/L$$

4-13.   A.   *Incorrect answer.* Giving the same dose would result in the same peak concentration of 14 mg/L.

      B.   *Incorrect answer.* Doubling the dose would result in a doubling of the steady-state peak concentration to 28 mg/L.

      C.   CORRECT ANSWER

$$X_{0 \ (new)} = \frac{C_{ss \ peak \ (new)}}{C_{ss \ peak \ (old)}} \times X_{0 \ (old)}$$

$$= \frac{(40 \ mg/L)}{(14 \ mg/L)} \times 500 \ mg$$

$$= (2.86) \times 500 \ mg$$

$$= 1430 \ mg$$

      D.   *Incorrect answer.* This dose would result in a steady-state peak concentration of 56 mg/L.

4-14.   A, B, C. *Incorrect answers*

   D.   CORRECT ANSWER. To answer this question, K must first be calculated:

$$K = (\ln C_{5\ hr} - \ln C_{peak}) / 5 = -0.206\ hr^{-1}$$

Then, use the following to calculate the trough plasma concentration:

$$C_{trough} = C_{peak} \times e^{-Kt} = 40\ mg/L \times e^{-0.21 hr^{-1} \times 8\ hr}$$

$$= 35\ mg/L \times 0.186 = 7.45\ mg/L$$

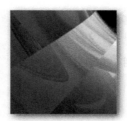 Discussion Points

D-1. Explain why, for most drugs, the increase in drug plasma concentrations resulting from a single dose will be the same magnitude, whether it is the first or tenth dose.

D-2. Explain why the plasma concentrations (maximum or minimum) remain the same for each dose after steady state is reached.

D-3. Explain why changing the dose or the dosing interval does not affect the time to reach steady state.

D-4. The peak plasma concentration achieved after the first IV dose of drug X is 25 mg/L. The drug's half-life is 3.5 hours, and it is administered every 12 hours. What will be the peak plasma concentration at steady state?

D-5. Discuss why the equations for the IV bolus model may not be relevant in clinical practice.

D-6. Discuss the advantages and disadvantages of using the one-compartment first-order model before steady state is attained.

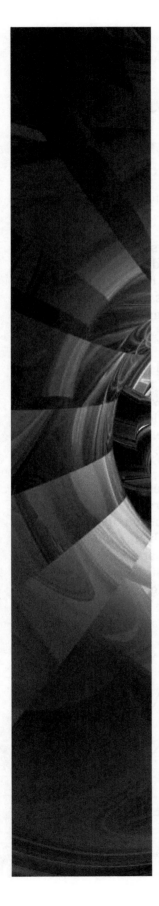

Relationships of Pharmacokinetic Parameters and Intravenous Intermittent and Continuous Infusions

OBJECTIVES

After completing Lesson 5, you should be able to:

1. Explain the relationships of pharmacokinetic parameters and how changes in each parameter affect the others.

2. Describe the relationship between the rate of continuous intravenous (IV) drug infusion, drug clearance, and steady-state plasma concentration.

3. Calculate plasma drug concentrations during and after continuous IV infusion.

4. Calculate an appropriate loading dose to achieve therapeutic range at onset of infusion.

5. Calculate peak and trough concentrations at steady state after intermittent IV infusions.

Relationships of Pharmacokinetic Parameters

Understanding the relationships of pharmacokinetic parameters is important to determine what will occur to the plasma concentration versus time curve when changes in any of the parameters arise. If we administer multiple IV doses of a drug that exhibits one-compartment, first-order elimination kinetics, we might find a plasma drug concentration versus time curve that resembles **Figure 5-1**. A thorough understanding of the basic components of the IV bolus and continuous infusion model will lead to a better understanding of the more commonly used steady-state IV intermittent model equations. Consequently, study this lesson with the knowledge that many of these equations will later be combined and changed to yield the final, more commonly used dosing equations as shown in the cases presented later. Changes in pharmacokinetic parameters often occur due to new illnesses. The new illness will often impact multiple pharmacokinetic parameters simultaneously. Next, we review the impact of changes in pharmacokinetic parameters and common illnesses that cause them.

Changes in Elimination Rate Constant

If the dose, volume of distribution, and dosing interval (τ) all remain the same, but the elimination rate constant (K) decreases (as with decreasing renal or hepatic

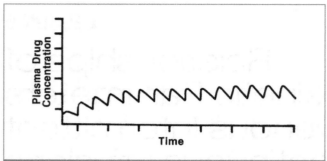

FIGURE 5-1.
Plasma drug concentrations after multiple intravenous doses.

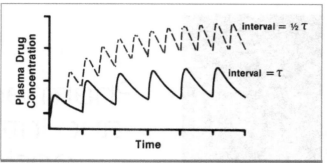

FIGURE 5-3.
Effect of decreased τ on plasma drug concentrations.

function), the curve should change as shown in **Figure 5-2**. With a lower K, we would see the following:

1. Peak and trough concentrations at steady state are higher than before.

2. The difference between peak and trough levels at steady state is smaller because the elimination rate is lower.

Because K is decreased in this situation, the half-life ($T\frac{1}{2}$) is increased; therefore, the time to reach steady state ($5 \times T\frac{1}{2}$) is also lengthened. This concept is important in designing dosing regimens for patients with progressing diseases of the primary organs of drug elimination (kidneys and liver).

Changes in Dosing Interval

For another example, suppose everything, including the elimination rate, remains constant, but the dosing interval (τ) is decreased. The resulting plasma drug concentration versus time curve would be similar to that in **Figure 5-3**. The peak and trough concentrations at steady state are increased. Also, the difference between peak and trough plasma

concentrations at steady state is smaller (only because the body is allowed less time to eliminate drug before receiving the next dose). Because K (and therefore $T\frac{1}{2}$) is the same, the time to reach steady state remains unchanged.

Changes in Dose

Now, suppose that K, V, and τ remain constant, but the dose (X_0) is increased. The plasma concentration versus time curve shown in **Figure 5-4** would result. The drug concentrations at steady state are higher, but there is no difference in the time required to reach steady state, as it is dependent only on $T\frac{1}{2}$ (and K).

With some drugs, it is preferable to give a smaller dose at more frequent intervals; with other drugs, the reverse is true. The disadvantage of larger, less frequent dosing is that the fluctuation from peak to trough concentrations is greater. Thus, the possibility of being in a toxic range just after a dose is given and in a subtherapeutic range before the next dose is given is also greater. The problem with smaller, more frequent doses is that such administration

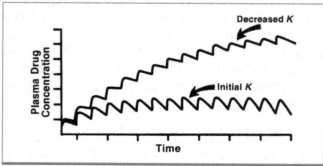

FIGURE 5-2.
Effect of decreased K (and therefore increased $T\frac{1}{2}$) on plasma drug concentrations.

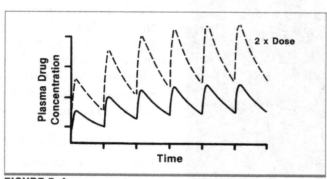

FIGURE 5-4.
Effect of increased dose on plasma drug concentrations.

may not be practical, even though plasma concentrations may be within the therapeutic range for a greater portion of the dosing interval.

Changes in Clearance and Volume of Distribution

A drug's half-life and elimination rate constant are determined by its clearance and volume of distribution (discussed in Lessons 2 and 3). These last two pharmacokinetic parameters determine the plasma drug concentrations that result from a dosing regimen, so changes in clearance or volume of distribution result in changes in steady-state plasma drug concentrations.

Volume of distribution and clearance may change independently. However, some disease states may alter both the clearance and the volume of distribution. An example is the effect of renal failure on aminoglycoside concentrations. The renal clearance of aminoglycosides decreases in patients with renal failure, and the volume of distribution may increase because of the fluid accumulation that occurs with oliguric renal failure.

There are many conditions that may increase or decrease volume of distribution. The volume of distribution of drugs that distribute primarily in body water increases in patients with conditions that cause fluid accumulation (e.g., renal failure, heart failure, liver failure with ascites, and inflammatory processes such as sepsis). As one would expect, dehydration results in a decreased volume of distribution for drugs of this type. Drugs that are highly bound to plasma protein (such as phenytoin) have a greater volume of distribution when protein binding is decreased by hypoalbuminemia or phenytoin-displacing agents (valproic acid, salicylic acid). If fewer proteins are available for binding, then to maintain equilibrium with the tissues, free drug moves from the plasma to the tissues, thus increasing the "apparent" volume of distribution.

Changes in the volume of distribution directly affect steady-state plasma drug concentrations. In general, if the drug dose, dosing interval (τ), and drug clearance are all unchanged but the volume of distribution decreases, there will be greater fluctuation of plasma concentrations with higher peak concentrations. Conversely, if the volume of

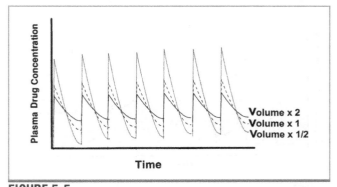

FIGURE 5-5.
Effect of changes in volume of distribution on plasma drug concentrations when clearance is kept constant.

distribution increases, there will be less fluctuation of plasma concentrations with a lower peak (**Figure 5-5**).

The effect of volume of distribution changes on plasma drug concentrations can be easily estimated for most drugs. When the volume of distribution increases, assuming there are no other changes, peak steady-state plasma drug concentrations decrease. Conversely, if the volume of distribution decreases, peak steady-state plasma drug concentrations increase. This is true for medications regardless of whether the medication is delivered via continuous infusion or by intermittent bolus dose. Using drug delivery by constant infusion, this can be demonstrated by the following equation:

$$C_{ss} = K_0 / KV$$

where K_0 = the rate of drug infusion (or administration). (***Note:*** This equation is derived in the section Continuous Infusion later in this lesson.)

There are a number of conditions that may increase or decrease drug clearance. Agents that change renal blood flow directly affect the clearance of drugs excreted by the kidneys. Renal clearance may decrease when agents that compete for active renal secretion are administered concomitantly (such as penicillin with probenecid). For drugs that are eliminated hepatically, clearance may be altered by drugs or conditions that increase or decrease

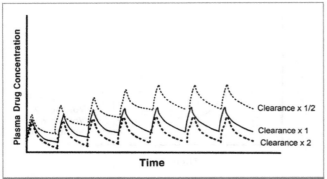

FIGURE 5-6.
Effect of changes in clearance on plasma drug concentrations.

liver blood flow. Some conditions (such as hepatitis or cirrhosis) also may decrease the capability of liver enzymes to metabolize drugs. Drug clearance may increase when organ function improves after healing, with concomitant drug administration, or under conditions that increase organ blood flow or the activity of metabolic enzymes.

Changes in drug clearance affect steady-state plasma drug concentrations. If the dose, dosing interval, and volume of distribution are all unchanged but clearance increases, plasma drug concentrations will decrease, because the drug is being removed at a faster rate. Conversely, if clearance decreases, plasma concentrations will increase, because the drug is being removed at a slower rate (**Figure 5-6**).

This can also be demonstrated by the modification of the equation presented above:

$$C_{ss} = K_0 / Cl_t$$

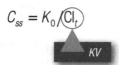

where K_0 = the rate of drug infusion and Cl_t = total body clearance. (**Note:** This equation is also derived in the section Continuous Infusion.)

As with volume of distribution, the effect of changes in clearance on plasma drug concentrations can be easily estimated for most drugs. For example, if drug clearance increases by a factor of two, the average steady-state plasma drug concentration decreases by half. Conversely, if drug clearance decreases by half, the average steady-state plasma drug concentration would increase by a factor of two.

Clinical Correlate

Two conditions that may substantially alter the volume of distribution are severe traumatic or burn injuries. Severely traumatized or burned patients often have a cytokine-induced, systemic inflammatory response syndrome (SIRS), which results in decreased plasma proteins (i.e., albumin) and thus an accumulation of fluid in tissues. An average-weight person (70 kg) may gain as much as 20 kg in fluid over a few days. In comparison to the extra fluid, the body has decreased albumin for binding, and with the accumulation of fluid due to this SIRS, free drug shifts from the plasma into the extravascular fluid, causing drugs that are primarily distributed into body water to have an increased volume of distribution.

Continuous Infusion

The remainder of this lesson describes the continuous infusion model and then shows how it can be combined with the IV bolus model, previously described, to yield the commonly used IV intermittent infusion model (i.e., IV piggyback). As stated earlier, repeated doses of a drug (i.e., intermittent infusions) result in fluctuations in the plasma concentration over time. For some drugs, maintenance of a consistent plasma concentration is advantageous because of a desire to achieve a consistent effect. To maintain consistent plasma drug concentrations, continuous IV infusions are often used. Continuous IV infusions provide continuous administration of drug. If administration is begun and maintained at a constant rate, the plasma drug concentration versus time curve in **Figure 5-7** will result.

The plasma concentrations resulting from the continuous IV infusion of drug are determined by the rate of drug input (rate of drug infusion, K_0), volume of distribution (V), and drug clearance (Cl_t).

The relationship among these parameters is:

$$C_t = \frac{K_0}{VK}(1 - e^{-Kt})$$

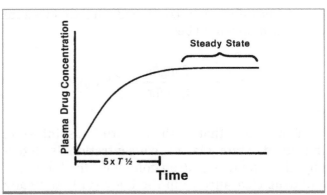

FIGURE 5-7.
Plasma drug concentrations over time with a continuous IV infusion.

where t is the time since the beginning of the drug infusion. This equation shows that the plasma concentration is determined by the rate of drug infusion (K_0) and the clearance of drug from the body (remember, $VK = Cl_t$). The equation is used to find a concentration at a time before steady state is reached.

The term $(1 - e^{-Kt})$ gives the fraction of steady-state concentration achieved by time t after the infusion is begun. For example, when t is a very low number just after an infusion is begun, $K_0(1 - e^{-Kt})$ is also very small. When t is very large, $(1 - e^{-Kt})$ approaches 1, so $K_0(1 - e^{-Kt})$ approaches K_0, and plasma concentration approaches steady state.

Suppose that a drug has a half-life of 8 hours (then $K = 0.087$ hr^{-1}). **Table 5-1** shows how the factor $(1 - e^{-Kt})$ changes with time. When $(1 - e^{-Kt})$ approaches 1 (at approximately five half-lives), steady-state concentrations are approximately achieved.

In Figure 5-7, steady state is attained where the horizontal portion of the curve begins. With a

drug such as theophylline given by continuous IV infusion, the average half-life in adults is approximately 7 hours. Therefore, it will take 35 hours (5 × 7 hours) to reach approximate steady-state plasma concentrations.

When steady state is achieved, the factor e^{-nKt} (see Lesson 4) approaches zero, and thus the factor $(1 - e^{-Kt})$ equals 1, and then:

$$C_{ss} = \frac{K_0}{Cl_t}(1 - e^{-\infty}) = \frac{K_0}{Cl_t}(1 - 0) = \frac{K_0}{Cl_t}$$

At steady state, the plasma concentration of drug is directly proportional to the rate of administration (assuming clearance is unchanged). If the infusion is increased, the steady-state plasma concentration (C_{ss}) will increase proportionally. Clearance is the pharmacokinetic parameter that relates the rate of drug input (dosing or infusion rate) to plasma concentration. The actual plasma concentration attained with a continuous IV infusion of drug depends on the following two factors:

1. rate of drug infusion (K_0)

2. clearance of the drug (Cl_t)

If we know from previous data that a patient receives IV theophylline (or aminophylline), which has a half-life of 6 hours ($K = 0.116$ hr^{-1}) and a volume of distribution of 30 L (clearance then equals 3.48 L/hr), we can predict the steady-state plasma concentration for a continuous IV theophylline infusion of 40 mg/hr:

$$C_{ss} = \frac{K_0}{Cl_t}(1 - e^{-\infty}) = \frac{K_0}{Cl_t}(1 - 0) - \frac{40\text{ mg/hr}}{3.48\text{ L/hr}} = 11.5\text{ mg/L}$$

If we wish to increase the steady-state theophylline plasma concentration to 14 mg/L, we would use the same equation to determine K_0:

$$14\text{ mg/L} = \frac{K_0}{30\text{ L} \times 0.116\text{ hr}^{-1}}$$

$$K_0 = (14\text{ mg/L})(30\text{ L} \times 0.116\text{ hr}^{-1}) = 48.7\text{ mg/hr}$$

Or, as concentration and infusion rate are directly proportional, the following equation may be used to

TABLE 5-1. Changes in Factor $(1 - e^{-Kt})$ Over Time

Time after Starting Infusion (hr)	Value of $(1 - e^{-Kt})$	Drug Half-Lives Elapsed
4	0.29	0.5
8	0.50	1.0
16	0.75	2.0
24	0.88	3.0
40	0.97	5.0
60	0.99	7.5

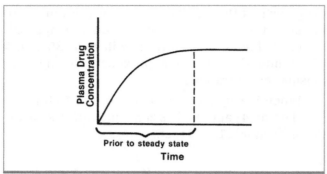

FIGURE 5-8.
Plasma drug concentrations over time with a continuous intravenous infusion.

find a new infusion rate to obtain a desired steady-state concentration:

$$K_{0(new)} = \frac{C_{ss\ (desired)}}{C_{ss\ (measured)}} \times K_{0(original)}$$

$$= \frac{14\ mg/L}{11.5\ mg/L} \times 40\ mg/hr$$

$$= 48.7\ mg/hr$$

With the continuous IV infusion method of drug administration, it is sometimes necessary to predict drug plasma concentrations at times other than at steady state. In the following section, we examine some of these situations (**Figure 5-8**).

The equation predicting plasma concentrations with continuous IV infusion can be used to estimate plasma drug concentrations at times before steady state, as stated previously in the lesson:

$$C_t = \frac{K_0}{VK}(1 - e^{-Kt})$$

(Remember, $VK = Cl_t$.)

For example, if Cl_t for a drug is known to be 4.5 L/hr (with $K = 0.15$ hr^{-1}), and this drug is given at a rate of 50 mg/hr, then the plasma concentration 8 hours after starting the infusion would be:

$$C_{8\ hr} = \frac{50\ mg/hr}{4.5\ L/hr}(1 - e^{-(0.15\ hr^{-1})(8\ hr)})$$

$$= \frac{50\ mg/hr}{4.5\ L/hr}(0.70)$$

$$= 7.8\ mg/L$$

If this infusion is continued, the steady-state concentration would be:

$$C_{ss} = \frac{K_0}{Cl_t} = \frac{50\ mg/hr}{4.5\ L/hr} = 11.1\ mg/L$$

Remember that with a continuous infusion, the steady-state plasma concentration is determined by the rate of drug going into the body (K_0) and drug clearance from the body (Cl_t). At steady state, the amount of drug going into the body per hour equals the amount of drug being removed per hour.

You have learned that it takes approximately five drug half-lives to reach steady state. Each time the infusion rate is changed, five half-lives will be required to attain a new steady-state concentration. For example, for a patient receiving IV theophylline at 20 mg/hr, the steady-state plasma concentration is 7.5 mg/L, and 25 hours is required to reach steady state ($T\frac{1}{2} = 5$ hours, $K = 0.139$ hr^{-1}). If the infusion rate is increased to 40 mg/hr, an additional 25 hours will be required to attain the new steady-state concentration of 15 mg/L (**Figure 5-9**). If a dosing rate is changed, it takes one half-life to reach 50% of the difference between the old concentration and the new, two half-lives to reach 75% of the difference, three half-lives to reach 87.5%, etc.

If we wish to calculate the plasma concentration before the new steady state is achieved, we can use the factor given before: $(1 - e^{-Kt})$, where t is the time after beginning the new infusion rate and the resulting fraction is the relative "distance" between the old and new steady-state concentrations. For

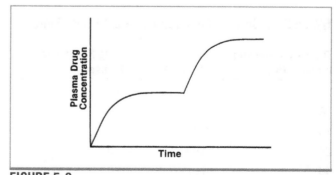

FIGURE 5-9.
Changing plasma drug concentrations with increased drug infusion rate.

the example above (where $K = 0.139$ hr^{-1}), 8 hours after the infusion rate is increased:

$$(1 - e^{-Kt}) = 1 - e^{(-0.139 \text{ hr}^{-1})(8 \text{ hr})}$$

$$= 0.67$$

So at 8 hours, the concentration would be approximately two-thirds (67%) of the way between 7.5 and 15 mg/L (about 12.5 mg/L).

If an infusion is stopped before steady state is reached, the concentration can be determined as follows:

$$C_t = (K_0/Cl_t)(1 - e^{-Kt})$$

where t = the duration of the infusion.

Another important situation occurs when a continuous infusion is stopped after steady state is achieved. To predict plasma drug concentrations at some time after the infusion is stopped (**Figure 5-10**), the concentration at steady state (C_{ss}) is treated as if it were a peak concentration after an IV injection (C_0). In this situation, plasma concentrations after C_0 are predicted by:

$$C_t = (C_0 e^{-Kt}) \quad \text{(See Equation 3-2.)}$$

where t in this case is time after C_0, which is the time after the infusion is stopped.

In the case of continuous infusions:

$$C_t = (C_{ss} e^{-Kt})$$

where t = time after the infusion is stopped.

If, as in the previous example, $K = 0.139$ hr^{-1} and $C_{ss} = 15$ mg/L, the plasma concentration 12 hours after discontinuing the infusion would be:

$$C_{12 \text{ hr}} = (15 \text{ mg/L})e^{(-0.139 \text{ hr}^{-1})(12 \text{ hr})}$$

$$= 15 \text{ mg/L} (0.19)$$

$$= 2.9 \text{ mg/L}$$

Loading Dose

As stated previously, after a continuous IV infusion of drug is begun, five drug half-lives are needed to achieve steady state. In many clinical situations, an

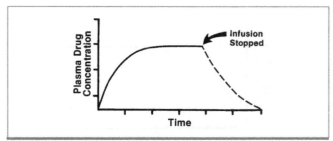

FIGURE 5-10.
Plasma drug concentrations after discontinuation of an intravenous infusion.

immediate effect of a drug is desired in a patient. In these situations, a loading dose is often administered at the initiation of the infusion to achieve an immediate therapeutic plasma concentration of the drug. By doing so, a serum concentration within therapeutic range of the drug is maintained from the outset of therapy. This loading dose is usually relatively large and may produce immediate therapeutic plasma concentrations (**Figure 5-11**). Note that a loading dose should not be used if substantial side effects occur with large doses of the drug. Also, sometimes clinicians prefer that drugs accumulate slowly rather than achieve therapeutic concentrations immediately so that the patient may have adequate time to develop tolerance to the initial side effects (e.g., tricyclic antidepressants).

The desired loading dose for many drugs can be derived from the definition of the volume of distribution. As shown previously, $V = X_0/C_0$ (see Equation 1-1) for a drug described by a one-compartment model. Rearranging this equation, we see that the

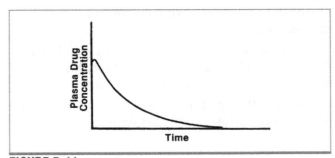

FIGURE 5-11.
Plasma drug concentrations resulting from an intravenous loading dose.

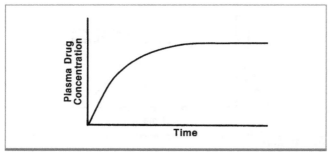

FIGURE 5-12.
Plasma drug concentrations over time resulting from a continuous intravenous infusion.

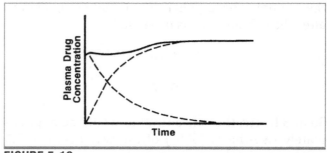

FIGURE 5-13.
Plasma drug concentrations resulting from an intravenous loading dose given with a continuous infusion.

loading dose equals the desired concentration multiplied by the volume of distribution:

$$X_0 = C_{0(desired)}V \quad \text{(See **Equation 1-1**.)}$$

Note that C_0 in this case is equivalent to the desired steady-state concentration.

We know that an IV loading dose produces plasma concentrations as shown in Figure 5-11, and the continuous infusion produces plasma concentrations as shown in **Figure 5-12**. If both the loading dose and the continuous IV infusion are given, the net effect should be a fairly steady plasma concentration, as depicted by the bold line in **Figure 5-13**. Before the constant IV infusion has reached steady state, the bolus loading dose has produced a nearly steady-state drug concentration, and when the drug from the loading dose is almost eliminated, the constant IV infusion should be approximately at steady state. With lidocaine, heparin, and theophylline, loading doses usually precede their continuous IV infusions, providing immediate as well as sustained effects that combine to produce a steady therapeutic plasma concentration.

Previously used equations can be combined to describe the plasma concentration resulting from a bolus injection with continuous infusion.

With an IV injection, the equation describing the plasma concentration after a dose is:

$$C_t = \frac{X_0}{V}e^{-Kt}$$

where:

t = time after dose

X_0 = initial loading dose

V = volume of distribution

K = elimination rate constant

With a continuous infusion, the plasma concentrations are described by:

$$C_t = \frac{K_0}{VK}(1 - e^{-Kt'})$$

where:

t' = time after beginning infusion

K_0 = rate of drug infusion

V = volume of distribution

K = elimination rate constant

When both the injection and infusion are administered together, the plasma concentration after beginning the regimen is calculated by adding the two equations:

$$C_t = \frac{X_0}{V}e^{-Kt} + \frac{K_0}{VK}(1 - e^{-Kt'})$$

For example, an adult patient is estimated to have a theophylline half-life of 8 hours ($K = 0.087$ hr^{-1}) and a V of 30 L. These estimates are obtained from known information about this patient or from published reports of similar patients. If the patient is given a loading dose of 400 mg of theophylline, and a continuous infusion of 35 mg/hr is begun at the same time, what will the plasma concentration be 24 hours later?

$$C_t = \frac{X_0}{V}e^{-Kt} + \frac{K_0}{VK}(1 - e^{-Kt'})$$

$$= \frac{400 \text{ mg}}{30 \text{ L}}e^{-0.087 \text{ hr}^{-1}(24 \text{ hr})} + \frac{35 \text{ mg/hr}}{30 \text{ L} \times 0.087 \text{ hr}^{-1}}(1 - e^{-0.087 \text{ hr}^{-1}(24 \text{ hr})})$$

$$= \frac{400 \text{ mg}}{30 \text{ L}}(0.124) + \frac{35 \text{ mg/hr}}{30 \text{ L} \times 0.087 \text{ hr}^{-1}}(0.876)$$

$$= 1.6 \text{ mg/L} + 11.7 \text{ mg/L} = 13.3 \text{ mg/L}$$

In clinical practice, drugs such as theophylline usually are not given by IV bolus injection, not even loading doses. Loading doses usually are given as short infusions (often 30–60 minutes). Taking this procedure into account, we can further modify the above equations to predict plasma concentrations.

For the loading dose:

$$C_{ss\,peak} = \frac{X_0/t}{VK}(1 - e^{-Kt})$$

where:

X_0 = dose (in this case, the loading dose)

t = infusion period (e.g., 0.5 hour)

K = elimination rate constant

V = volume of distribution

Multiple Intravenous Infusions (Intermittent Infusions)

In Lesson 4, we discussed multiple-dose IV bolus drug administration. With multiple-dose IV bolus administration, we assumed that the drug was administered by rapid IV injection. However, rapid IV injections are often associated with increased risks of adverse effects.

Therefore, many drugs administered intravenously are infused over a 30- to 60-minute time period; some drugs may require a longer infusion time. This method of giving multiple doses by infusion at specified intervals (τ), called *intermittent IV infusion*, changes the plasma concentration profile from what would be seen with multiple rapid IV injections. Therefore, a new model must be created

to predict plasma drug concentrations after multiple-dose intermittent IV infusions. This model combines the approaches just presented for multiple-dose injections and continuous infusions.

Let's assume that a drug is given intravenously over 1 hour every 8 hours. For the first in a series of IV infusions lasting 60 minutes each, the plasma concentrations will be similar to those observed during the first 60 minutes of a continuous infusion. Then, when the infusion is stopped, plasma concentrations will decline in a first-order process, just as after IV injections (**Figure 5-14**).

The peak (or maximum) plasma concentration after the first infusion ($C_{max\,1}$) is estimated by:

$$C_{max\,1} = \frac{K_0}{VK}(1 - e^{-Kt})$$

where:

C = concentration in plasma

K_0 = rate of drug infusion (dose/time of infusion)

V = volume of distribution

K = elimination rate constant

t = time (duration) of infusion

This equation was used above to describe plasma drug concentrations with continuous infusion before steady state.

The trough concentration after the first dose (C_{min1}) occurs at the end of the dosing interval (τ) directly before the next dose.

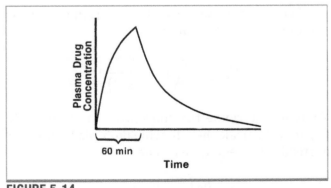

FIGURE 5-14.
Plasma drug concentrations resulting from a short intravenous infusion.

$C_{\min 1}$ is calculated by multiplying $C_{\max 1}$ by $e^{-K(\tau-t)}$ or $C_{\min 1} = C_{\max 1}\, e^{-K(\tau-t)}$.

This equation can be rewritten as follows:

$$C_{\min 1} = \left(\frac{K_0}{VK}\right)(1-e^{-Kt})(e^{-K(\tau-t)})$$

By the principle of superposition (see Lesson 4), $C_{\max 2}$ can be estimated:

$$C_{\max 2} = C_{\max 1} + C_{\min 1}$$

$$= \frac{K_0}{VK}(1-e^{-Kt}) + \frac{K_0}{VK}(1-e^{-Kt})(e^{-K(\tau-t)})$$

$$= \frac{K_0}{VK}(1-e^{-Kt})(1+e^{-K(\tau-t)})$$

$C_{\min 2}$ can be calculated:

$$C_{\min 2} = C_{\max 2} \times e^{-K(\tau-t)}$$

$$= \frac{K_0}{VK}(1-e^{-Kt})(1+e^{-K(\tau-t)})(e^{-K\tau})$$

$$= \frac{K_0}{VK}(1-e^{-Kt})(e^{-K\tau}+e^{-2K\tau})$$

This expansion of the equation can continue as in Lesson 4 until n number of infusions have been given:

$$C_{\max n} = \frac{K_0}{VK}\left[\frac{(1-e^{-Kt})(1-e^{-nK\tau})}{(1-e^{-K\tau})}\right]$$

As n becomes very large, $(1-e^{-nK\tau})$ approaches 1, and the equation becomes:

5-1 $$C_{ss\,\max} = \frac{K_0}{VK}\left[\frac{(1-e^{-Kt})}{(1-e^{-K\tau})}\right]$$

Then, to determine the concentration at any time (t') after the peak, the following multiple IV infusion at steady state equation can be used:

$$C = \frac{K_0}{VK}\left[\frac{(1-e^{-Kt})}{(1-e^{-K\tau})}\right]e^{-Kt'}$$

where t' = total hours drug was allowed to be eliminated.

A practical example for this equation is shown in Equation 5-2 to determine the $C_{\min}$ or trough concentration of a drug given by intermittent infusion:

5-2 $$C_{ss\,\min} = \frac{K_0}{VK}\left[\frac{(1-e^{-Kt})}{(1-e^{-K\tau})}\right]e^{-Kt'}$$

where $t' = \tau - t$.

The equation for $C_{ss\,\min}$ is very important in clinical practice. It can be used to predict plasma concentrations for multiple intermittent IV infusions of any drug that follows first-order elimination (assuming a one-compartment model). It also can be used to predict plasma concentrations at any time between $C_{\max}$ and $C_{\min}$, where t' equals the time between the end of the infusion and the determination of the plasma concentration. For application of this method, refer to cases that include IV intermittent infusions, which will show a step-by-step process for dose calculations.

Clinical Correlate

Here is one way we can illustrate the relationship of the equations described in this section: Suppose a patient with severe renal dysfunction receives a 100-mg dose of gentamicin, and a peak concentration, drawn at the end of the infusion, is reported by the laboratory as 8 mg/L. No additional doses are administered, and a repeat serum concentration drawn 24 hours later is reported as 3 mg/L. Before we can administer a second dose of gentamicin in this patient, we want to wait until the serum concentration is 1 mg/L. How much longer must we wait until this occurs?

The first step in solving this question is to determine the patient's K, which can be calculated using the equation that follows. Instead of using the variable $C_{\min}$, we use the variable C_t, which in this case represents the concentration 24 hours after the first level is drawn:

$$C_t = C_{peak}e^{-Kt}$$

$$3 \text{ mg} / L = (8 \text{ mg} / L)e^{-K(24 \text{ hr})}$$

$$\frac{3 \text{ mg/L}}{8 \text{ mg/L}} = e^{-K(24 \text{ hr})}$$

$$0.375 = e^{-K(24 \text{ hr})}$$

$$\ln 0.375 = -K(24 \text{ hr})$$

$$-0.981 = -K(24 \text{ hr})$$

$$\frac{0.981}{24 \text{ hr}} = K$$

$$K = 0.041 \text{ hr}^{-1}$$

Knowing K, we can calculate the time (t) required for the concentration to decrease to 1 mg/L. C_t will now be our desired concentration of 1 mg/L:

$$C_t = C_{peak}e^{-Kt}$$

$$1.0 \text{ mg} / L = (8 \text{ mg} / L)e^{(-0.041 \text{ hr}^{-1})t}$$

$$\frac{1.0 \text{ mg/L}}{8 \text{ mg/L}} = e^{(-0.041 \text{ hr}^{-1})t}$$

$$0.125 = e^{(-0.041 \text{ hr}^{-1})t}$$

$$\ln 0.125 = (-0.041 \text{ hr}^{-1})t$$

$$-2.08 = (-0.041 \text{ hr}^{-1})t$$

$$\frac{-2.08}{-0.041 \text{ hr}^{-1}} = t$$

$$t = 50.7 \text{ hours}$$

Therefore, it will take slightly longer than 2 days after the peak concentration for the serum concentration to decrease to 1 mg/L.

Clinically Important Equations Identified in This Chapter

1. $X_0 = C_{0(desired)}V$

   This is **Equation 1-1** rearranged.

   X_0 is the Loading Dose, sometimes abbreviated as LD.

2. $C_{ss \, max} = \dfrac{K_0}{VK}\left[\dfrac{(1 - e^{-Kt})}{(1 - e^{-K\tau})}\right]$ **Equation 5-1**

3. $C_{ss \, min} = \dfrac{K_0}{VK}\left[\dfrac{(1 - e^{-Kt})}{(1 - e^{-K\tau})}\right]e^{-Kt'}$ **Equation 5-2**

   where $t' = \tau - t$.

   This equation may be rewritten as

   $$C_{ss \, trough} = C_{ss \, peak} \times e^{-K(\tau - t)}$$

   or

   $$C_{ss \, min} = C_{ss \, max} \times e^{-K(\tau - t)}$$

REVIEW QUESTIONS

5-1. For a drug regimen, if the elimination rate (K) of a drug is increased while V, X_0, and τ remain constant, the peak and trough concentrations will _____.

A. Increase

B. Decrease

5-2. An increase in drug dose will result in higher plasma concentrations at steady state but will not change the time to reach steady state.

A. True

B. False

5-3. Which of the following dosing techniques results in greater fluctuations between peak and trough plasma levels?

A. Small doses very frequently

B. Large doses relatively less frequently

C. Continuous infusion at a consistent rate

5-4. When the volume of distribution decreases (and clearance remains the same), steady-state plasma concentrations will have more peak-to-trough variation.

A. True

B. False

5-5. When drug clearance increases (while volume of distribution remains unchanged), steady-state plasma concentrations will _____.

A. Increase

B. Decrease

5-6. How many half-lives are required to reach steady-state concentration when a medication is administered via continuous infusion?

A. Two

B. Three

C. Five

D. Ten

5-7. If you reduce the infusion rate of a drug by 25% (assume that clearance remains constant), you should expect to see the drug's steady-state concentration _____.

A. Fall by 10%

B. Fall by 25%

C. Fall by 50%

D. Remain constant

5-8. Theophylline is administered to a patient at 50 mg/hr via a constant IV infusion. If the patient has a total body clearance for theophylline of 45 mL/min, what should this patient's steady-state plasma concentration be?

A. 14.6 mg/L

B. 18.5 mg/L

B. 20.1 mg/L

C. 1.1 mg/L

5-9. With a continuous IV infusion of drug, the steady-state plasma concentration is directly proportional to _____.

A. Clearance

B. Volume of distribution

C. Drug infusion rate

D. K

5-10. If a drug is given by continuous IV infusion at a rate of 18 mg/hr and produces a steady-state plasma concentration of 9 mg/L, what infusion rate will result in a new C_{ss} of 15 mg/L?

A. 30 mg/hr

B. 35 mg/hr

C. 50 mg/hr

D. 75 mg/hr

5-11. For a continuous infusion, given the equation $C = K_0(1 - e^{-Kt})/Cl_t$, at steady state the value for t approaches infinity, and e^{-Kt} approaches 1.

A. True

B. False

This case applies to **Questions 5-12 and 5-13**. A patient is to be started on a continuous infusion of a drug. To achieve an immediate effect, a loading dose is administered over 30 minutes and then the continuous infusion will begin. From a previous regimen of the same drug, you estimate that the patient's $K = 0.04$ hr^{-1} and $V = 24$ L. Assume that none of this drug has been administered in the last month, so the plasma concentration before therapy is 0 mg/L.

5-12. If the $C_{ss(desired)}$ is 15 mg/L, what should the loading dose be?

 A. 14.4 mg

 B. 200 mg

 C. 360 mg

 D. 1000 mg

5-13. What rate of infusion (K_0) should result in a C_{ss} of 15 mg/L?

 A. 0.9 mg/hr

 B. 14.4 mg/hr

 C. 60 mg/hr

 D. 360 mg/hr

Refer to this equation when working on **Questions 5-14 through 5-16**:

$$C = \frac{K_0}{VK}\left[\frac{(1-e^{-nKt})}{(1-e^{-K\tau})}\right]e^{-Kt'}$$

5-14. A patient is to be given 120 mg of gentamicin IV over 1 hour every 12 hours. If the patient is assumed to have a K of 0.12 hr^{-1} and a V of 18 L, how long will it take to reach steady state?

 A. 6 hours

 B. 11 hours

 C. 18 hours

 D. 29 hours

5-15. For the patient in Question 5-14, what will the peak plasma concentration be at steady state?

 A. 6.6 mg/L

 B. 8.3 mg/L

 C. 10.6 mg/L

 D. 14.4 mg/L

5-16. For the patient in Question 5-15, calculate the trough plasma concentration at steady state.

 A. 0.54 mg/L

 B. 1.42 mg/L

 C. 1.92 mg/L

 D. 2.3 mg/L

ANSWERS

5-1. A. *Incorrect answer*

 B. CORRECT ANSWER. This can be determined by examination of the equation from Lesson 4:

$$C_{ss\,peak} = \frac{X_0}{V}\left[\frac{1}{(1-e^{-K\tau})}\right]$$

 If V is constant and K is increased, this means that Clearance ($K*V$) is lower and the average steady-state concentration will be lower and the peak and trough will be decreased.

5-2. A. CORRECT ANSWER. The time to reach steady state is determined by K.

 B. *Incorrect answer*

5-3. A. *Incorrect answer*. Because volume is consistent, a small dose produces less change in peak values, and the shorter dose interval allows less time for clearance (less change in trough).

B. CORRECT ANSWER. Because the interval is longer, more time for elimination results in lower trough concentrations and therefore greater fluctuation in serum drug concentrations.

C. *Incorrect answer.* This would produce the smallest fluctuation in concentration for the reasons described in A.

5-4.   A. CORRECT ANSWER. A smaller volume of distribution with unchanged clearance will result in the same amount of drug distributing in a lesser volume, which would result in greater peak-to-trough variation.

B. *Incorrect answer*

5-5.   A. *Incorrect answer*

B. CORRECT ANSWER. When clearance increases, plasma concentrations will decrease because drug is administered at the same rate (dose and dosing interval) but is removed at a higher rate.

5-6.   A. *Incorrect answer.* Only 75% of the steady-state concentration would be reached by two half-lives.

B. *Incorrect answer.* Only 87.5% of the steady-state concentration would be reached by three half-lives.

C. CORRECT ANSWER. At five half-lives, approximately 97% of the steady-state concentration has been reached.

D. *Incorrect answer.* Steady state is achieved, but this is much longer than necessary.

5-7.   A, C, D. *Incorrect answers*

B. CORRECT ANSWER. Assuming a medication has first-order (linear) elimination, the serum drug concentration should change in direct relationship to the change in dose.

5-8.   A, C, D. *Incorrect answers*

B. CORRECT ANSWER. The equation $C_{ss} = K_0/Cl_t$ should be used. The value for K_0 is 50 mg/hr. The value for Cl_t must be converted from 45 mL/min to 2.7 L/hr.

5-9.   A, B, D. *Incorrect answers*

C. CORRECT ANSWER. The steady-state concentration is directly proportional to the drug infusion rate for medications with first-order pharmacokinetics.

5-10.   A. CORRECT ANSWER. Because the medication is administered as a continuous infusion we can use $C_{ss} = K_0/Cl_t$ and available data to solve for Cl_t.

9 mg/L = (18 mg/hr)/Cl_t so Cl_t = (18 mg/hr)/(9 mg/L) = 2 L/hr. With this a new K_0 can be calculated using the same equation.

$C_{ss} = K_0/Cl_t$ where K_0 is unknown.

15 mg/hr = K_0/(2 L/hr)

K_0 = (15 mg/hr)(2 L/hr)

= 30 mg/L

B, C, D. *Incorrect answers*

5-11.   A. CORRECT ANSWER. As t becomes larger, the term e^{-Kt} becomes smaller, and the term $1 - e^{-Kt}$ approaches 1.

B. *Incorrect answer*

5-12.   A, B, D. *Incorrect answers*

C. CORRECT ANSWER. The loading dose is determined by multiplying the desired concentration (12 mg/L) by the volume of distribution:

$C_{ss(desired)} \times V$ = 15 mg/L × 24 L = 360 mg

Note that the units cancel out to yield milligrams.

5-13.   A, C, D. *Incorrect answers*

B. CORRECT ANSWER. The infusion rate is related to Cl_t and C_{ss} as follows:

$C_{ss} = K_0/Cl_t$.

Cl_t can be determined by multiplying

$V \times K$ = 0.96 L/hr.

So, rearranging,

$K_0 = C_{ss} \times Cl_t$ = 15 mg/L × 0.96 L/hr = 14.4 mg/hr.

5-14. A, B, C. *Incorrect answers*

D. CORRECT ANSWER. One half-life is calculated as follows:

$$T\tfrac{1}{2} = 0.693/K$$

Steady state is reached by five half-lives, or 29 hours.

5-15. A, B, D. *Incorrect answers*

C. CORRECT ANSWER. At steady state, the following equation would be used:

$$C_{ss\,max} = \frac{K_0(1 - e^{-Kt})}{VK(1 - e^{-K\tau})}$$

$$= \frac{(120 \text{ mg/hr})(0.113)}{(2.16 \text{ L/hr})(0.73)}$$

$$= 8.57 \text{ mg/L}$$

5-16. A, C, D. *Incorrect answers*

B. CORRECT ANSWER. The trough concentration is calculated from the peak value as follows:

$$C_{trough} = C_{peak} \times e^{-K(\tau - t)}$$

$$= 8.6 \text{ mg/L} \times e^{-0.12 \text{ hr}^{-1}(12 \text{ hr} - 1 \text{ hr})}$$

$$= 8.6 \text{ mg/L} \times 0.267 = 2.3 \text{ mg/L}$$

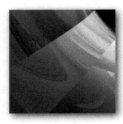

Discussion Points

D-1. With the continuous IV infusion model of drug administration, what two factors determine the steady-state plasma concentration?

D-2. What is the purpose of administering a loading dose of a drug?

D-3. What is the following portion of the multiple-dose equation called, and why is it called that?

$$1/(1 - e^{-K\tau})$$

D-4. Given the following equation for a drug given by intermittent infusion, what does t' represent?

$$C_{ss\,min} = \frac{K_0}{VK}\left[\frac{(1-e^{-Kt})}{(1-e^{-K\tau})}\right]e^{-Kt'}$$

D-5. Explain how changing the dosing interval (τ) influences the time to reach steady state when multiple doses are administered.

D-6. If clearance is reduced to 25% of the initial rate and all other factors (such as dose, dosing interval, and volume of distribution) remain constant, how will steady-state plasma concentrations change?

D-7. Explain why, for most drugs, the increase in drug plasma concentrations resulting from a single dose will be the same magnitude whether it is the first or the tenth dose.

Two-Compartment Models

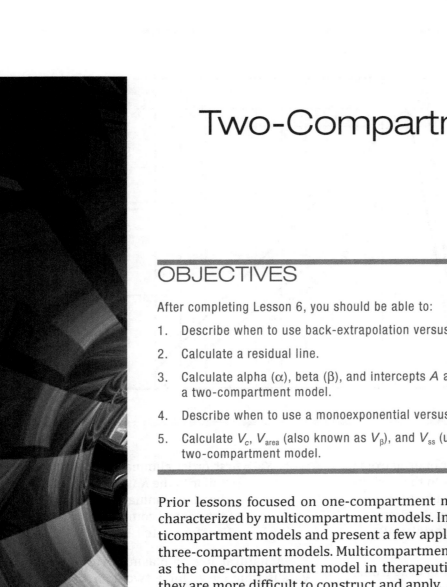

OBJECTIVES

After completing Lesson 6, you should be able to:

1. Describe when to use back-extrapolation versus method of residuals.

2. Calculate a residual line.

3. Calculate alpha (α), beta (β), and intercepts A and B for a drug conforming to a two-compartment model.

4. Describe when to use a monoexponential versus a biexponential equation.

5. Calculate V_c, V_{area} (also known as V_β), and V_{ss} (using both methods) for a two-compartment model.

Prior lessons focused on one-compartment models, but many drugs are better characterized by multicompartment models. In this lesson, we briefly discuss multicompartment models and present a few applications. Drugs may exhibit two- or three-compartment models. Multicompartment models are not used as frequently as the one-compartment model in therapeutic drug monitoring, partly because they are more difficult to construct and apply.

Generally, multicompartment models are applied when the natural log of plasma drug concentration versus time curve is not a straight line after an intravenous (IV) dose or when the plasma concentration versus time profile cannot be characterized by a single exponential function (i.e., $C_t = C_0 e^{-Kt}$). When the natural log of plasma drug concentration versus time curve is not a straight line, a multicompartment model must be constructed to describe the change in concentration over time (**Figure 6-1**).

Of the multicompartment models, the two-compartment model is most frequently used. This model usually consists of a central compartment of the well-perfused tissues (such as the liver and kidneys) and a peripheral compartment of less well-perfused tissues (such as muscle and fat). **Figure 6-2** shows a diagram of the two-compartment model after an IV bolus dose, where:

X_0 = dose of drug administered

X_c = amount of drug in central compartment

X_p = amount of drug in peripheral compartment

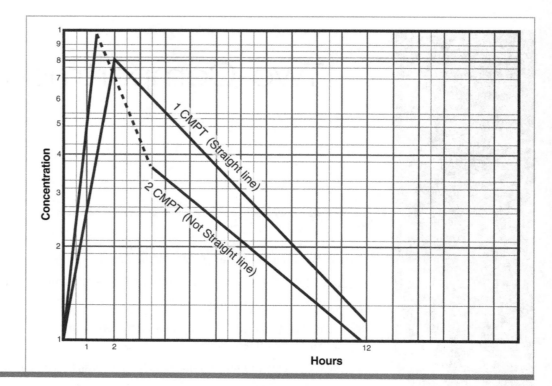

FIGURE 6-1.
Concentration versus time plot for one- versus two-compartment (CMPT) model.

K_{12} = rate constant for transfer of drug from the central compartment to the peripheral compartment. (The subscript 12 indicates transfer from the first [central] to the second [peripheral] compartment.)

K_{21} = rate constant for transfer of drug from the peripheral compartment to the central compartment. (The subscript 21 indicates transfer from the second [peripheral] to the first [central] compartment.

Note: Both K_{12} and K_{21} are called *microconstants* and are assumed to be first order.)

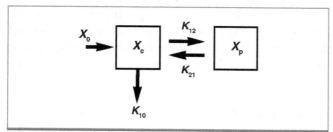

FIGURE 6-2.
A two-compartment model.

K_{10} = first-order elimination rate constant (similar to the K used previously), indicating elimination of drug out of the central compartment into urine, feces, etc.

A natural log of plasma drug concentration versus time curve for a two-compartment model shows a curvilinear profile—a curved portion followed by a straight line. This bi-exponential curve can be described by two exponential terms (**Figure 6-3**). The phases of the curve may represent rapid distribution to organs with high blood flow (central compartment) and slower distribution to organs with less blood flow (peripheral compartment).

After the IV injection of a drug that follows a two-compartment model, the drug concentrations in all fluids and tissues associated with the central compartment decline more rapidly in the distribution phase than during the post-distribution phase. After some time, a pseudoequilibrium is attained between the central compartment and the tissues and fluids of the peripheral compartment; the plasma drug concentration versus time profile is then characterized as a linear process when plotted

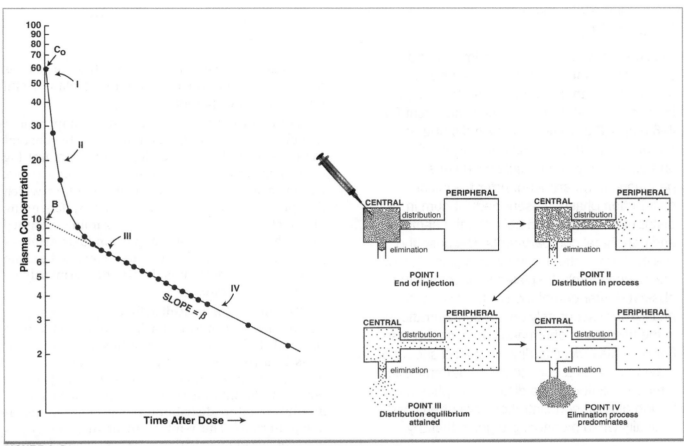

FIGURE 6-3.

Four stages of drug distribution and elimination after rapid IV injection. Points I, II, III, and IV (*right*) correspond to the points on the plasma concentration curve (*left*). **Point I:** The injection has just been completed, and drug density in the central compartment is highest. Drug distribution and elimination have just begun. **Point II:** Midway through the distribution process, the drug density in the central compartment is falling rapidly, mainly because of rapid drug distribution out of the central compartment into the peripheral compartment. The density of drug in the peripheral compartment has not yet reached that of the central compartment. **Point III:** Distribution equilibrium has been attained, and drug densities in the central and peripheral compartments are approximately equal. Drug distribution in both directions continues to take place, but the ratio of drug quantities in the central and peripheral compartments remains constant. At this point, the major determinant of drug disappearance from the central compartment becomes the elimination process; previously, drug disappearance was determined mainly by distribution. **Point IV:** During this elimination phase, the drug is being "drained" from both compartments out of the body (via the central compartment) at approximately the same rate.

Source: Reprinted with permission from Greenblatt DJ, Shader RI. *Pharmacokinetics in Clinical Practice*. Philadelphia, PA: WB Saunders; ©1985.

on semilog paper (i.e., terminal or linear elimination phase). For many drugs (e.g., aminoglycosides), the distribution phase is very short (e.g., minutes). If plasma concentrations are measured after this phase is completed, the central compartment can be ignored and a one-compartment model adequately represents the plasma concentrations observed.

Other drugs (e.g., vancomycin, digoxin) have a longer distribution phase (hours). If plasma concentrations of these drugs are determined within the first few hours after a dose is given, the nonlinear (multiexponential) decline of drug concentrations must be considered when calculating half-life and other parameters.

Clinical Correlate

Digoxin is a drug that, when administered as a short IV infusion, is best described by a two-compartment model. After the drug is infused, the distribution phase is apparent for 4–6 hours (**Figure 6-4**). Digoxin distributes out of plasma (the central compartment) and extensively into muscle tissue (the peripheral compartment). After the initial distribution phase, a pseudoequilibrium in distribution is achieved between the central and peripheral compartments. Because the site of digoxin effect is in muscle (specifically, the myocardium), the plasma concentrations observed after completion of the distribution phase more accurately reflect concentrations in the tissue and pharmacodynamic response. For patients receiving digoxin, blood should be drawn for plasma concentration determination after completion of the distribution phase; thus, trough digoxin concentrations are often used clinically when monitoring digoxin therapy.

Vancomycin is another drug that follows a two-compartment model with an initial 2- to 4-hour α-distribution phase followed by a linear terminal elimination phase. As described later in the vancomycin cases (see Lesson 13), peak vancomycin concentrations must be drawn approximately 2 hours after the end of a vancomycin infusion to avoid obtaining a peak concentration during the initial distribution phase (see Figure 13-3).

Calculating Two-Compartment Parameters

In this section, we apply mathematical principles to the two-compartment model to calculate useful pharmacokinetic parameters.

From discussion of the one-compartment model, we know that the elimination rate constant (K) is estimated from the slope of the natural log of plasma drug concentration versus time curve. However, in a two-compartment model, in which that plot is curvilinear, the slope varies, depending on which portion of the curve is examined (**Figure 6-5**). The slope of the initial portion is determined primarily by the distribution rate, whereas the slope of the terminal portion is determined primarily by the elimination rate.

The linear (or post-distributive) terminal portion of this curve may be back-extrapolated to time zero (t_0). The negative slope of this line is referred to as *beta* (β), and like K in the one-compartment model, β is an elimination rate constant. β is the terminal elimination rate constant, which means it applies after distribution has reached pseudoequilibrium. The y-intercept of this line (B) is used in various equations for two-compartment parameters.

As in the one-compartment model, a half-life (the β half-life) can be calculated from β:

$$T\tfrac{1}{2} = \frac{0.693}{\beta} \qquad T\tfrac{1}{2} = \frac{0.693}{K}$$

Throughout the time that drug is present in the body, distribution takes place between the central

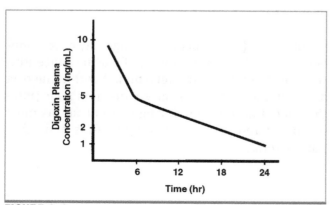

FIGURE 6-4.
Digoxin plasma concentration versus time.

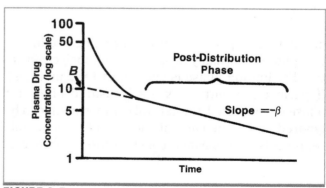

FIGURE 6-5.
Plasma drug concentrations with a two-compartment model after an IV bolus dose.

and peripheral compartments. We can calculate a rate of distribution using the method of residuals, which separates the effects of distribution and elimination. This method estimates the effect of distribution on the overall plasma concentration curve and uses the difference between the effect of elimination and the actual plasma concentrations to determine the distribution rate.

To apply the method of residuals, we use the back-extrapolated line used to determine β and *B* (**Figure 6-6**). If *w*, *x*, *y*, and *z* are actual, determined concentration time points, let *w′*, *x′*, *y′*, and *z′* represent points on the new (extrapolated) line at the same times that the actual concentrations were observed. These newly generated points represent the effect of elimination alone, as if distribution had been instantaneous. Subtraction of the extrapolated points from the corresponding actual points (*w – w′*, *x – x′*, etc.) yields a new set of plasma concentration points for each time point. If we plot these new points, we generate a new line, the residual line (**Figure 6-7**). The negative slope of the residual line is referred to as *alpha* (α), and α is the distribution rate constant for the two-compartment system. The *y*-intercept of the residual line is *A*.

Let's proceed through an example, applying the method of residuals. Draw the plot for the following example on semilog graph paper. A dose of drug is administered by rapid IV injection, and the concentrations shown in **Table 6-1** result.

The last four points form a straight line (similar to Figure 6-5), so a line can be back-extrapolated to connect them to the *y*-axis. Then, for the first five points, extrapolated values can be estimated at each time (0.25, 0.5, 1, 1.5, and 2 hours), where the

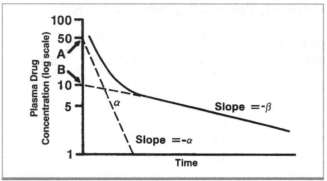

FIGURE 6-7.
Determination of the residual line.

time intersects the new line (similar to Figure 6-6). Subtracting the extrapolated values from the actual plasma concentrations yields a new set of residual concentration points, similar to those values shown in **Table 6-2**.

On the same semilog paper, plot the residual concentrations versus time and draw a straight line connecting all of the new points (similar to Figure 6-7). Determine that the slope of that plot equals -1.8 hours^{-1}.

$$\text{Slope } (\alpha) = \frac{\ln C_1 - \ln C_0}{t_1 - t_0} = \frac{(\ln 3 - \ln 18.5)}{(1.5 \text{ hr} - 0.5 \text{ hr})} = -1.8 \text{ hr}^{-1}$$

(distribution rate)

(See **Equation 3-1**.)

When the negative is dropped, this slope equals α; we observe from the plot that the intercept

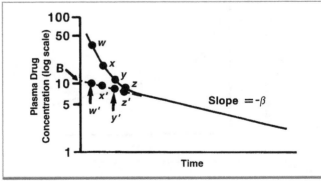

FIGURE 6-6.
Method of residuals.

TABLE 6-1. Plasma Drug Concentrations after Rapid Intravenous Injection

Time after Dose (hr)	Plasma Concentration (mg/L)
0.25	43
0.5	32
1	20
1.5	14
2	11
4	6.5
8	2.8
12	1.2
16	0.52

TABLE 6-2. Residual Concentration Points

Time after Dose (hr)	Plasma Concentration (mg/L)		
	Actual	Extrapolated	Residual
0.25	43	14.5	28.5
0.5	32	13.5	18.5
1	20	12.3	7.7
1.5	14	11	3
2	11	10	1

(*A*) of the residual line is 45 mg/L. We also can estimate β (0.21 hour^{-1}) from the slope of the terminal straight-line portion.

$$\text{Slope } (\beta) = \frac{\ln C_1 - \ln C_0}{t_1 - t_0} = \frac{(\ln 2.8 - \ln 6.5)}{(8 \text{ hr} - 4 \text{ hr})} = -0.21 \text{ hr}^{-1}$$

(elimination rate)

Looking at the extrapolated portion of the line yields a value for *B* (15 mg/L).

Note that α must be greater than β, indicating that drug removal from plasma by distribution into tissues proceeds at a greater rate than does drug removal from plasma by eliminating organs (e.g., kidneys and liver). The initial portion of the plot is steeper than the terminal portion.

Biexponential Equation and Volumes of Distribution

The estimations of *A, B,* α, and β performed previously are useful for predicting plasma concentrations of drugs characterized by a two-compartment model. For a one-compartment model (**Figure 6-8**), we know that the plasma concentration (*C*) at any time (*t*) can be described by:

$$C_t = C_0 \, e^{-Kt} \quad \text{(See Equation 3-2.)}$$

where C_0 is the initial concentration, and *K* is the elimination rate. The equation is called a *monoexponential equation* because the line is described by one exponent.

The two-compartment model (**Figure 6-9**) is the sum of two linear components, representing

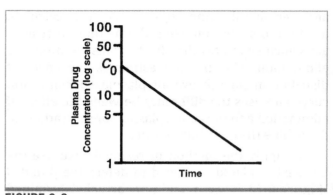

FIGURE 6-8.
Plasma drug concentrations with a one-compartment model after an IV bolus dose (first-order elimination).

distribution and elimination (**Figure 6-10**), so we can determine drug concentration (*C*) at any time (*t*) by adding those two components. In each case, *A* or *B* is used for C_0, and α or β is used for *K*. Therefore:

$$C_t = Ae^{-\alpha t} + Be^{-\beta t}$$

This equation is called a *biexponential equation*, because two exponents are incorporated.

For the two-compartment model, different volumes of distribution parameters exist: the central compartment volume (V_c), the volume by area (V_{area}, also known as V_β), and the steady-state volume of distribution (V_{ss}). Each of these volumes relates to different underlying assumptions.

As in the one-compartment model, a volume can be calculated by:

$$V_c = \frac{\text{dose}}{A + B} = \frac{\text{dose}}{C_0}$$

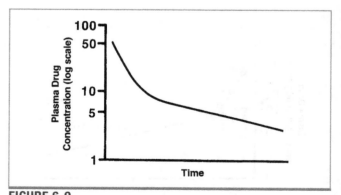

FIGURE 6-9.
Plasma drug concentrations with a two-compartment model after an IV bolus dose (first-order elimination).

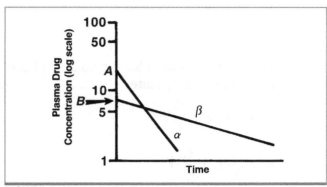

FIGURE 6-10.
Linear components of a two-exponential (two-compartment) model.

For the two-compartment model, this volume would be equivalent to the volume of the central compartment (V_c). The V_c relates the amount of drug in the central compartment to the concentration in the central compartment. In the two-compartment model, C_0 is equal to the sum of intercepts A and B.

If another volume (V_{area} or V_β) is determined from the area under the plasma concentration versus time curve and the terminal elimination rate constant (β), this volume is related as follows:

$$V_{area} = V_\beta = \frac{dose}{\beta \times AUC} = \frac{Cl}{\beta}$$

This calculation is affected by changes in clearance (Cl). The V_{area} relates the amount of drug in the body to the concentration of drug in plasma in the post-absorption and post-distribution phases.

A final volume is the volume of distribution at steady state (V_{ss}). Although it is not affected by changes in drug elimination or clearance, it is more difficult to calculate.

One way to estimate V_{ss} is to use the two-compartment microconstants:

$$V_{ss} = V_c + \frac{K_{12}}{K_{21}} V_c$$

or it may be estimated by:

$$V_{ss} = \frac{dose \left(\dfrac{A}{\alpha^2} + \dfrac{B}{\beta^2} \right)}{\left(\dfrac{A}{\alpha} + \dfrac{B}{\beta} \right)^2}$$

using A, B, α, and β.

Because different methods can be used to calculate the various volumes of distribution of a two-compartment model, you should always specify the method used. When reading a pharmacokinetic study, pay particular attention to the method for calculating the volume of distribution.

Clinical Correlate

Here is an example of one potential problem when dealing with drugs exhibiting biexponential elimination: If plasma concentrations are determined soon after an IV dose is administered (during the distribution phase), and a one-compartment model is assumed, then the patient's drug half-life would be underestimated, and β would be overestimated (**Figure 6-11**). Recall that:

$$\text{Slope } (\beta \text{ or } K) = \frac{\ln C_1 - \ln C_0}{t_1 - t_0}$$

A steeper slope equals a faster rate of elimination resulting in a shorter half-life.

If a terminal half-life is being calculated for drugs such as vancomycin, you must be sure that the distribution phase is completed (approximately 3–4 hours after the dose) before drawing plasma levels.

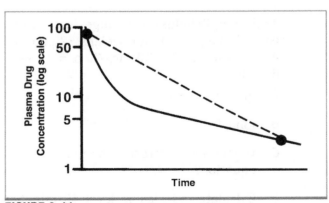

FIGURE 6-11.
Biexponential elimination.

REVIEW QUESTIONS

6-1. In the two-compartment model, what does C_0 represent?

 A. It is equal to the sum of intercepts A and B.

 B. It relates the amount of drug in the body to the concentration of drug in plasma in the post-absorption and post-distribution phase.

 C. It is the volume of distribution at steady state.

 D. It represents the dose of drug administered.

6-2. When determining the terminal half-life for a multicompartmental drug such as vancomycin, which of the following must be assured?

 A. The distribution phase has not started before drawing plasma levels.

 B. The distribution phase is completed before drawing plasma levels.

 C. The absorption phase is complete before drawing plasma levels.

 D. The absorption phase has not started before drawing plasma levels.

6-3. Which of the drugs listed does not follow the two-compartment model?

 A. Cephalothin

 B. Vancomycin

 C. Gabapentin

 D. Digoxin

6-4. A 550-mcg IV bolus dose of digoxin is administered to a patient who weighs 52 pounds. A = 62 mcg/L, B = 30 mcg/L, α = 15 hr^{-1}, β = 4 hr^{-1}.

 A. Find V_c.

 B. Find $T\frac{1}{2}$.

 C. What does β represent in the $T\frac{1}{2}$ equation?

 D. Calculate the plasma level 45 minutes after the dose was administered.

6-5. What is the equation for the volume of distribution at steady state?

 A. $V_{ss} = T\frac{1}{2} + \dfrac{K_{12}}{K_{21}} V_c$

 B. $V_{ss} = V_c + \dfrac{K_{12}}{K_{31}} V_c$

 C. $V_{ss} = V_c + \dfrac{K_{12}}{K_{21}} V_c$

 D. $V_{ss} = V_c + \dfrac{K_{12}}{K_{21}} C_0$

6-6. An IV dose of drug A was just administered, and the plasma concentration was determined at this time. A one-compartment model was assumed; however, the drug actually exhibits biexponential elimination. Drug A's half-life would be _____ and β would be _____.

 A. underestimated; overestimated

 B. overestimated; underestimated

 C. the same; overestimated

 D. underestimated; the same

6-7. Which of the following drug(s) is/are best described by a two-compartment model?

 A. Aminoglycosides

 B. Digoxin

 C. Vancomycin

 D. None of the above

6-8. The equation describing elimination after an IV bolus dose of a drug characterized by a two-compartment model requires two exponential terms.

 A. True

 B. False

6-9. A patient is given a 500-mg dose of drug by IV injection, and the following plasma concentrations result:

Plasma Concentration (mg/L)	Time after Dose (hr)
62	0.25
49	0.5
31	0.75
22.5	1
18.7	1.5
13.2	2
11.4	3
9.1	4
4.8	6
1.9	8
1	10

Which one of the following answers has the best estimates for α and β?

A. 4.12 hr^{-1}, 0.61 hr^{-1}

B. 1.98 hr^{-1}, 0.15 hr^{-1}

C. 3.59 hr^{-1}, 0.348 hr^{-1}

D. 0.98 hr^{-1}, 1.67 hr^{-1}

ANSWERS

6-1. B, C, D. *Incorrect answers*

A. CORRECT ANSWER. The impact of multiple volume of distributions must be accounted for to estimate C_0.

6-2. A, C, D. *Incorrect answers*

B. CORRECT ANSWER. The distribution phase is completed (approximately 3–4 hours after the dose) before drawing plasma levels.

6-3. A, B, D. *Incorrect answers*

C. CORRECT ANSWER

6-4. A. $V_c = \dfrac{dose}{A+B} = \dfrac{dose}{C_0}$

$V_c = \dfrac{550}{62+30} = 5.978 \text{ liters}$

B. $T\frac{1}{2} = \dfrac{0.693}{\beta} = \dfrac{0.693}{4} = 0.17325 \text{ hours}$

C. It represents the terminal elimination rate constant.

D. $C_t = Ae^{-\alpha t} + Be^{-\beta t}$

$C_t = 62e^{-15(0.75)} + 30e^{-4(0.75)}$

$C_t = 1.494$ micrograms per milliliter

6-5. A, B, D. *Incorrect answers*

C. CORRECT ANSWER $V_{ss} = V_c + \dfrac{K_{12}}{K_{21}} V_c$

6-6. A. CORRECT ANSWER.

B, C, D. *Incorrect answers*

6-7. A, D. *Incorrect answers.* Although aminoglycosides do have a distribution phase, it is relatively short (minutes rather than hours), allowing modeling via a single-compartment model.

B and C. CORRECT ANSWERS. Vancomycin and digoxin are examples of medications that have a longer distribution phase (>1 hour) and are best described by a two-compartment model.

6-8. A. CORRECT ANSWER. One exponent is needed for distribution phase and the other for elimination or post-distribution phase.

B. *Incorrect answer*

6-9.   A, B, D. *Incorrect answers*

C.   CORRECT ANSWER. See table below. Your numbers may vary slightly.

Time (hr)	Actual (mg/L)	Extrapolated (mg/L)	Residual (mg/L)
0.25	62	25	37
0.5	49	23.5	25.5
0.75	31	22	9
1	22.5	20	2.5
1.5	18.7	17	1.7

The slope of the residual line is determined to calculate α. Two residual points are selected, such as 0.25 and 1 hour:

$$\text{slope} = \frac{\Delta x}{\Delta y} = \frac{\ln C_2 - \ln C_1}{t_2 - t_1}$$

$$= \frac{\ln 2.5 - \ln 37}{1.0 \text{ hr} - 0.25 \text{ hr}}$$

$$= \frac{0.916 - 3.61}{0.75 \text{ hr}}$$

$$= -3.59 \text{ hr}^{-1}$$

$$\alpha = -\text{slope} = -3.59 \text{ hr}^{-1}$$

The β can be determined from the slope of the terminal straight-line portion of the plot. For example, the points at 3 and 10 hours may be selected:

$$-\text{slope} = \frac{\Delta x}{\Delta y} = \frac{\ln C_2 - \ln C_1}{t_2 - t_1}$$

$$= \frac{\ln 1 - \ln 11.4}{10 \text{ hr} - 3 \text{ hr}}$$

$$= \frac{0 - 2.43}{7 \text{ hr}} = \frac{-2.43}{9 \text{ hr}}$$

$$= -0.348 \text{ hr}^{-1}$$

$$\beta = -\text{slope} = 0.348 \text{ hr}^{-1}$$

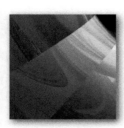 Discussion Points

D-1. In the biexponential elimination equation, what does a steeper slope indicate?

D-2. How would you describe the slope in a two-compartment model?

D-3. When the natural log of plasma drug concentration versus time curve is not a straight line, what does this mean?

D-4. Describe what may happen if phenytoin is given at higher than therapeutic doses.

D-5. Describe what "steady state" means in your own words.

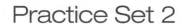

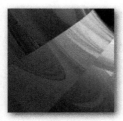

The following problems are for your review. Definitions of symbols and key equations are provided here:

K = elimination rate constant

C_0 = plasma drug concentration just after a single intravenous injection

e = base for the natural log function = 2.718

τ = dosing interval

K_0 = rate of dose administration (may be expressed as milligrams per hour in the sense of a continuous infusion or as drug dose divided by infusion time for intermittent infusions)

V = volume of distribution

C_{peak} = peak plasma drug concentration at steady state

C_{trough} = trough plasma drug concentration at steady state

t = duration of intravenous infusion

For multiple-dose, intermittent, intravenous bolus injection at steady state:

$$C_{peak} = \frac{X_0}{V}\left(\frac{1}{1-e^{-K\tau}}\right)$$

$$C_{trough} = C_{peak}e^{-K\tau}$$

For multiple-dose, intermittent, intravenous infusion:

$$C_{peak} = \frac{K_0}{VK}\left(\frac{1-e^{-Kt}}{1-e^{-K\tau}}\right)$$

$$C_{trough} = C_{peak}e^{-K(\tau-t)}$$

For continuous infusion before steady state is reached:

$$C = \frac{K_0}{VK}(1-e^{-Kt})$$

For continuous infusion at steady state:

$$C_{ss} = \frac{K_0}{VK} = \frac{K_0}{Cl_t}$$

QUESTIONS

The following applies to **Questions PS2-1 to PS2-6**: An 85-kg patient is started on a continuous intravenous infusion of theophylline at 45 mg/hr. At 72 hours after beginning the infusion, the plasma concentration is 15 mg/L.

PS2-1. If we assume that this concentration is at steady state, what is the theophylline clearance?

   A. 3 L/hr

   B. 0.33 L/hr

   C. 3.3 L/hr

   D. 33 L/hr

PS2-2. If the volume of distribution is estimated to be 24 L, what is the half-life?

   A. 1.7 hours

   B. 5.54 hours

   C. 13.3 hours

   D. 18 hours

PS2-3. As we know V and K, what would the plasma concentration be 15 hours after beginning the infusion?

   A. 3.2 mg/L

   B. 4.8 mg/L

   C. 8.1 mg/L

   D. 12.7 mg/L

PS2-4. If the infusion is continued for 5 days and then discontinued, what would the plasma concentration be 18 hours after stopping the infusion?

A. 1.58 mg/L

B. 3.27 mg/L

C. 8.1 mg/L

D. 1.33 mg/L

PS2-5. If the infusion is continued for 4 days at 45 mg/hr and the steady-state plasma concentration is 15 mg/L, what rate of drug infusion would likely result in a concentration of 18 mg/L?

A. 48 mg/hr

B. 50 mg/hr

C. 54 mg/hr

D. 60 mg/hr

PS2-6. After the increased infusion rate in PS2-5 is begun, how long would it take to reach a plasma concentration of 18 mg/L?

A. 6.3 hours

B. 12.6 hours

C. 18.9 hours

D. 27.7 hours

The following pertains to **Questions PS2-7 to PS2-10**: A 75-kg patient is started on 100 mg of gentamicin every 8 hours given as 1-hour infusions.

PS2-7. If this patient is assumed to have an average V of 18 L and a normal gentamicin half-life of 3 hours, what will be the peak plasma concentration at steady state?

A. 4.3 mg/L

B. 5.89 mg/L

C. 8.72 mg/L

D. 10.4 mg/L

PS2-8. After the seventh dose, a peak plasma concentration (drawn at the end of the infusion) is 5.9 mg/L, and the trough concentration (drawn right before the sixth dose) is 0.4 mg/L. What is the patient's actual gentamicin half-life?

A. 0.385 hour

B. 1 hour

C. 1.25 hours

D. 1.8 hours

PS2-9. What would be the volume of distribution? [*Hint*: Rearrange **Equation 5-1**]

A. 11.1 L

B. 14.75 L

C. 15.5 L

D. 22.0 L

PS2-10. For this patient, what dose should be administered to reach a new steady-state peak gentamicin concentration of 8 mg/L?

A. 107 mg

B. 115 mg

C. 128 mg

D. 135 mg

ANSWERS

PS2-1. A. CORRECT ANSWER. $Cl_t = K_0/C_{ss} =$ 45 mg/hr/15 mg/L = 3 L/hr

B. *Incorrect answer.* You may have inverted the formula.

C, D. *Incorrect answers*

PS2-2. A, C, D. *Incorrect answers*

B. CORRECT ANSWER. First, K can be calculated from the equation $Cl_t = KV$.

Rearranged:

$K = Cl_t/V = 3.0$ L/hr/24 L $= 0.125$ hr^{-1}

Then:

$T\frac{1}{2} = 0.693/K = 5.54$ hr

PS2-3. A, B, C. *Incorrect answers*

D. CORRECT ANSWER. To calculate the plasma concentration with a continuous infusion before steady state is reached, the following equation can be used:

$$C = \frac{K_0}{VK}(1 - e^{-Kt})$$

where $t = 15$ hours. Then:

$$C = \frac{45 \text{ mg/hr}}{24 \text{ L} \times 0.125 \text{ hr}^{-1}}(1 - e^{-0.125 \text{ hr}^{-1}(15 \text{ hr})})$$

$$= \frac{45 \text{ mg/hr}}{24 \text{ L} \times 0.125 \text{ hr}^{-1}}(0.847)$$

$$= 12.71 \text{ mg/L}$$

PS2-4. B, C, D. *Incorrect answers*

A. CORRECT ANSWER. If the continuous intravenous infusion is continued for 5 days, steady state would have been reached, so the plasma concentration would be 15 mg/L. When the infusion is stopped, the declining drug concentration can be described just as after an intravenous injection:

$$C_t = C_{ss}e^{-Kt}$$

where:

C_t = plasma concentration after infusion has been stopped for t hour

C_{ss} = steady-state plasma concentrations from continuous infusion, and K = elimination rate constant

So, when $t = 18$ hours:

$$C_{18 \text{ hr}} = (15 \text{ mg/L})(e^{-0.125 \text{ hr}^{-1}(18 \text{ hr})})$$

$$= (15 \text{ mg/L})(0.105)$$

$$= 1.58 \text{ mg/L}$$

PS2-5. A, B, D. *Incorrect answers*

C. CORRECT ANSWER. The patient's theophylline clearance equals 3.0 L/hr. Then remember that at steady state:

$$C_{ss} = K_0/Cl_t$$

or, rearranged:

$$C_{ss} \times Cl_t = K_0$$

If the desired C_{ss} equals 18 mg/L, then:

$$K_0 = 18 \text{ mg/L} \times 3.0 \text{ L/hr}$$

$$= 54 \text{ mg/hr}$$

PS2-6. A, B, C. *Incorrect answers*

  D. CORRECT ANSWER. Whenever the infusion rate is changed to a new rate (increased or decreased), it will take approximately five half-lives to achieve a new steady state. So it will take 5 × 5.54 hours = 27.7 hours.

PS2-7. B. CORRECT ANSWER. First, recall that the multiple-dose infusion equation should be used:

$$C_{peak} = \frac{K_0(1-e^{-Kt})}{VK(1-e^{-K\tau})}$$

where K_0 = 100 mg/1 hr (because the dose is given over 1 hour). As given, V = 18 L, τ = 8 hours, and $T\frac{1}{2}$ = 3 hours. So:

$$K = \frac{0.693}{3 \text{ hr}} = 0.231 \text{ hr}^{-1}$$

Then:

$$C_{peak} = \frac{(100 \text{ mg/hr})(1-e^{-0.231 \text{ hr}^{-1}(1 \text{ hr})})}{(18 \text{ L} \times 0.231 \text{ hr}^{-1})(1-e^{-0.231 \text{ hr}^{-1}(8 \text{ hr})})}$$

$$= \frac{(100 \text{ mg/hr})(0.206)}{(18 \text{ L} \times 0.231 \text{ hr}^{-1})(0.842)}$$

$$= 5.89 \text{ mg/L}$$

Your answer may vary slightly due to differences in rounding during calculations.

A, C, D. *Incorrect answers*

PS2-8. A, B, C. *Incorrect answers*

  D. CORRECT ANSWER. The half-life can be calculated from the concentrations given. Recall that there are two concentrations on a straight line, where K is the slope of the line. The slope equals the change in the y-axis divided by the change in the x-axis. The time between the end of one infusion and the start of the next is 7 hours (because the dose is given over a 1-hour infusion and the peak is taken at the end of the infusion. Therefore:

$$K = -slope = -\frac{\Delta y}{\Delta x}$$

$$= -\frac{(\ln 0.4 \text{ mg/L} - \ln 5.9 \text{ mg/L})}{0 - 7 \text{ hr}}$$

$$= \frac{[-0.92 - (1.775)]}{-7 \text{ hr}} =$$

$$= 0.385 \text{ hr}^{-1}$$

Then:

$$T\frac{1}{2} = \frac{0.693}{K} = \frac{0.693}{0.385 \text{ hr}^{-1}} = 1.8 \text{ hr}$$

PS2-9. A, C, D. *Incorrect answers*

B. CORRECT ANSWER. To calculate V, the multiple-dose infusion equation (**Equation 5-1**) can be used, where:

$$C_{peak} = \frac{K_0(1-e^{-Kt})}{VK(1-e^{-K\tau})}$$

and:

C_{peak} = 5.9 mg/L

K_0 = 100 mg/hr

K = 0.385 hr^{-1}

t = 1 hour

τ = 8 hours

By substituting, we get:

$$5.9 \text{ mg/L} = \frac{(100 \text{ mg/hr})(1-e^{-0.385 \text{ hr}^{-1}(1 \text{ hr})})}{(V \times 0.385 \text{ hr}^{-1})(1-e^{-0.385 \text{ hr}^{-1}(8 \text{ hr})})}$$

Rearranging gives:

$$V = \frac{(100 \text{ mg/hr})(1-e^{-0.385 \text{ hr}^{-1}(1 \text{ hr})})}{(5.9 \text{ mg/L} \times 0.385 \text{ hr}^{-1})(1-e^{-0.385 \text{ hr}^{-1}(8 \text{ hr})})}$$

$$= \frac{(100 \text{ mg/hr})(0.320)}{(5.9 \text{ mg/L} \times 0.385 \text{ hr}^{-1})(0.954)}$$

$$= 14.75 \text{ L}$$

Your number may vary slightly due to differences in rounding during calculations.

PS2-10. A, B, C. *Incorrect answers*

D. CORRECT ANSWER. To calculate a new dose, we would use the same previous equation but would now include the known V and desired C_{peak}, and then solve for K_0:

$$K_0 = \frac{C_{peak}VK(1-e^{-K\tau})}{(1-e^{-Kt})}$$

$$= \frac{(8 \text{ mg/L})(14.75 \text{ L})(0.385 \text{ hr}^{-1})(0.954)}{(0.320)}$$

$$= 135 \text{ mg over 1 hour}$$

So, in practical terms, we would likely round up and give a 140-mg dose (due to availability of how the product comes), and this would be infused over 1 hour to attain a peak of approximately 8.3 mg/L. (Because we rounded the dose up, the actual peak will be slightly higher than the 8 mg/L that the exact dose of 135 mg would have provided).

8 mg/L/135 mg = X /140 mg

X = 8.3 mg/L

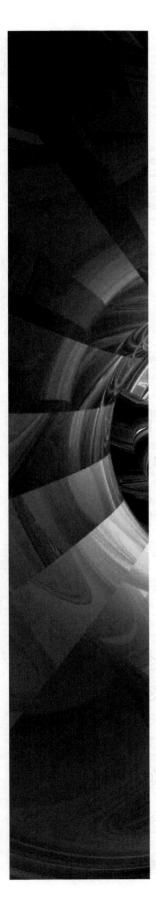

Biopharmaceutics: Absorption

OBJECTIVES

After completing Lesson 7, you should be able to:

1. Define and understand the factors that comprise the term *biopharmaceutics.*

2. Describe the effects of the extent and rate of absorption of a drug on plasma concentrations and area under the curve (AUC).

3. Name factors that can affect a drug's oral bioavailability, and explain the relationship of bioavailability to drug absorption and AUC.

4. Calculate an *F* factor for a drug given its intravenous (IV) and oral absorption time versus concentration AUCs.

5. Use the oral absorption model to calculate pharmacokinetic parameters.

6. Describe the pharmacokinetic differences and clinical utility of controlled-release products and the several techniques used in formulating controlled-release drugs.

7. Calculate dose and clearance of controlled-release products given plasma concentration, volume of distribution, and elimination rate constant.

Introduction to Biopharmaceutics

The effect of a drug depends not only on the drug's characteristics but also on the nature of the body's systems. The drug enters the body by some route of administration and is subjected to processes such as absorption, distribution, metabolism, and excretion (**Figure 7-1**).

The concepts used in pharmacokinetics enable us to understand what happens to a drug when it enters the body. Unless a drug is given by the IV or transcutaneous route, it must be absorbed into the systemic circulation to exert its effect. After entering the systemic circulation, the drug is distributed to various tissues and fluids. While the drug is distributing into tissues and producing an effect, the body is working to eliminate the drug and terminate its effect.

A term often used in conjunction with pharmacokinetics is *biopharmaceutics,* which is the study of the relationship between the nature and intensity of a drug's effects and various drug formulations or administration factors. These factors include the drug's chemical nature, inert formulation substances, pharmaceutical processes used to manufacture the dosage form, and routes of administration.

For an orally administered drug, the absorption process depends on the drug dissociating from its dosage form, dissolving in body fluids, and then diffusing

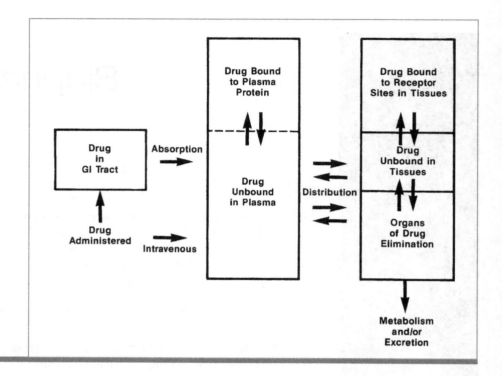

FIGURE 7-1.
Disposition of drug in the body.

across the biologic membrane barriers of the gut wall into the systemic circulation (**Figure 7-2**). Different drugs or different formulations of the same drug can vary considerably in both the rate and extent of absorption. The extent of absorption depends on the nature of the drug itself (e.g., its solubility and pKa) as well as the physiologic environment (pH, gastrointestinal [GI] motility, and muscle vascularity). Most drugs given orally are not fully absorbed into the systemic circulation. The difference in absorption rates of drugs has important therapeutic implications. Assuming that concentration correlates with effect, if one drug is absorbed at a faster rate than another similar drug, the first drug may produce a higher peak concentration, which may lead to a clinical effect sooner than the second drug (**Figure 7-3**).

When drug absorption is delayed (usually through manipulation of the rate of drug release from the formulation), a prolonged or sustained effect can be produced. For certain drugs such as select oral analgesics and hypnotics, rapid absorption is preferable. For other agents, such as antiarrhythmics and bronchodilators, a slower rate of

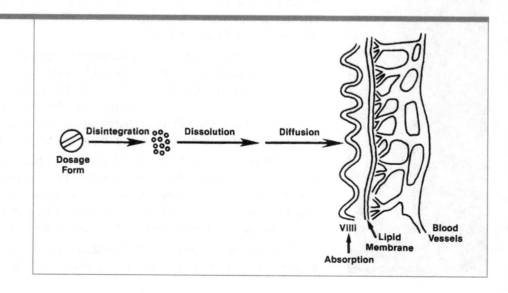

FIGURE 7-2.
Processes involved in drug absorption after oral administration.

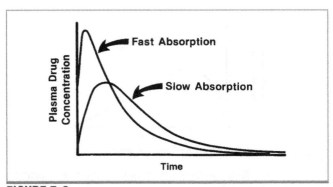

FIGURE 7-3.
Typical effect of absorption rate on plasma drug concentrations.

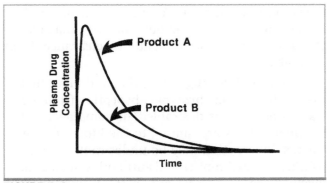

FIGURE 7-4.
Typical effect of different extents of absorption on plasma drug concentrations.

absorption with a stable effect over a longer time may be desirable.

A term used to express bioavailability is F. It is a number less than or equal to 1 that indicates the fraction of drug reaching the systemic circulation. Bioavailability is often erroneously referred to as the *fraction of a drug absorbed*; however, it actually represents the fraction of a drug that reaches the systemic circulation. Factors that can affect F include not only absorption, but that fraction of drug that escapes both presystemic (i.e., intestinal wall) and systemic first-pass metabolism. The F term gives no indication of how fast a drug is absorbed. Proper studies of drug product bioavailability examine both the rate and extent of absorption.

For instance, for oral formulations of a drug:

$$F = \frac{\text{amount of drug reaching systemic circulation}}{\text{total amount of drug}}$$

Usually, F is determined by comparing the AUC for the oral dosage form with the AUC for IV administration of the same dose. The AUC for IV administration is used, because when a drug is given intravenously, it bypasses absorption and reflects the absolute bioavailability. The total amount of drug goes into the systemic circulation. As an example, digoxin tablets have an F value of 0.70, while digoxin elixir has a value of 0.80. This indicates that for digoxin, more of the drug reaches systemic circulation when administered as the elixir. Factors that can affect a drug's oral bioavailability include the drug's absorption characteristics, drug metabolism within the intestinal wall, and hepatic first-pass metabolism of a drug.

Therefore, overall oral bioavailability can be described by the following equation, which shows the combination of all of these factors:

$$F_{\text{oral}} = F_{\text{abs}} \times F_{\text{gut}} \times F_{\text{hepatic}}$$

A product with poor bioavailability is not completely absorbed into the systemic circulation or is eliminated by the liver before it reaches the systemic circulation. Differences in bioavailability may be evident between two products (A and B) containing the same drug but producing different plasma concentrations (**Figure 7-4**). Although these products may contain the same amount of drug, their formulations are different (e.g., tablet and capsule). Different formulations may have different absorption characteristics and result in different plasma concentrations. Because product B is not absorbed to the same extent as product A, lower plasma concentrations result for product B.

The AUC of a plasma drug concentration versus time plot reflects the total amount of drug reaching the systemic circulation. Because bioavailability describes the extent of drug eventually reaching the systemic circulation, comparison of the AUCs of various dosage forms of a drug would compare their relative bioavailabilities.

In Figure 7-4, a drug is given in a similar dose (e.g., 100 mg) in two different oral dosage products (A and B). The AUC for product A is greater than that for product B, indicating that the bioavailability of product A is greater than that of product B. When comparing AUCs to assess bioavailability, we assume that the clearance of drug with each dosage form is the same, so differences in the AUC are directly related to the amount of drug that enters the systemic circulation. For a specific drug, the AUC is determined by the amount of drug that enters the systemic circulation and its clearance from circulation.

In discussing drug absorption and bioavailability, we should recognize that absorption from the GI tract is not always desirable. For some agents, the intended effects are limited to the lumen of the GI tract, so absorption may be undesirable. Examples would be anthelmintics and antibiotics, such as neomycin, given to decrease gut bacterial counts.

Clinical Correlate

Absorption of a drug whose bioavailability is low due to a low *F* factor is erratic and is more likely to be affected by disease-related changes in absorption such as rapid GI transit times and short bowel syndromes.

Bioavailability

Next we will examine a one-compartment model in which the drug is given orally and absorbed from the GI tract. This example would also apply to intramuscular administration as the drug must undergo absorption from the muscle to produce a therapeutic effect.

Let us assume the following:

- The drug is 100% absorbed ($F = 1$).

- The absorption rate is much greater than the elimination rate.

- Distribution to all tissues and fluids is instantaneous (a one-compartment model).

- The drug follows first-order elimination (**Figure 7-5**).

Continuous measurement of plasma drug concentrations would probably produce a plot similar

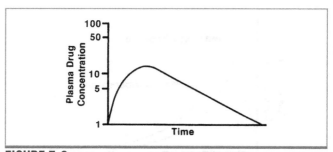

FIGURE 7-6.
Typical plasma drug concentration versus time curve resulting from an oral formulation.

to that shown in **Figure 7-6** when plotted using semilog graph paper. By knowing *F* to be 1 in this example and the drug concentrations over time, we can calculate the pharmacokinetic parameters of elimination rate (*K*), volume of distribution (*V*), half-life (*T½*), and total clearance (Cl$_t$). In many cases, the actual *F* is not known, so these parameters can be calculated only in terms of their relationship to *F* (e.g., Cl$_t$/*F*, *V*/*F*). But first, let's examine the plot more closely. The initial uphill portion of the graph indicates drug absorption. Of course, elimination of drug also begins as soon as some drug is in the body. But in the initial portion of the curve (*A*), the rate of drug absorption is greater than the rate of elimination, so there is an increase in the plasma drug concentration (**Figure 7-7**). As the amount of drug in the GI tract (or in the muscle with intramuscular administration) decreases, the rate of absorption begins to taper off; at point *B*, the rate of absorption equals the rate of elimination. On the downhill portion of the curve (*C*), elimination predominates, and absorption is nearly complete.

If the drug follows first-order elimination, the terminal portion of the plasma drug concentration versus time curve should theoretically be a straight line on semilog graph paper (**Figure 7-8**). The slope of the straight-line portion of the curve is related to

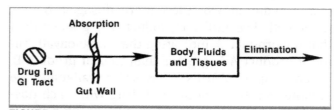

FIGURE 7-5.
First-order elimination.

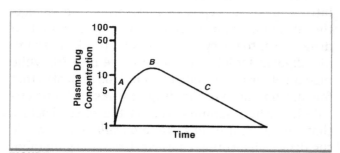

FIGURE 7-7.
Effects of both absorption and elimination on concentration versus time curve.

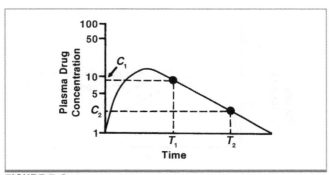

FIGURE 7-8.
Determination of slope (and K) from terminal portion of plasma drug concentration curve.

the elimination rate constant (K). To calculate K or $T\frac{1}{2}$, we use the techniques described previously, but the calculations are made from the terminal portion (straight-line portion) of the curve.

$$slope = \frac{\ln C_2 - \ln C_1}{t_2 - t_1} = -K$$

(See **Equation 3-1.**)

$$T\frac{1}{2} = \frac{0.693}{K}$$

(See **Equation 3-3.**)

For most drugs, absorption after oral administration is usually nearly complete by 1–2 hours. Plasma concentrations drawn after that time should reflect the effect of elimination. For sustained-release products, however, significant drug absorption can continue for considerably longer than 2 hours.

Let's calculate the volume of distribution after oral or intramuscular administration. This calculation can be performed as follows:

$$V = \frac{\text{amount of drug administered}}{K \times \text{AUC}}$$

(assuming $F = 1$), using the trapezoidal rule to calculate the AUC.

Terms in the equation

$$\frac{mg}{hr^{-1} \times (mg/L) \times hr}$$

can be canceled, leaving us with a unit for volume of distribution in liters, which is referred to as the V_{area}.

Once we have the values of volume of distribution (V) and elimination rate constant (K), the total body clearance (Cl_t) can be calculated as follows:

$$Cl_t = V \times K \quad \text{(See **Equation 3-4.**)}$$

When drug is absorbed from outside the systemic circulation, as with oral and intramuscular doses, the peak plasma drug concentration occurs sometime after time zero rather than at time zero, as with an IV drug injection. The peak plasma concentration occurs at the point at which the amount eliminated and the amount absorbed are equal (**Figure 7-9**).

Clinical Correlate

When a drug is administered via a route with slower absorption, such as after an intramuscular injection, it will have a smaller peak concentration and a slightly longer duration of action than the IV administration of the same drug. Because of the slower absorption of intramuscularly administered drugs, it will take longer to reach peak concentrations than with IV administration. Consequently, a therapeutic peak concentration may not be attained. To obtain a correct peak concentration time for intramuscularly administered drugs, the measurement must be made in the appropriate time frame. For example, a drug that reaches its peak concentration after 1 hour should not be sampled after 20 minutes; otherwise, a false value will be obtained, because absorption is not complete. In addition, because intramuscular absorption occurs more slowly, allowing significant drug elimination to occur before absorption is complete, peak concentrations after an intramuscular injection can yield a lower value than that seen with IV administration. The *time to peak* is the time corresponding with that peak concentration. The time required to reach the peak plasma concentration depends on the relative rates of absorption and elimination. A rapidly absorbed drug has a short time to peak concentration.

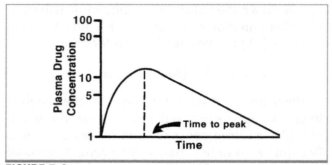

FIGURE 7-9.
Time to peak for oral or intramuscular concentration versus time curve.

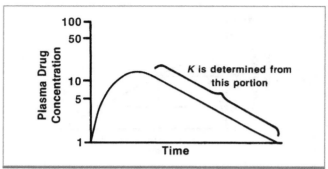

FIGURE 7-10.
Plasma drug concentration versus time for a typical oral formulation.

Oral Absorption Model

The elimination rate constant has been denoted by the symbol K. The absorption rate constant will be represented by K_a. This value indicates the fraction of drug present at the absorption site, usually the GI tract, that is absorbed per unit of time. The usual measurement of K_a is the percentage of drug absorbed per unit of time. If K_a is greater than one in a time unit, almost all of the drug would be absorbed over that time interval.

A high K_a (over 1.0 hr^{-1}) indicates rapid absorption. For this explanation, we assume that first-order absorption or elimination rates do not change with time. Although the rates do not change, the amount of drug absorbed or eliminated changes.

Clinical Correlate

Some drug absorption rates (K_a) change when large doses are administered as a single oral dose—the percentage of the total dose absorbed is smaller with a large dose than with a smaller dose of the same drug. Gabapentin (Neurontin), which is actively absorbed via the gut's L-amino acid transport system, is a common example of this absorption phenomenon. Consequently, the daily dose must sometimes be given in divided doses, depending on the total daily dose desired.

With an orally administered drug, K is measured by the slope of the terminal portion of the plasma drug concentration versus time curve, the time when absorption no longer has an appreciable effect (**Figure 7-10**). In the first part of the curve (the uphill portion), absorption is occurring, but K_a cannot be measured directly, because the curve demonstrates the effects of both absorption and elimination.

Elimination processes begin immediately after the drug is given. A steeper uphill portion indicates a K_a much greater than K, but visual inspection does not provide an accurate assessment of K_a.

One way to calculate K_a is to use the *method of residuals*, which estimates the plasma drug concentration plot if absorption were instantaneous and then uses the difference between the actual and estimated concentrations to determine K_a. Using back-extrapolation, we first estimate the straight-line portion of the curve (**Figure 7-11**). The extrapolated portion represents the effect of elimination alone—as if absorption had been instantaneous.

Let us suppose that A, B, and C are actual measured concentrations and that A', B', and C' are extrapolated concentrations for the same times

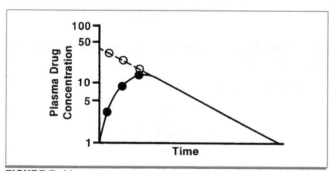

FIGURE 7-11.
Back-extrapolation.

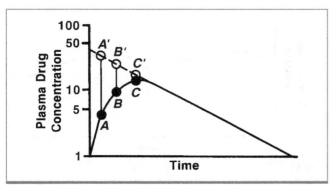

FIGURE 7-12.
Back-extrapolated concentrations.

(**Figure 7-12**). Points on the extrapolated line can be determined visually from the graph or with the following equation:

$$C = (y\text{-intercept}) \times e^{-Kt}$$

Subtraction of the actual points on the uphill portion from the corresponding points on the extrapolated line (e.g., $A' - A$, $B' - B$, and $C' - C$) will yield a new set of plasma drug concentrations for each time point. These values can be plotted with the appropriate times, and a line is then drawn that best fits the new points. This new line is called the *residual* (**Figure 7-13**).

The slope of the line for these new points gives an estimate of the absorption rate. Just as the negative slope of the terminal portion of the plasma concentration curve equals K, the negative slope of the residual line equals K_a.

The technique of residuals attempts to separate the two processes of absorption and elimination. These concepts become important when different dosage forms of a drug are evaluated. They can also be used to evaluate the absorption of different brands of the same drug in the same dosage form. A higher K_a indicates a faster absorption rate. This factor is only one component of such evaluations, but it is often important to know how rapidly a drug is made available to the systemic circulation. An overriding assumption of this technique for calculating K_a is that $K_a >>> K$.

Determination of K and K_a can also be used to predict the resulting plasma drug concentrations after an oral drug dose. If K, K_a, and the intercepts of the back-extrapolated line from the drug elimination phase (B) and the residual line (A) are known, the plasma drug concentration (C), which represents the y-intercept, at any time after a single dose (t) can be calculated:

$$C = Be^{-Kt} - Ae^{-K_a t}$$

Although this equation is similar to the one for a single IV injection in a one-compartment model described previously, it accounts for drug yet to be absorbed ($-Ae^{-K_a t}$).

Plasma drug concentration can also be calculated for any given single dose (X_0) when K and K_a are known and estimates of the bioavailability (F) and volume of distribution (V) are available:

$$C_t = \frac{FX_0 K_a}{V(K_a - K)}(e^{-Kt} - e^{-K_a t})$$

C_t = concentration at time t

F = bioavailability

X_o = amount of drug given orally

K_a = absorption rate constant

V = volume of distribution

K = elimination rate constant

t = time after dose has been given

Just as with multiple IV doses, multiple oral doses result in increasing drug concentrations until steady state is reached (**Figure 7-14**). If K, K_a, V, and F are known, the steady-state plasma drug concentration at any time (t) after a dose (X_0) is given can also be calculated:

$$C_t = \frac{FX_0 K_a}{V(K_a - K)}\ \frac{1}{1 - e^{-K\tau}}e^{-Kt} - \frac{1}{1 - e^{-K_a \tau}}e^{-K_a t}$$

These equations are presented to demonstrate that plasma drug concentrations after oral doses can be predicted, but they are infrequently applied in clinical practice.

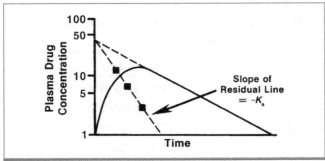

FIGURE 7-13.
Residual line.

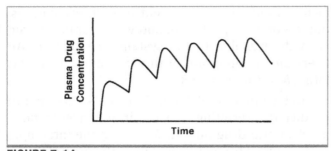

FIGURE 7-14.
Plasma drug concentration versus time for a typical oral formulation given in multiple doses.

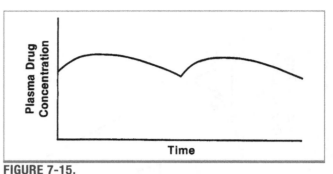

FIGURE 7-15.
Typical plasma drug concentration versus time curve at steady state for a controlled-release oral formulation.

Controlled-Release Products

In our discussions of drug absorption so far, it was assumed that the drug formulations used were relatively rapidly absorbed from the GI tract into the systemic circulation. In fact, many drugs are absorbed relatively rapidly from the GI tract. With rapid drug absorption, a peak plasma concentration of drug is evident soon after drug administration (often within 1 hour), and plasma concentrations may decline relatively soon after dose administration, particularly with drugs having short elimination half-lives. When drugs are eliminated rapidly from the plasma, a short dosing interval (e.g., every 6 hours) may be required to maintain plasma concentrations within the therapeutic range.

To overcome the problem of frequent dosage administration with drugs having short elimination half-lives, products have been devised that release drugs into the GI tract at a controlled rate. These controlled-release or sustained-release products usually allow for less frequent dosage administration. As opposed to the first-order absorption that occurs with most rapidly absorbed oral drug products, some controlled-release drug products approximate zero-order drug absorption. With zero-order absorption, the amount of drug absorbed in a given time remains constant for much of the dosing interval. The result of zero-order absorption is a more consistent plasma concentration (**Figure 7-15**).

Many types of controlled-release drug products have been produced. Products from different manufacturers (e.g., theophylline products) that contain the same drug entity may have quite different absorption properties, resulting in different plasma concentration versus time curves.

Controlled-release formulations incorporate various techniques to slow drug absorption. These techniques include the application of coatings that delay absorption; the use of slowly dissolving salts or esters of the parent drug; the use of ion-exchange resins that release drug in either acidic or alkaline environments; and the use of gel, wax, or polymeric matrices. Examples of available drugs in controlled-release formulations are shown in **Table 7-1**.

Two features of controlled-release products must be considered in therapeutic drug monitoring:

1. When multiple doses of a controlled-release drug product are administered, before reaching steady state, the difference between peak and trough plasma concentrations is not as great as would be evident after multiple doses of rapidly absorbed drug products (**Figure 7-16**).

2. Because the drug may be absorbed for most of a dosing interval, an elimination phase may not be as apparent—that is, the log of plasma drug concentration versus time curve may not be linear for any part of the dosing interval.

Because, with controlled-release formulations, the drug may be absorbed continuously from the GI

TABLE 7-1. Examples of Controlled-Release Formulations

Drug	Formulation
Potassium chloride	Wax matrix tablet
Theophylline	Coated pellets in tablet
Decongestants	Coated pellets in capsule
Aspirin	Microencapsulation
Nifedipine	Osmotic pump

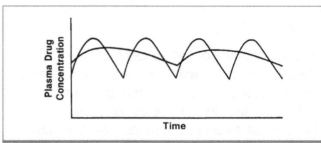

FIGURE 7-16.
Plasma drug concentrations over time with controlled-release and rapid-release products.

tract over the dosing interval, it may not be possible to calculate a drug's half-life.

Clinical Correlate

The peak and trough concentrations of controlled-release products generally differ very little, so plasma drug concentration sampling is generally done at the approximate midpoint of any dosing interval to approximate the average steady-state concentration.

Some predictions can be made about plasma drug concentrations with controlled-release preparations.

For preparations that result in continued release of small drug doses, the plasma drug concentration can be estimated as follows:

$$\text{average steady-state plasma concentration} = \frac{\text{dose} \times \text{fraction reaching systemic circulation}}{\text{dosing interval} \times \text{clearance}}$$

or:

$$\overline{C} = \frac{X_0 \times F}{\tau \times Cl_t}$$

(See **Equation 4-3.**)

Given this equation, the dose, the amount entering the systemic circulation, the dosing interval, and the clearance can be used to predict the average steady-state plasma drug concentration. Also, if the average plasma drug concentration is estimated

(determined approximately halfway through a dosing interval), drug clearance can be determined using the same formula. Finally, the effect of changing the dose or dosing interval on plasma drug concentration can be estimated.

For example, if it is known from previous regimens that a patient has a theophylline half-life of 7 hours ($K = 0.1$ hr^{-1}) and a volume of distribution of 30 L, what dose of a sustained-release preparation given every 12 hours will be required to achieve an average plasma concentration of 12 mg/L? Assume that the product is 90% absorbed.

First, theophylline clearance must be estimated as follows:

$$Cl_t = K \times V$$

$$= 0.1 \text{ hr}^{-1} \times 30 L$$

$$= 3 L/hr$$

Then the known variables can be applied:

$$\overline{C} = \frac{X_0 \times F}{\tau \times Cl_t}$$

$$12 \text{ mg/L} = \frac{X_0 \times 0.9}{12 \text{ hr} \times 3 \text{ L/hr}}$$

Rearranging gives:

$$X_0 = \frac{3 \text{ L/hr} \times 12 \text{ hr} \times 12 \text{ mg/L}}{0.9}$$

$$= 480 \text{ mg given every 12 hr}$$
(may be rounded to 500 mg)

This same equation could be used to estimate drug clearance if a steady-state plasma drug concentration at the midpoint of a dosing interval is known.

Another feature of sustained-release dosage products is that the drug dose is directly related to the AUC, just as for rapidly absorbed products. If rapid- and sustained-release products of the same drug are absorbed to the same extent, then the resulting AUC at steady state for a similar time will be equivalent for each product if the same daily dosages are given. For example, if 500 mg of a sustained-release drug product is given every 12 hours and 250 mg of a rapidly absorbed formulation of the same drug is given every 6 hours, the AUC over 12 hours (two dosing intervals for the rapidly absorbed product) should be the same. Again, the assumption is that the bioavailability (*F*) is the same for each product.

The AUC after administration of a controlled-release dosage formulation is related to drug dosage; the relating factor is drug clearance, as discussed previously:

$$AUC = \frac{dose \times F}{clearance}$$

(See **Equation 3-5.**)

or:

$$clearance = \frac{dose \times F}{AUC}$$

If the AUC, dose administered, and fraction reaching the systemic circulation are known, drug clearance can be estimated. Remember, AUC is expressed as milligrams per liter times hours (mg/L × hr).

The considerations for controlled-release dosage forms will become increasingly important as more drugs are being formulated into preparations that can be administered at convenient intervals (daily or even less frequently).

Clinical Correlate

The importance of the absorption rate depends to some extent on the type of illness being treated and the pharmacodynamics actions of the drug. For example, when treating acute pain, it is usually desirable to use an analgesic that is rapidly absorbed (i.e., has a high absorption rate constant) so that drug effect may begin as soon as possible. For chronic diseases, such as hypertension, it is more desirable to have a product that results in a lower absorption rate and more consistent drug absorption over time so that blood pressure does not change over the dosing interval.

Clinically Important Equation Identified in This Chapter

$$\overline{C} = \frac{X_0 \times F}{\tau \times Cl_t}$$

This is a revision of Equation 4-3 in which *F* is incorporated into the equation.

REVIEW QUESTIONS

7-1. Which of the following statements best describes K_a?

A. Rate at which the drug is eliminated from circulation

B. Fraction of the drug dose that reaches systemic circulation

C. Rate at which the drug is absorbed into systemic circulation

D. Concentration at which rate of absorption equals rate of elimination

7-2. The amount of drug that enters systemic circulation is _____.

A. Bioavailability

B. Half-life

C. Volume of distribution

D. Elimination rate

7-3. The bioavailability of a drug formulated is influenced by _____.

A. Rate dissolution

B. Extent of dissolution

C. Gastrointestinal motility

D. All of the above are correct.

7-4. What is the clearance for a drug that has a bioavailability of 70%, an AUC of 200 (mg/L) × hr following administration of a 200 mg dose?

7-5. A 750-mg dose of sustained release dose form of drug X is given to a patient every 12 hours which has a bioavailability of 0.8. Assume $V = 40$ L and $K = 0.5$ hr^{-1}. What is the concentration at steady state?

Use the following information for **Questions 6-10**

You wish to convert a patient from IV to oral form of drug Y which has a bioavailability of 0.75. You want to maintain steady state level of 10 mg/L. From published data, you estimate V and K for this drug to be 10 L and 0.18 hr^{-1}, respectively.

7-6. Calculate the clearance of drug Y.

7-7. Calculate the dose of drug Y to reach steady state of 10 mg/L if given every 8 hours.

7-8. You have calculated a dose for drug Y in question 7. You know that drug Y is available in 100-mg, 200-mg, and 300-mg dosage forms. Using the information you previously calculated, select a dosage form for drug Y and recommend a regimen. Next, predict the serum drug concentration the recommended regimen will yield.

7-9. Calculate the AUC based on the dose from last question.

7-10. Calculate the dose of drug Y if the patient is only taking the medication every 12 hours to reach the same steady state.

7-11. If the elixir of drug X has larger K_a than the K_a for the tablet form of drug X (same dose administered and same K) therefore the elixir will reach the peak level slower that the tablet.

A. True

B. False

7-12. A drug has the following properties: $V = 20$ L, $K = 0.3$ hr^{-1}, $F = 0.8$

If the patient took 100 mg of this drug every 6 hour s, what would be his steady-state concentration?

7-13. If drug X has a bioavailability of 0.6 what oral dose would produce the same AUC as a 150 mg IV dose for drug X?

7-14. The target steady-state concentration for drug Y is 25 mg/L and it is available as 100-mg tablet. The drug has a bioavailability of 0.9 and clearance is 0.3L/hr. How often should the patient take a 100-mg tablet to reach steady-state concentration?

7-15. The AUC of drug A is 25 mg/L × hr and the drug is 45 percent bioavailable. If 50 mg of the drug is administered, what is the clearance of the drug?

ANSWERS

7-1.   A, B, D. *Incorrect answers*. A. Defines K not K_a. B. The definition for F. D. Defines steady-state.

      C.   CORRECT ANSWER

7-2.   B, C, D. *Incorrect answers*

      A.   CORRECT ANSWER

7-3.   A, B, C. *Incorrect answers*. All are correct as individual responses.

      D.   CORRECT ANSWER

7-4. $\text{Clearance} = \dfrac{\text{dose} \times F}{\text{AUC}}$

$$Cl = \dfrac{200\,mg \times 0.7}{\dfrac{200\,mg}{L} \times hr}$$

$$Cl = 0.7 \text{ L/hr}$$

7-5. $\overline{C} = \dfrac{X_0 \times F}{\tau \times Cl_t}$

$$\overline{C} = \dfrac{750\,mg \times 0.8}{12\,hr \times 40\,L \times \dfrac{0.5^{-1}}{hr}}$$

$$\overline{C} = 2.5 \text{ mg/L}$$

7-6. $Cl_t = K \times V$

$$Cl_t = 0.18 \text{ hr}^{-1} \times 10 \text{ L}$$

$$Cl_t = 1.8 \text{ L/hr}$$

7-7. $\overline{C} = \dfrac{X_0 \times F}{\tau \times Cl_t}$

$$10 = \dfrac{X_0\,mg/L \times 0.75}{8\,hr \times 1.8\,L/hr}$$

Dose = 192 mg every 8 hours

7-8.   The dose could be rounded to 200 mg.

The estimated steady-state concentration can be estimated using the same equation.

$$\overline{C} = \dfrac{X_0 \times F}{\tau \times Cl_t}$$

$$\overline{C} = \dfrac{200\,mg \times 0.75}{8\,hr \times 1.8\,L/hr}$$

$$\overline{C} = \dfrac{150\,mg}{14.40\,L}$$

The estimated steady-state concentration would equal 10.4 mg/L.

7-9. $AUC = \dfrac{\text{dose} \times F}{\text{clearance}}$

$$AUC = \dfrac{200\,mg \times 0.75}{1.8\,L/hr}$$

$$AUC = 83.3 \text{ mg} \times \text{hr/L}$$

7-10. $\overline{C} = \dfrac{X_0 \times F}{\tau \times Cl_t}$

$$10\,mg/L = \dfrac{X_0 \times 0.75}{12\,hr \times 1.8\,L/hr}$$

Dose = 288 mg

7-11.   A.   *Incorrect answer*

      B.   CORRECT ANSWER. The question asks about peak achieved. The time to peak is influence by K_a as well as K (elimination). The larger K_a indicates more rapid absorption resulting in more rapid peak concentration.

7-12. $\overline{C} = \dfrac{X_0 \times F}{\tau \times Cl_t}$

$$\overline{C} = \dfrac{100\,mg \times 0.8}{6\,hr \times 20\,L \times 0.3\,hr^{-1}}$$

$$\overline{C} = 2.22 \text{ mg/L}$$

7-13.   150 mg = dose × 0.6

Dose = 250 mg

7-14. $\overline{C} = \dfrac{X_0 \times F}{\tau \times Cl_t}$

$25 \text{ mg/L} = \dfrac{100 \text{ mg} \times 0.9}{\tau \times 0.3 \text{ L/hr}}$

$\tau = 12$ hours

7-15. $AUC = \dfrac{\text{dose} \times F}{\text{clearance}}$

$25 \text{ mg/L} \times \text{hr} = \dfrac{50 \text{ mg} \times 0.45}{\text{clearance}}$

Clearance = 0.9 L/hr

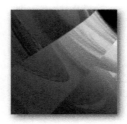

Discussion Points

D-1. If 500 mg of Drug X is administered by continuous infusion every 24 hours and a steady-state serum level is reported as 22 mg/L. Assuming $F = 1$, calculate the clearance for this drug.

D-2. Using the clearance value from discussion point D-1, calculate a new dose administered by continuous infusion every 24 hours that would result in a steady-state serum level of 30 mg/L.

D-3. Look up the bioavailability for the tablet and elixir dosage forms of Lanoxin. Plot representation concentration versus time curves for these two products at the same dose. Discuss all pharmacokinetic differences observed from these plots.

D-4. For discussion point D-3, discuss potential advantages and disadvantages of these two dosage forms. Also, list specific situations in which one dosage form might be preferred or not preferred in a clinical dosing situation.

D-5. Find bioavailability data for at least two different brands of the same drug (brand versus generic, if possible) and describe the bioavailability comparisons made for each product.

D-6. For the drug products researched in discussion point D-5 above, research the U.S. Food and Drug Administration's bioequivalence statement. Can these drugs be generically substituted, and if so, what data are used to support this claim?

D-7. Plot (not to scale) the concentration versus time curves for 100 mg of the following four oral formulations of a drug and then rank (from highest to lowest) their relative peak concentrations and AUCs. Describe the effects of variation in these two factors (K_a and F) on the concentration versus time curves.

A. $F = 1, K_a = 1 \text{ hr}^{-1}$

B. $F = 0.7, K_a = 1 \text{ hr}^{-1}$

C. $F = 1, K_a = 0.4 \text{ hr}^{-1}$

D. $F = 0.7, K_a = 0.4 \text{ hr}^{-1}$

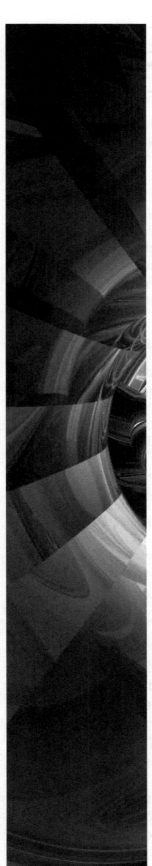

Drug Distribution and Protein Binding

OBJECTIVES

After completing Lesson 8, you should be able to:

1. Describe the major factors that affect drug distribution.

2. Explain the relative perfusion (i.e., high or low) characteristics of various body compartments (e.g., kidneys, fat tissue, and lungs).

3. Describe the three main proteins that bind various drugs.

4. List the major factors that affect drug protein binding.

5. Describe the dynamic processes involved in drug protein binding.

6. Compare perfusion-limited distribution and permeability-limited distribution.

7. Calculate the volume of distribution based on drug protein binding data.

Once a drug begins to be absorbed, it undergoes various transport processes, which deliver it to body areas away from the absorption site. These transport processes are collectively referred to as *drug distribution* and are evidenced by the changing concentrations of drug in various body tissues and fluids.

Information concerning the concentration of a drug in body tissues and fluids is limited to a few instances in time (i.e., we know the precise plasma drug concentration only at the few times that blood samples are drawn). Usually, we measure only plasma concentrations of drug, recognizing that the drug can be present in many body tissues.

For most drugs, distribution throughout the body occurs mainly by blood flow through organs and tissues. However, many factors can affect distribution, including the following:

- Differing characteristics of body tissues
- Disease states that alter physiology
- Lipid solubility of the drug
- Regional differences in physiologic pH (e.g., stomach and urine)
- Extent of protein binding of the drug

Body Tissue Characteristics

To understand the distribution of a drug, the characteristics of different tissues must be considered. Certain organs, such as the heart, lungs, and kidneys, are highly perfused with blood; fat tissue and bone (not the marrow) are much less perfused. Skeletal muscle is intermediate in blood perfusion. The importance of these differences in perfusion is that for most drugs, the rate of delivery from the circulation to a particular tissue depends greatly on the blood flow to that tissue. This is called *perfusion-limited distribution*. Drugs apparently distribute more rapidly to areas with higher blood flow. If the blood flow rate increases, the distribution of the drug to the tissue increases.

Highly perfused organs rapidly attain drug concentrations approaching those in the plasma; less well-perfused tissues take more time to attain such concentrations. Furthermore, certain anatomic barriers inhibit distribution, a concept referred to as *permeability-limited distribution*. This situation occurs for polar drugs diffusing across tightly knit lipoidal membranes. It is also influenced by the oil/water partition coefficient and degree of ionization of a drug. For example, the blood–brain barrier limits the amount of drug entering the central nervous system from the bloodstream. This limitation is especially great for highly ionized drugs and for those with large molecular weights.

After a drug begins to distribute to tissue, the concentration in tissue increases until it reaches an equilibrium at which the amounts of drug entering and leaving the tissue are the same. The drug concentration in a tissue at equilibrium depends on the plasma drug concentration and the rate at which drug distributes into that tissue. In highly perfused organs, such as the liver, the distribution rate is relatively high; for most agents, the drug in that tissue rapidly equilibrates with the drug in plasma. For tissues in which the distribution rate is lower (e.g., fat), reaching equilibrium may take much longer (**Figure 8-1**).

Disease States Affecting Distribution

Another major factor affecting drug distribution is the effect of various disease states on body physiology. In several disease states, such as liver, heart, and renal failure, the cardiac output and/or perfusion of blood to various tissues is altered. A decrease in perfusion to the tissues results in a lower rate of

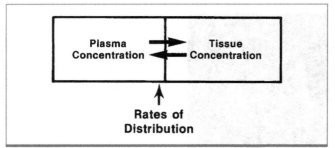

FIGURE 8-1.
Distribution rates.

distribution and, therefore, a lower drug concentration in the affected tissues relative to the plasma drug concentration. When the tissue that receives poor perfusion is the primary eliminating organ, a lower rate of drug elimination results, which then may cause drug accumulation in the body.

Lipid Solubility of the Drug

The extent of drug distribution in tissues also depends on the physicochemical properties of the drug as well as the physiologic functions of the body. A drug that is highly lipid soluble easily penetrates most membrane barriers, which are mainly lipid based, and distributes extensively to fat tissues. Drugs that are very polar and therefore hydrophilic (e.g., aminoglycosides) do not distribute well into fat tissues. This difference becomes important when determining loading dosage requirements of drugs in overweight patients. If total body weight is used to estimate dosage requirements and the drug does not distribute to adipose tissue, the dose can be overestimated.

Clinical Correlate

In general, volume of distribution is based on ideal body weight for drugs that do not distribute well into adipose tissue and on total body weight for drugs that do. If a drug distributes partially into fat, an adjusted body weight between the patient's actual and ideal body weights is often used. Vancomycin is one notable exception to this rule; the patient's total body weight is usually used to calculate volume of distribution for vancomycin.

Regional Differences in Physiologic pH

Another factor affecting drug distribution is the different physiologic pHs of various areas of the body. The difference in pH can lead to localization of drug in tissues and fluids. A drug that is predominantly in its ionized state at physiologic pH (7.4) does not readily cross membrane barriers and probably has a limited distribution. An example of this phenomenon is excretion of drugs in breast milk. Only un-ionized drug can pass through lipid membrane barriers into breast milk. Alkaline drugs, which would be mostly un-ionized at pH 7.4, pass into breast tissue. Once in breast tissue, the alkaline drugs ionize because breast tissue has an acidic pH; therefore, the drugs become trapped in this tissue. This same phenomenon can occur in the urine.

Due to the nature of biologic membranes, drugs that are un-ionized (uncharged) and have lipophilic (fat-soluble) properties are more likely to cross most membrane barriers. Several drugs (e.g., amphotericin) are formulated in a lipid emulsion to deliver the active drug to its intended site while decreasing toxicity to other tissues.

Physiologic Model

It is difficult to conceptualize the effect that the factors discussed above have on the volume of distribution of a drug. Many of these factors can be incorporated into a relatively simple physiologic model. This model describes the critical components that influence a drug's volume of distribution.

The following equation represents this physiologic model and provides a conceptual perspective of the volume of distribution:

$$V = V_p + V_t(F_p/F_t)$$

where:

V = volume of distribution

V_p = plasma volume

V_t = tissue volume

F_p = fraction of unbound drug in the plasma

F_t = fraction of unbound drug in the tissue

From this model, it is evident that the volume of distribution is dependent on the volume of the plasma (3–5 L), the volume of the tissue, the fraction of unbound drug in the plasma, and the fraction of unbound drug in the tissue. Changes in any of these parameters can influence a drug's volume of distribution. We use this equation to help us understand why the volume of distribution of a drug may have changed as a consequence of drug interactions or disease states. Usually, changes in the volume of distribution of a drug can be attributed to alterations in the plasma or tissue protein binding of the drug. This topic is discussed in the next section, Protein Binding.

The clinical consequence of changes in the volume of distribution of a drug in an individual patient is obvious. An example of this would be the use of drug loading doses. Because the initial plasma concentration of the drug (C_0) is primarily dependent on the size of the loading dose and the volume of distribution (C_0 = loading dose/V), changes in either of these parameters could significantly alter the C_0 achieved. Therefore, one must carefully consider the loading dose of a drug for a patient whose volume of distribution is believed to be unusual.

Phenytoin is an example of a drug that can be used to illustrate the effects of changes in the factors that determine volume of distribution. For a typical 70-kg person, the volume of distribution for phenytoin is approximately 45 L. Generally, the unbound fraction of this drug in plasma is approximately 0.1 (90% bound to albumin). If we assume that the plasma volume is 5 L, the tissue volume is 80 L, and the fraction unbound in tissue is 0.2, we can estimate how changes in plasma unbound fraction affect volume of distribution:

$$V = V_p + V_t(F_p/F_t)$$

$$= 5\,L + 80\,L\,(0.1/0.2)$$

$$= 45\,L$$

If the plasma fraction unbound increases to 0.2, which is possible for patients with hypoalbuminemia, the volume of distribution would change as shown:

$$V = V_p + V_t(F_p/F_t)$$

$$= 5\,L + 80\,L\,(0.2/0.2)$$

$$= 85\,L$$

So, by changing protein binding in the plasma, the volume of distribution has almost doubled.

Protein Binding

Another factor that influences the distribution of drugs is binding to tissues (nucleic acids, ligands, calcified tissues, and adenosine triphosphatase) or proteins (albumins, globulins, alpha-1-acid glycoprotein, and lipoproteins). It is the unbound or free portion of a drug that diffuses out of plasma. Protein binding in plasma can range from 0% to 99% of the total drug in the plasma and varies with different drugs. The extent of protein binding may depend on the presence of other protein-bound drugs and the concentrations of drug and proteins in the plasma.

The usual percentages of binding to plasma proteins for some commonly used agents are shown in **Table 8-1**. Theoretically, drugs bound to plasma proteins are usually not pharmacologically active. To exert an effect, the drug must dissociate from protein (**Figure 8-2**).

Although only unbound drug distributes freely, drug binding is rapidly reversible (with few exceptions), so some portion is always available as free drug for distribution. The association and dissociation process between the bound and unbound states is very rapid and, we assume, continuous (**Figure 8-3**).

A drug's protein-binding characteristics depend on its physical and chemical properties. Hydrophobic drugs usually associate with plasma proteins.

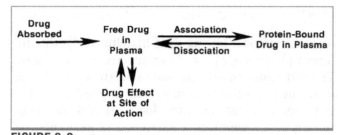

FIGURE 8-2.
Free drug is available to interact with receptor sites and exert effects.

The binding of a drug to plasma proteins will primarily be a function of the affinity of the protein for the drug.

The percentage of protein binding of a drug in plasma can be determined experimentally as follows:

$$\% \text{ protein binding} = \frac{[\text{total}] - [\text{unbound}] \times 100}{[\text{total}]}$$

where [*total*] is the total plasma drug concentration (unbound drug + bound drug) and [*unbound*] refers to the unbound or free plasma drug concentration.

Another way of thinking about the relationship between free and total drug concentration in the plasma is to consider the fraction of unbound drug in the plasma (F_p). F_p is determined by the following relationship:

$$F_p = \frac{[\text{unbound}]}{[\text{total}]}$$

TABLE 8-1. Protein Binding

Drug	Binding (%)
Ampicillin	18
Chloramphenicol	53
Digoxin	25
Gentamicin	<10
Lidocaine	70
Phenytoin	89
Vancomycin	30

Source: Reprinted with permission from Shargel L, Yu ABC. *Applied Biopharmaceutics and Pharmacokinetics.* 3rd ed. Norwalk, CT: Appleton & Lange; ©1996:594–95.

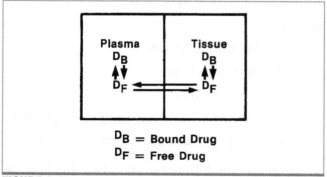

FIGURE 8-3.
Association and dissociation process.

Although the protein binding of a drug will be determined by the affinity of the protein for the drug, it will also be affected by the concentration of the binding protein. Two frequently used methods for determining the percentage of protein binding of a drug are equilibrium dialysis and ultrafiltration.

Three plasma proteins are primarily responsible for the protein binding of most drugs. They are shown in **Table 8-2** with their normal plasma concentration ranges.

Although only the unbound portion of drug exerts its pharmacologic effect, most drug assays measure total drug concentration—both bound and unbound drug. Therefore, changes in the binding characteristics of a drug could affect pharmacologic response to the drug. For example, the anticonvulsant and toxic effects of phenytoin are more closely related to the concentration of free drug in plasma than to the concentration of total drug in plasma. In most patients, the free phenytoin concentration is approximately 10% of the total concentration. However, in patients with low serum albumin concentrations, a lower fraction of phenytoin is bound to protein, and the free portion is up to 20% of the total concentration (**Table 8-3**). With hypoalbuminemia, therefore, a patient with a total phenytoin concentration of 15 mg/L may experience side effects (nystagmus and ataxia) usually seen at a total concentration of 30 mg/L. In these patients, a lower total phenytoin concentration may be effective in controlling seizures.

TABLE 8-2. Plasma Protein Plasma Concentrations

Protein	Normal Concentration	Type of Drugs Bound	Example
Albumin	3.5–4.5 g/L	Anionic, cationic	Phenytoin
Alpha-1-acid glycoprotein	0.4–1 g/L	Cationic	Lidocaine
Lipoproteins	Variable	Lipophilic	Cyclosporine

Source: Reprinted with permission from Shargel L, Yu ABC. *Applied Biopharmaceutics and Pharmacokinetics.* 3rd ed. Norwalk, CT: Appleton & Lange; ©1996:93.

TABLE 8-3. Phenytoin Concentration with Regard to Serum Albumin Concentration

	Normal (10%)	Hypoalbuminemia (e.g., 20% free)
Total	15	15
Unbound	1.5	3

Clinical Correlate

For certain drugs that are highly protein bound and have a narrow therapeutic index, it may be useful to obtain an unbound plasma drug concentration rather than a total plasma drug concentration. This will more accurately reflect the true concentration of active drug. An example of this is phenytoin. In the past, not all institutions had the capability to perform "free phenytoin" level laboratory tests in house, so calculation of true phenytoin concentration based on a total phenytoin concentration was necessary to make clinical assessments. Today, most hospital laboratories are able to measure "free phenytoin levels" from serum so that the most accurate unbound phenytoin concentration can be known. The therapeutic range differs depending on which laboratory measurement is used (total 10–20 mg/L; free 1–2 mg/L). Total phenytoin concentrations (reported by the laboratory) must also be adjusted in patients with significant renal impairment. (Adjusted formulas to be used in these patients can be found in the Phenytoin section of Lesson 15.)

The implications of protein binding are not fully understood. The extent of protein binding does not consistently predict tissue distribution or half-life of highly bound drugs. In other words, because an agent has a high fraction bound to protein does not mean it achieves poor tissue penetration.

Protein binding must be considered in the interpretation of plasma drug concentration data.

A considerable amount of intra- and interpatient variability exists in the plasma concentration of binding proteins (albumin and alpha-1-acid glycoprotein) as well as their affinity for a specific drug. A major contributor to this variability is the presence of a disease or altered physiologic state, which can affect the plasma concentration or affinity of the binding protein. For example, albumin concentrations are decreased with hepatic failure, renal dysfunction, burns, stress/trauma, and pregnancy. Alpha-1-acid glycoprotein concentrations are increased with myocardial infarction, renal failure, arthritis, surgery, or stress/trauma. In addition, concomitant administration of a displacer drug (i.e., an agent that competes with the drug of interest for common protein binding sites) can alter the protein binding of a drug. Examples of displacer drugs include salicylic acid and valproic acid.

Changes in plasma protein binding of drugs can have considerable influence on therapeutic or toxic effects that result from a drug regimen. Provided in the following text are practical considerations regarding plasma protein binding, with examples of specific agents for which these considerations are important to therapeutics.

The following questions should be considered when assessing the clinical importance of protein binding for a given drug:

- Does the drug possess a narrow therapeutic index?

- Is a high fraction of the drug bound to plasma protein?

- Which plasma protein is primarily responsible for binding, and does it account for the majority of the drug's binding variability?

Answers to these questions will help you establish a basis on which to evaluate the clinical significance of changes in plasma protein binding due to drug–drug or drug–disease state interactions.

In addition to having an impact on the interpretation of a drug's steady-state plasma concentration data, changes in plasma and tissue protein binding can have a major influence on clearance and volume of distribution. The remainder of this lesson discusses the effect that changes in a drug's protein binding will have on the apparent volume of distribution of a drug. The ramifications of altered protein binding on drug clearance are discussed in Lesson 9.

The consequence of protein binding changes on volume of drug distribution was implied in this equation shown earlier in this lesson:

$$V = V_p + V_t(F_p/F_t)$$

where:

V = volume of distribution

V_p = plasma volume

V_t = tissue volume

F_p = fraction of unbound drug in the plasma

F_t = fraction of unbound drug in the tissue

How can the administration of other drugs, diseases, or an altered physiologic state alter a drug's volume of distribution? The unbound fraction in the plasma and tissue is dependent on both the quantity (concentration) and quality (affinity) of the binding proteins; therefore, changes in these parameters can alter the volume of distribution. Four examples are briefly discussed to demonstrate the potential consequences of altered protein binding on a drug's volume of distribution.

EXAMPLE 1.

Plasma Protein Binding Drug Interaction: Effect of Valproic Acid Administration on Volume of Distribution of Phenytoin

Assuming that V_p and V_t are unchanged as a consequence of valproic acid administration, let's consider the effect of valproic acid on the protein binding of phenytoin. Both phenytoin and valproic acid are highly protein bound (approximately 90%) to the same site on the plasma albumin molecule. When these drugs are administered concomitantly, the protein binding of phenytoin is reduced (e.g., from 90% to 80%). This is an example of displacement, or reduction in the protein binding of a drug due to competition from another drug (i.e., the displacer). In this case, valproic acid has a higher affinity for the plasma protein binding site on the albumin molecule and competitively displaces phenytoin, resulting in a higher fraction of unbound phenytoin.

What is the consequence of phenytoin having a higher unbound fraction due to plasma protein binding displacement by valproic acid?

The previous equation would predict that an increase in the unbound fraction in the plasma would result in an increase in phenytoin's volume of distribution and result in a lower plasma drug concentration:

$$V_p(\leftrightarrow) + V_t(\leftrightarrow)\frac{F_p(\uparrow)}{F_t(\leftrightarrow)} = V(\uparrow)$$

EXAMPLE 2.

Tissue Binding Drug Interaction: Effect of Quinidine Administration on Volume of Distribution of Digoxin

As in Example 1, we assume that V_p and V_t are unchanged as a result of quinidine administration. Digoxin is negligibly bound to plasma proteins (approximately 25%), whereas 70% to 90% of quinidine is bound to plasma albumin and alpha-1-acid glycoprotein. Digoxin normally has a very large apparent volume of distribution (4–9 L/kg), which suggests extensive tissue distribution. Digoxin is significantly associated with cardiac muscle tissue, as demonstrated by a 70:1 cardiac muscle to plasma digoxin concentration ratio, which explains why its volume of distribution exceeds any normal physiologic space.

When these drugs are administered concomitantly, the tissue binding of digoxin is reduced. This is also an example of displacement, but in this case, quinidine has a higher affinity for the tissue protein binding site and displaces digoxin, resulting in a high unbound fraction in the tissue. What are the consequences of digoxin having a higher unbound fraction in the tissue due to quinidine displacement? The equation given previously predicts that an increase in the unbound fraction in the tissue would result in a decrease in the volume of distribution of digoxin, thus increasing digoxin's plasma drug concentration:

$$V_p(\leftrightarrow) + V_t(\leftrightarrow)\frac{F_p(\leftrightarrow)}{F_t(\uparrow)} = V(\downarrow)$$

Drug–drug interactions are not the only way a drug's apparent volume of distribution can be altered. In Example 3, we next consider the effect of a disease state (chronic renal failure) on the volume of distribution of phenytoin and digoxin.

EXAMPLE 3.

Effect of Disease State on Volume of Distribution: Renal Failure and Volume of Distribution of Phenytoin

Assuming that V_p and V_t are unchanged as a consequence of renal failure, let's consider the consequences of this disease state on the protein binding of phenytoin. Phenytoin's plasma protein binding is dependent on both the quantity and quality of albumin. Because chronic renal failure reduces albumin concentrations as well as albumin's affinity for phenytoin, it is not surprising that the plasma protein binding of phenytoin could be reduced from approximately 90% to 80%. What is the consequence of phenytoin's higher unbound fraction (0.2 [renal failure] versus 0.1 [normal]) due to renal failure?

The following equation predicts that an increase in the unbound fraction in the plasma would result in an increase in the volume of distribution of phenytoin, which would increase the concentration of the active unbound phenytoin able to cross the blood–brain barrier. This increase could result in supratherapeutic unbound concentrations, even when the total concentration is within normal limits:

$$V_p(\leftrightarrow) + V_t(\leftrightarrow)\frac{F_p(\uparrow)}{F_t(\leftrightarrow)} = V(\uparrow)$$

EXAMPLE 4.

Effect of Disease State on Volume of Distribution: Renal Failure and Volume of Distribution of Digoxin

As in Example 3, we assume that V_p and V_t are unchanged as a consequence of renal failure. Because digoxin is negligibly bound to plasma proteins, changes in its concentration should not be of clinical significance. However, renal failure does reduce the cardiac muscle-to-plasma digoxin concentration ratio to 30:1. What is the consequence of digoxin's higher unbound fraction in the tissue due to renal failure? The following equation predicts that an increase in the unbound fraction in the tissue would result in a decrease in the volume of distribution of digoxin and may cause an increased plasma digoxin drug concentration:

$$V_p(\leftrightarrow) + V_t(\leftrightarrow)\frac{F_p(\leftrightarrow)}{F_t(\uparrow)} = V(\downarrow)$$

In all of these examples, the volume of distribution of the drug in question was altered as a consequence of a drug–drug or drug–disease state interaction. Consequently, the calculation of their loading dose ($X_0 = C_0 V$) is influenced by changes in a drug's plasma or tissue protein binding. This must be considered in the development of a patient's drug dosing regimen.

REVIEW QUESTIONS

8-1. Drugs that are very water soluble tend to distribute poorly into body tissues.

A. True

B. False

8-2. Drugs that are predominantly ionized at physiologic pH (7.4) have greater distribution when compared to drugs that are primarily un-ionized.

A. True

B. False

8-3. Highly perfused tissue has lower drug distribution (compared to those with poor perfusion).

A. True

B. False

8-4. Estimate the volume of distribution for a drug when the volume of plasma and tissue are 6 and 34 L, respectively, and the fraction of drug unbound in plasma and tissue are 0.70 and 0.60, respectively.

A. 18.5 L

B. 34.7 L

C. 45.7 L

D. 50 L

8-5. The portion of drug that is bound to plasma protein is pharmacologically inactive.

A. True

B. False

8-6. Penetration of drug into tissues is related to the extent to which a drug is bound to plasma proteins.

A. True

B. False

8-7. Cationic drugs and weak bases are more likely to bind to _____.

A. Globulin

B. Alpha-1-acid glycoprotein

C. Lipoprotein

D. A and C

8-8. Anionic drugs and weak acids are more likely to bind to _____.

A. Albumin

B. Globulin

C. Alpha-1-acid glycoprotein

D. Lipoprotein

8-9. Predict how the volume of distribution (V) would change if the unbound fraction of phenytoin in plasma increased from 80% to 90%. Assume that unbound fraction in tissues (F_t) and volumes of plasma (V_p) and tissues (V_t) are unchanged.

A. Increase

B. No change

C. Decrease

D. Cannot be predicted with the information provided

8-10. A new drug has a tissue volume (V_t) of 20 L, an unbound fraction in plasma (F_p) of 9%, and an unbound fraction in tissues (F_t) of 5%. What will be the resulting volume of distribution if the plasma volume (V_p) is reduced from 12 to 5 L?

A. 25 L

B. 41 L

C. 48 L

D. 52 L

8-11. How is the volume of distribution (V) of digoxin likely to change if a patient has been taking both digoxin and quinidine, and the quinidine is discontinued? Assume that plasma volume (V_p), tissue volume (V_t), and unbound fraction of drug in plasma (F_p) are unchanged.

A. Increase

B. No change

C. Decrease

D. Cannot be predicted with the information provided

ANSWERS

8-1. A. CORRECT ANSWER. Hydrophilic drugs are more likely to remain in vascular space.
   B. *Incorrect answer*

8-2. A. *Incorrect answer*
   B. CORRECT ANSWER. Hydrophilic drugs are more likely to remain in vascular space.

8-3. A. *Incorrect answer*
   B. CORRECT ANSWER. Highly perfused tissue provides greater opportunity for drug to cross into tissue.

8-4. A, B, D. *Incorrect answers*
   C. CORRECT ANSWER

$$V = V_p + V_t\left(\frac{F_p}{F_t}\right)$$

$$= 6\,L + 34\,L\left(\frac{0.70}{0.60}\right) = 45.7\,L$$

8-5. A. CORRECT ANSWER
   B. *Incorrect answer*

8-6. A. CORRECT ANSWER
   B. *Incorrect answer*

8-7. A, C, D. *Incorrect answers*
   B. CORRECT ANSWER

8-8. A. CORRECT ANSWER
   B, C, D. *Incorrect answers*

8-9. B, C, D. *Incorrect answers*
   A. CORRECT ANSWER. If fraction unbound increases, then V will also increase:

$$V = V_p + V_t\left(\frac{F_p}{F_t}\right)$$

If F_p is decreased,

$$V_p(\leftrightarrow) + V_t(\leftrightarrow)\frac{F_p(\uparrow)}{F_t(\leftrightarrow)} = V(\uparrow)$$

8-10. A, C, D. *Incorrect answers*
   B. CORRECT ANSWER. Solve the equation using V_p = 8 L, then resolve using 4 L, and compare:

$$V = V_p + V_t\left(\frac{F_p}{F_t}\right)$$

$$= 12\,L + 20\,L\left(\frac{0.09}{0.05}\right) = 48\,L$$

If V_p is decreased to 5 L,

$$V = 5\,L + 20\,L\left(\frac{0.09}{0.05}\right) = 41$$

8-11. A. CORRECT ANSWER. Remember, when quinidine is administered concomitantly with digoxin, quinidine competes with digoxin for tissue binding sites and increases the unbound fraction of digoxin in the tissues (F_t). Therefore, assuming V_p and V_t remain unchanged, the effect of quinidine is as follows:

$$V_p(\leftrightarrow) + V_t(\leftrightarrow)\frac{F_p(\leftrightarrow)}{F_t(\uparrow)} = V(\downarrow)$$

When quinidine is discontinued, the unbound fraction of digoxin in the tissues (F_t) decreases as the tissue binding sites formerly occupied by quinidine become available.

$$V_p(\leftrightarrow) + V_t(\leftrightarrow)\frac{F_p(\leftrightarrow)}{F_t(\downarrow)} = V(\uparrow)$$

Therefore, the volume of distribution will increase.

   B, C, D. *Incorrect answers*

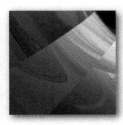

Discussion Points

D-1. Describe how knowledge of a drug's distribution and lipid solubility affects the calculation of a drug's loading dose. Clinically, what type of loading dose adjustments can be made to account for these factors?

D-2. A patient has a total plasma phenytoin concentration of 15 mcg/mL with a serum albumin concentration of only 2.2 g/dL. Estimate this patient's bound and unbound phenytoin concentration.

D-3. In the same patient as described in discussion point D-2, calculate a new total phenytoin concentration that would yield a therapeutic unbound phenytoin concentration.

D-4. Draw representative concentration versus time curves for: (*a*) a drug that diffuses into highly vascularized tissue before equilibrating in all body compartments, and (*b*) a drug that distributes equally well into all body compartments. Describe how these curves differ, and discuss potential clinical implications.

D-5. Discuss major physiologic and physiochemical factors that affect a drug's distribution, and comment on how these factors can affect the pharmacokinetic variable *apparent volume of distribution*.

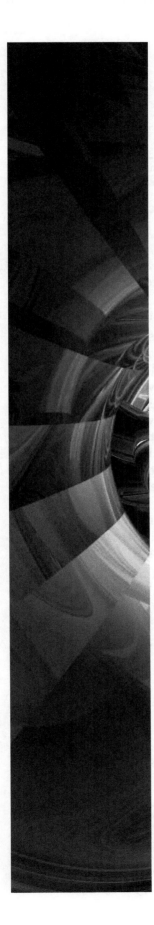

Drug Elimination Processes

OBJECTIVES

After completing Lesson 9, you should be able to:

1. Describe the impact of disease and altered physiologic states on the clearance and dosing of drugs.

2. Identify the various routes of drug metabolism and excretion.

3. Explain the two general types (Phase I and II) of drug metabolism.

4. Define the methods of hepatic drug metabolism and the approaches used to quantitate and characterize this metabolism.

5. Describe the effects of a drug's hepatic extraction ratio on that drug's removal via the liver's first-pass metabolism.

6. Explain the various processes involved in renal elimination (i.e., filtration, secretion, and reabsorption).

7. Define both the physiologic and mathematical relationship of drug clearance to glomerular filtration.

Drug Elimination

The liver and kidneys are the two major organs responsible for eliminating drugs from the body. Although both organs share metabolic and excretory functions, the liver is principally responsible for metabolism and the kidneys for elimination. The importance of these organs cannot be overestimated in determining the magnitude and frequency of drug dosing. Additionally, an appreciation of the anatomy and physiology of these organs will provide insight into the impact of disease and altered physiologic states, as well as concomitant drug administration, on the clearance and dosing of drugs.

The physical and chemical properties of a drug are important in determining drug disposition. For example, lipophilic drugs (compared with hydrophilic drugs) tend to have the following properties:

- Bound to a greater extent to plasma proteins
- Distributed to a greater extent throughout the body
- Metabolized to a greater extent in the liver

Hydrophilic drugs, particularly ionized species, tend to have the following properties:

- More limited distribution

- More rapid elimination (often by renal excretion)

Drug elimination from the body can be very complex. Metabolism (also known as biotransformation) involves conversion of the administered drug into another substance. Metabolism can result in the formation of either an active or inactive metabolite, which may then be excreted either faster or slower than the parent compound. The various consequences of hepatic biotransformation include active drug to inactive metabolite, active drug to active metabolite, and inactive drug to active metabolite.

Two examples of drugs with active metabolites are carbamazepine and its active metabolite carbamazepine-10, 11-epoxide and prednisone and its active metabolite prednisolone. For both drugs, the metabolites formed are active and may contribute significantly to the patient's pharmacologic response. Consequently, the plasma concentration of an active metabolite must be considered in addition to that of the parent compound when predicting overall pharmacologic response. In addition, many drugs are actually prodrugs, which require activation to their active forms. An example of a prodrug is sulfasalazine, which is a prodrug that is cleaved by colonic bacterial reductases to the antibacterial agent sulfapyridine and the anti-inflammatory agent 5-aminosalicylic acid.

Let's next explore two introductory concepts with regard to metabolite pharmacokinetics. Consider the following situation:

$$\text{drug X} \xrightarrow[K_h]{\text{liver}} \text{metabolite Y} \xrightarrow[K_r]{\text{kidney}} \text{excreted Y}$$

where drug X represents the intravenous (IV) bolus administration of the compound and K_h and K_r represent the elimination rate constants for hepatic metabolism of drug X and renal excretion of metabolite Y, respectively.

Figure 9-1 shows the decline in plasma concentration of parent drug X (assuming a one-compartment model after IV administration). Now consider the profile of metabolite Y after the same dose of drug X (**Figure 9-2**). If the excretion rate constant of metabolite Y (K_r) is much greater than the elimination rate constant of drug X (K_h), the terminal slope of the natural log of concentration of metabolite Y

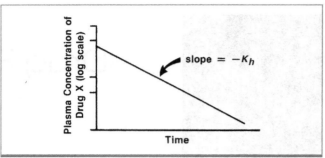

FIGURE 9-1.
Plasma concentration versus time curve for drug X, primarily metabolized by the liver.

versus time plot will be K_h and not K_r. This result occurs because the plasma concentration of metabolite Y is determined by the rate of formation from drug X (the slower rate constant).

On the other hand, if K_r is much less than K_h, the terminal slope of the plasma metabolite Y concentration versus time plot will be K_r (**Figure 9-3**). In this case, the relatively slow renal elimination of metabolite Y determines the resulting plasma concentrations. Although the liver is the major organ of drug biotransformation, the intestines, kidneys, and lungs may also metabolize some drugs. Before we can develop the concepts of drug metabolism, we must first examine the anatomy, physiology, and fundamental functions of the liver. The adult liver weighs 1400–1600 g and is uniquely situated between the gastrointestinal (GI) tract and the systemic circulation (**Figure 9-4**).

The basic functional unit of the liver is the liver lobule (**Figure 9-5**). The human liver contains approximately 50,000–100,000 such lobules. The liver lobule is constructed around a central vein, which empties into the hepatic veins and the vena

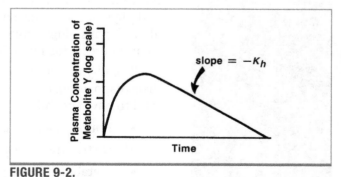

FIGURE 9-2.
Plasma concentrations of metabolite Y (from drug X) when the elimination rate constant (K_r) of metabolite Y is greater than the rate constant for metabolism (K_h) of drug X.

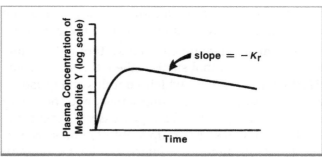

FIGURE 9-3.
Plasma concentrations of metabolite Y (from drug X) when the elimination rate constant (K_r) of metabolite Y is less than the rate constant for metabolism (K_h) of drug X.

cava. Therefore, the hepatic cells (hepatocytes), which are principally responsible for metabolic functions (including drug metabolism), are exposed to portal blood.

The liver (ultimately the liver lobule) receives its blood supply from two separate sources: the portal vein and the hepatic artery. The liver receives approximately 1100 mL/min of blood from the portal vein and 350 mL/min of blood from the hepatic artery. Consequently, blood flow in a normal 70-kg adult is approximately 1450 mL/min.

After entering the liver, blood flows in the veins and arteries of the portal triads, enters the sinusoidal spaces of the liver, and exits via the central

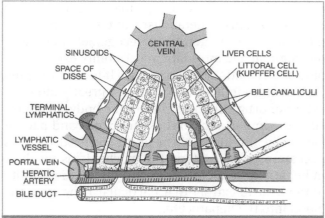

FIGURE 9-5.
Basic structure of a liver lobule showing the hepatic cellular plates, blood vessels, bile-collecting system, and lymph flow system composed of the spaces of Disse and interlobular lymphatics.

Source: Reproduced with permission from Guyton AC. *Textbook of Medical Physiology.* 7th ed. Philadelphia, PA: WB Saunders; © 1986.

hepatic vein. In the sinusoids, the drug is transferred from the blood to the hepatocytes, where it is metabolized or excreted unchanged into the biliary system (**Figure 9-6**).

The liver is involved in numerous functions, including storage and filtration of blood, secretion and excretion processes, and metabolism. In clinical

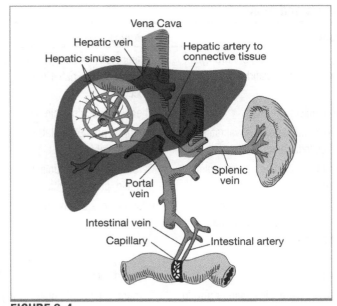

FIGURE 9-4.
Portal and hepatic circulations.

Source: Reproduced with permission from Guyton AC. *Textbook of Medical Physiology.* 7th ed. Philadelphia, PA: WB Saunders; ©1986.

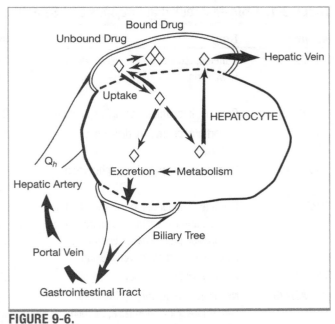

FIGURE 9-6.
Representation of drug metabolism and excretion by the hepatocyte. Q_h = hepatic blood flow.

pharmacokinetics, we are primarily interested in the last role, drug metabolism, and the factors that influence it. It is generally recognized that wide interpatient and intrapatient variability exists in the biotransformation of most drugs. It is also accepted that changes in liver function may greatly alter the extent of drug elimination from the body. To appreciate the importance of these functions and patient factors in the metabolism of a specific drug, it is necessary to understand the mechanisms involved in hepatic drug metabolism and the relative ability of the liver to extract that particular drug from the blood into the hepatocyte.

Hepatic metabolism occurs in two phases called *biotransformation* and *conjugation*:

1. *Phase I, biotransformation*—Drugs undergo oxidation, reduction, or hydrolysis to become more hydrophilic.

2. *Phase II, conjugation*—Drugs receive a molecular attachment (i.e., glucuronate) that facilitates transport within the body.

Drugs may be subjected to either type of reaction, but commonly drugs undergo Phase I (i.e., preparatory) reactions followed by Phase II reactions. The majority of drug–drug or drug–nutrient interactions occur during Phase I (biotransformation)

and involve either the inhibition or induction of the CYP isoenzyme involved in the drug's metabolism.

The major hepatic enzyme system responsible for Phase I metabolism is called the *cytochrome P450 enzyme system*, which contains many isoenzyme subclasses with varying activity and specificity in Phase I drug metabolism processes. Cytochrome P450 isoenzymes are grouped into families according to their genetic similarities. Enzymes with greater than 40% of their genes in common are considered to be from the same family and are designated by an Arabic number (e.g., 1, 2, 3), and those enzymes within each family that contain greater than 55% common genes are given a subfamily designation using a capital letter (e.g., A, B, C). Finally, those enzymes with greater than 97% common genes are further classified with another Arabic number and often represent a very specific drug-metabolizing enzyme. The cytochrome P450 enzymes most important in human drug metabolism are CYP1, CYP2, and CYP3. In addition to the action on specific drug substrates, these isoenzymes can also be either induced or inhibited by other drugs, thus increasing or decreasing the plasma concentration of the drug they metabolize. This can have clinical significance for drugs whose concentration-dependent effects are significantly affected by enzyme inhibition or induction. **Table 9-1** lists common

TABLE 9-1. Drug-Metabolizing Enzymes and Selected Inhibitors and Inducers

Isozyme	Drug	Inhibitors	Inducers
CYP1A2	Caffeine, tacrine, theophylline, lidocaine, R-warfarin	Cimetidine, ciprofloxacin, erythromycin, fluvoxamine, tacrine, zafirlukast	Omeprazole, tobacco, carbamazepine, nafcillin, broccoli
CYP2B6	Cocaine, ifosfamide, cyclophosphamide	Chloramphenicol	Phenobarbital, rifampin
CYP2C9	S-warfarin, phenytoin, diclofenac, piroxicam	Amiodarone, fluconazole, lovastatin, clopidogrel, leflunomide	Rifampin, phenobarbital, secobarbital
CYP2C19	Diazepam, omeprazole, mephenytoin	Fluvoxamine, fluoxetine, omeprazole, oxcarbazepine	Carbamazepine, prednisone, rifampin, phenobarbital
CYP2D6	Codeine, haloperidol, dextromethorphan, tricyclic antidepressants, phenothiazines, metoprolol, propranolol, risperidone, paroxetine, sertraline, venlafaxine	Bupropion, cinacalcet, quinidine, fluoxetine, sertraline, amiodarone, propoxyphene	Rifampin, dexamethasone
CYP2E1	Acetaminophen, alcohol	Disulfiram	Isoniazid, alcohol
CYP3A3/4/5/7	Nifedipine, verapamil, cyclosporine, carbamazepine, astemizole, tacrolimus, midazolam, alfentanil, diazepam, loratadine, ifosfamide, cyclophosphamide	Erythromycin, cimetidine, clarithromycin, fluvoxamine, fluoxetine, ketoconazole, itraconazole, isoniazid, grapefruit juice, metronidazole, ritonavir, indinavir	Carbamazepine, rifampin, phenytoin, phenobarbital, St. John's wort

drug-metabolizing isoenzymes and the drugs most commonly affected, as well as other drugs that can inhibit or induce the activity of these isoenzymes.

Another point regarding Phase I biotransformation reactions is that select drugs may be metabolized by more than one cytochrome P450 isoenzyme. An example is tricyclic antidepressants. Most of these agents are hydroxylated by CYP2D6; however, *N*-demethylation is probably mediated by a combination of CYP2C19, CYP1A2, and CYP3A4. Acetaminophen, another example, appears to be metabolized by both CYP1A2 and CYP2E1.

Phase II reactions, also called *synthetic* (or *conjugation*) *reactions*, result in very polar compounds that are easily excreted in the urine. Examples of drugs that undergo Phase I or Phase II reactions are shown in **Table 9-2**.

Understanding whether a drug undergoes Phase I or Phase II biotransformation may be helpful in predicting how it will be affected by a certain disease state. For example, liver disease and the aging process appear to reduce the elimination of drugs that undergo Phase I metabolism more than those dependent on conjugation (Phase II) reactions. This fact raises a significant question: at what point does liver disease significantly alter

Phase I metabolic processes? No single test can accurately estimate liver drug-metabolism capacity. High values for alkaline phosphatase, aspartate aminotransferase (AST), and alanine aminotransferase (ALT) usually indicate acute cellular damage and not poor liver drug-metabolism capacity. On the other hand, abnormal values that may be more suggestive of the liver's ability to function are elevated serum bilirubin concentrations, low serum albumin concentrations, and a prolonged prothrombin time. The Child-Pugh Score, a widely utilized clinical assessment tool for liver disease, may also be used to evaluate a patient's ability to metabolize drugs eliminated by the liver. A score of 8 to 9 indicates the need to initiate therapy at moderately decreased initial doses (~25%) for drugs primarily (≥60%) metabolized hepatically, while a score of ≥10 suggests a significant decrease (~50%) in initial doses of drugs primarily metabolized by the liver.

Membrane transport proteins are membrane-spanning substances that facilitate drug transport across the intestinal tract, excretion into the bile and urine, distribution across the blood–brain barrier and drug uptake into target cells. A major transport protein is P-glycoprotein. Commonly utilized agents that are affected by this protein include clopidogrel, digoxin, diltiazem, glyburide, and morphine. Increased or decreased expression of this substance can alter absorption, elimination, and serum concentrations of relevant drugs. Other membrane-transporter families include organic anion transporters (OAT family), the organic anion transporting polypeptides (OATP family), and the organic cation transporters (OCT family).

Biotransformation

Biotransformation processes are affected by many factors. The functioning of metabolic enzyme systems may be quite different at the extremes of age. Historically, neonates were at risk of toxicity from chloramphenicol because they do not conjugate this drug efficiently. Also, the social habits of a patient may affect drug elimination. Alcohol use and smoking may increase hepatic clearance of some drugs by inducing metabolic enzymes. Obviously, disease states such as cirrhosis and conditions that decrease liver blood flow (e.g., heart failure) significantly affect drug metabolism. Finally, concomitant drug use may affect drug metabolism. Certain drugs, such as phenytoin,

TABLE 9-2. Drugs Undergoing Phase I or II Metabolizing Reactions

Phase I Reactions	Examples
Oxidation:	
Hydroxylation	Cyclosporine, ibuprofen, phenytoin, acetaminophen (also Phase II)
Dealkylation	Diazepam, imipramine, tamoxifen
Deamination	Amphetamine, diazepam
Sulfoxidation	Chlorpromazine, cimetidine, omeprazole
Reduction	Sulfasalazine, chloramphenicol
Hydrolysis	Aspirin, carbamazepine, enalapril

Phase II Reactions	Examples
Glucuronidation	Acetaminophen (also Phase I), lorazepam, morphine, chloramphenicol
Methylation	Captopril, levodopa, methyldopa
Acetylation	Clonazepam, corticosteroids, dapsone, isoniazid, sulfonamides

rifampin, and phenobarbital, may induce hepatic enzymes, whereas other drugs, such as cimetidine, fluconazole, and valproic acid, may inhibit them.

Even in healthy individuals, in the absence of hepatic enzyme inducers or inhibitors, the ability to metabolize drugs may vary considerably due to individual genetic makeup. Genetic polymorphism can affect the individual response to a drug. For example, approximately one third of Caucasians carry at least one variant allele for the gene that encodes CYP2C9 involved in the metabolism of warfarin. Presence of this polymorphism increases the anticoagulant effect of warfarin, thus requiring lower warfarin doses. Investigators have also shown that two distinct subpopulations have varying capacities for drug acetylation (Phase II reaction) as a result of genetic polymorphism. Fast acetylators have a greater rate of elimination for drugs such as isoniazid and hydralazine. For slow acetylators, the usual doses of these agents may result in excessive plasma concentrations and, therefore, increased drug toxicities. Further discussions regarding genetic alteration of drug metabolism can be found in Lesson 11.

Hepatic Clearance

Now let's focus on hepatic drug metabolism and the approaches used to quantitate and characterize this process. Depending on physical and chemical properties, each drug is taken up or extracted by the liver to different degrees. Knowledge of the affinity of a drug for extraction by the liver is important in anticipating the influence of various factors on drug metabolism. Generally, drugs are characterized as possessing a low to high affinity for extraction by the liver. Briefly, drugs with a low hepatic extraction (<20%) tend to be more available to the systemic circulation and have a low systemic clearance. Drugs with a high hepatic extraction (>80%) tend to be less available to the systemic circulation and have a high systemic clearance. Drugs with extraction ratios between 20 and 80 are termed *intermediate-extraction drugs*. These points will become more apparent as we develop a mathematical model to relate a drug's hepatic clearance to hepatic physiology.

The efficiency of the liver in removing drug from the bloodstream is referred to as the *extraction ratio* (*E*), the fraction of drug removed during one pass through the liver. The value of *E* theoretically ranges from 0 to 1. With high-extraction drugs, *E* is closer to 1, and with low-extraction drugs, *E* is

closer to zero. The reader may wish to refer to the discussion of *E* in Lesson 2.

In Lesson 1, we learned that the concentration of drug in the body was dependent on the dose of the drug administered and the volume into which the agent was distributed. This was represented by the following equation:

$$C = \frac{X}{V}$$

where:

C = concentration

X = dose

V = volume

(See **Equation 1-1.**)

In Lesson 2, we further discovered that steady-state plasma drug concentrations are affected by several variables, including the rate at which a drug is administered and the drug's clearance. This relationship is demonstrated in the following equation, which was reviewed in lesson 5.

$$C_{ss} = \frac{K_0}{Cl_t}$$

where:

Cl_t = the total body clearance of the drug

K_0 = the drug infusion rate

C_{ss} = the steady-state plasma drug concentration

The factors that determine the extraction ratio and its relationship to overall hepatic clearance can be shown mathematically as the following:

$$E = \frac{Cl_i}{Q_h + Cl_i}$$

(See **Equation 2-2.**)

where:

Cl_i = intrinsic clearance

Q_h = hepatic blood flow

Because $Cl_h = Q_h \times E$, then:

$$Cl_h = \frac{Q_h \times Cl_i}{Q_h + Cl_i}$$

The systemic clearance of a drug relates dosing rate to a steady-state plasma drug concentration.

The systemic clearance of a drug equals the hepatic clearance when the liver is the sole organ responsible for elimination. Another way of looking at this relationship is to remember that clearance terms are additive. Therefore:

$$Cl_t = Cl_h + Cl_r + Cl_{other\ organs} \quad \text{(see Equation 2-1)}$$

and Cl_t is equal to Cl_h when Cl_r and $Cl_{other\ organs}$ are minimal.

For a drug that is totally dependent on the liver for its elimination, a number of useful mathematical models show critical relationships between systemic drug clearance and various physiologic functions.

These models consider three factors:

1. The liver's innate ability to remove unbound drug from plasma irreversibly

2. The fraction of drug unbound in the blood

3. Hepatic blood flow

One practical and useful model is called the *jar*, *venous equilibrium*, or *well-stirred model*:

$$Cl_h = \frac{Q_h F_p Cl_i}{Q_h + F_p Cl_i}$$

where:

Cl_h = hepatic drug clearance

F_p = fraction of free drug in plasma

Cl_i = intrinsic clearance (which is based on unbound drug concentration)

Q_h = hepatic blood flow

In the well-stirred method, it should be understood that this model represents the maximum ability of the enzymatic processes of the liver without physiological constraints (i.e., "liver in a beaker"). Thus, this equation allows us to approximate what is happening in the liver but knowing that the true extent of metabolism is influenced by other things that we can't fully capture in a mathematical equation.

Recall that Cl_h equals Cl_t for drugs eliminated only by the liver. Therefore, changes in any of the parameters defined in the previous equation will have a considerable impact on Cl_t and, consequently, the steady-state drug plasma concentration produced by a given dosing regimen. In a normal 70-kg individual, Q_h (portal vein plus hepatic artery blood flows) should approach 1500 mL/min. Obviously,

changes in Q_h would change the rate of drug delivery to the liver and have an impact on Cl_h. However, the magnitude of that impact would depend on the liver's ability to extract the drug. F_p is incorporated into the relationship because only free or unbound drug is available to be metabolized by the hepatocytes. Finally, intrinsic clearance (Cl_i) represents the liver's innate ability to clear unbound drug from intracellular water via metabolism or biliary excretion. Changes in Cl_i should have a profound effect on hepatic clearance. However, as with Q_h, the extent and magnitude of such an effect would depend on the extraction characteristics of the drug.

Examination of the equation for the venous equilibrium model at the extremes of intrinsic clearance values provides insight into the influences of hepatic blood flow and intrinsic clearance on drug dosing. For high intrinsic clearance drugs, Cl_i is much greater than Q_h; Q_h becomes insignificant when compared to Cl_i. Hepatic clearance of drugs with high extraction ratios (> 0.8) is dependent on hepatic blood flow only. It is not influenced by protein binding or enzymes.

Therefore, when Cl_i is large, Cl_h equals Q_h, or hepatic clearance equals hepatic blood flow. Hepatic clearance is essentially a reflection of the delivery rate (Q_h) of the drug to the liver; changes in blood flow will produce similar changes in clearance. Consequently, after IV administration, the hepatic clearance of highly extracted compounds (e.g., lidocaine and propranolol) is principally dependent on liver blood flow and independent of both free fraction and intrinsic clearance. This particular commonly used model is best applied to intravenously administered drugs, as orally absorbed drugs with high extraction ratios may act more like low-extraction drugs. Other models may work better in these cases.

For low intrinsic clearance drugs, Q_h is much greater than Cl_i. Therefore, the hepatic clearance of compounds with a low extraction ratio (e.g., phenytoin) is virtually independent of hepatic blood flow. Hepatic clearance for these drugs becomes a reflection of the drug's intrinsic clearance and the free fraction of drug in the plasma.

Some examples of individual intrinsic clearances are given in **Table 9-3**. However, there is no clear-cut division between the classes described; additional factors may need to be considered when predicting drug disposition.

TABLE 9-3. High-, Intermediate-, and Low-Extraction Drugs

High Intrinsic Clearance ($Cl_i \gg Q_h$)	Intermediate Intrinsic Clearance	Low Intrinsic Clearance ($Cl_i \ll Q_h$)
Propranolol	Aspirin	Warfarin
Lidocaine	Quinidine	Phenytoin
Propoxyphene	Desipramine	Isoniazid
Morphine		Theophylline
Meperidine		Diazepam
Nitroglycerin		Procainamide
Isoproterenol		Antipyrine
Pentazocine		Phenobarbital
Verapamil		Erythromycin

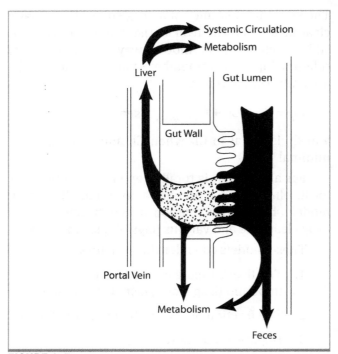

FIGURE 9-7.
Routes of drug disposition with oral drug administration.

Clinical Correlate

If the liver's ability to metabolize a drug is increased, possibly due to enzyme induction, then the extraction ratio (E) is also increased. However, the magnitude of change in E depends on the initial value of the intrinsic clearance of the drug.

If Cl_i is small (low intrinsic clearance drug), then E is initially small. Increasing Cl_i causes an almost proportional increase in extraction and hepatic clearance. However, if Cl_i and E are already high, a further increase in intrinsic clearance does not greatly affect the extraction ratio or hepatic drug clearance.

First-Pass Effect

An important characteristic of drugs having a high extraction ratio (e.g., propranolol) is that, with oral administration, a significant amount of drug is metabolized before reaching the systemic circulation (**Figure 9-7**). Drug removal by the liver after absorption is called the *first-pass effect*. The result can be that the amount of drug reaching the systemic circulation is considerably less than the dose given.

The first-pass effect becomes obvious when we examine comparable IV and oral doses of a drug with a high extraction ratio. For propranolol, plasma concentrations achieved after oral doses of 40–80 mg are equivalent to those achieved after IV doses of 1–2 mg. The difference in required dosage is not explained by low oral absorption but by liver first-pass metabolism. Anatomically, the liver receives the blood supply from the GI tract via the portal vein before its entrance into the general circulation via the hepatic vein. Therefore, the liver can metabolize or extract a certain portion of the drug before it reaches the systemic circulation. Also, enzymes in the gut wall can metabolize the drug before it reaches the liver.

Because the blood supply draining the GI tract passes through the liver first, the fraction of an oral dose (F) that reaches the general circulation (assuming the dose is 100% absorbed across the gut wall) is given by

$$F = 1 - E$$

Remember, E is the extraction ratio that indicates the efficiency of the organ eliminating a drug. For example, if the drug is 100% absorbed across the gut wall and the liver extracts 70% before it reaches the systemic circulation, 30% of the dose finally reaches the bloodstream. Therefore:

$$E = 0.7$$
$$F = 1 - E$$
$$= 0.3$$

Again, F is the fraction of drug reaching the systemic circulation.

Effects of Disease States and Drug Interactions on Hepatically Metabolized Drugs

It is important to appreciate the effect that a potential drug or disease state interaction may have on the pharmacologic response of a drug that is principally eliminated by the liver. Therefore, we will consider the potential impact that changes in Q_h, F_p, and Cl_i will have on the steady-state concentration of both total and free drug concentration. Remember, we will assume that Cl_t (total body clearance) equals Cl_h (hepatic clearance) and that steady-state free drug concentration is the major determinant of pharmacologic response.

When trying to assess clinical implications, always consider the following:

- Route of administration (IV versus oral)
- Extraction ratio (high [>0.8] versus low [<0.2])
- Protein binding (high [>80%] versus low [<50%])

$$Cl_h = \frac{Q_h F_p Cl_i}{Q_h + F_p Cl_i}$$

and

$$C_{ss(total)} = \frac{K_0}{Cl_t} \text{ or } \frac{K_0}{Cl_h}$$

Then, substituting for $C_{ss(total)}$

$$C_{ss(free)} = F_p \times C_{ss(total)} = F_p \times \frac{K_0}{Cl_h}$$

where:

Cl_h = hepatic drug clearance

F_p = fraction of drug unbound in plasma

K_0 = the drug infusion rate

In the following three examples, we apply the previously described hepatic extraction equation to several cases involving a specific disease state effect on drug interaction.

EXAMPLE 1.

Effect of Addition of Enzyme Inhibitor on Pharmacologic Response of Theophylline

Theophylline (which is metabolized primarily by CYP1A2 of the hepatic cytochrome P450 system) was administered to a patient via a constant IV infusion and produced a steady-state total plasma concentration of 15 mg/L (therapeutic range, 5–15 mg/L). Ciprofloxacin, a known inhibitor of the hepatic cytochrome P450 enzyme system (primarily 1A2), was later added to this patient's drug dosing regimen. Ciprofloxacin reduces the intrinsic clearance of theophylline by 25% to 30%. What impact should ciprofloxacin administration have on this patient's pharmacologic response (assume a 30% reduction in clearance)?

Considerations

- Theophylline (in this example) is administered via a constant intravenous infusion (K_0).
- Theophylline has a low extraction ratio.
- Theophylline possesses low protein binding.

Because theophylline has a low extraction ratio and is not extensively bound to proteins,

$$Cl_h = F_p \times Cl_i$$

and

$$C_{ss(total)} = \frac{K_0}{Cl_h} \text{ or } \frac{K_0}{F_p Cl_i}$$

Then substituting for $C_{ss(total)}$

$$C_{ss(free)} = F_p \times C_{ss(total)} = F_p \times \frac{K_0}{F_p Cl_i} = \frac{K_0}{Cl_i}$$

Impact on $C_{ss(total)}$

Because K_0 and F_p are unchanged and Cl_i is reduced by 30%, $C_{ss(total)}$ should increase by 30%.

Impact on $C_{ss(free)}$

Because K_0 is unchanged and Cl_i is reduced by 30%, $C_{ss(free)}$ should increase by 30%.

Consequence

You should anticipate significant side effects as a consequence of a higher free steady-state concentration of theophylline (**Figure 9-8**). The dosing rate of theophylline should be reduced by 30% in this example.

EXAMPLE 2.

Effect of Decreased Protein Binding of Phenytoin Due to Renal Failure

Phenytoin (which is metabolized primarily by CYP2C9/10 of the hepatic cytochrome P450 mixed function oxidase system) was administered to a patient by intermittent IV administration and produced a steady-state total plasma concentration of 15 mg/L (therapeutic range: 10–20 mg/L). The patient unexpectedly experienced acute renal failure. Renal failure is known to reduce the plasma protein binding of phenytoin from approximately 90% to about 80% but has minimal effect on phenytoin's intrinsic clearance.

What impact should renal failure have on this patient's pharmacologic response?

Considerations

- Phenytoin is administered by intermittent IV administration.
- Phenytoin has a low extraction ratio.
- Phenytoin possesses high protein binding.
- Because phenytoin has a low extraction ratio and is extensively bound to proteins, $Cl_h = F_p \times Cl_i$

$$C_{ss(total)} = \frac{K_0}{Cl_h} \text{ or } \frac{K_0}{F_p Cl_i}$$

Substituting for $C_{ss(total)}$

$$C_{ss(free)} = F_p \times C_{ss(total)} = F_p \times \frac{K_0}{F_p Cl_i} = \frac{K_0}{Cl_i}$$

Impact on $C_{ss(total)}$

Because K_0 and Cl_i are unchanged and F_p is doubled, $C_{ss(total)}$ should decrease by half.

Impact on $C_{ss(free)}$

Because K_0 and Cl_i are unchanged, $C_{ss(free)}$ should remain unchanged.

Consequence

You should anticipate no significant change in this patient's pharmacologic response (despite a significant drop in phenytoin's steady-state total concentration) because steady-state free drug concentrations remain unchanged (**Figure 9-9**). However, the total concentration necessary to achieve this therapeutic unbound concentration will be less than the normal reference range for phenytoin.

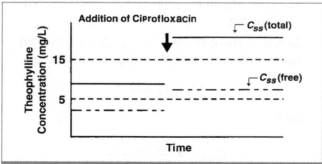

FIGURE 9-8.
Changes in free and total steady-state plasma theophylline concentrations with the addition of ciprofloxacin.

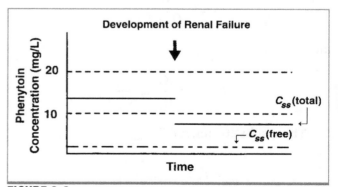

FIGURE 9-9.
Change in total steady-state plasma phenytoin concentration due to renal failure.

EXAMPLE 3.

Effects of Increased Protein Binding of Lidocaine Due to Myocardial Infarction

Lidocaine (which is metabolized primarily by CYP1A2 of the hepatic cytochrome P450 mixed function oxidase system) was administered to a patient for a life-threatening ventricular arrhythmia via a constant IV infusion, producing a steady-state total plasma concentration of 4 mg/L (therapeutic range: 1.5–5 mg/L). The next day, the patient had a myocardial infarction. Myocardial infarctions are known to significantly increase the concentration of alpha-1-acid glycoprotein (a serum globulin) and the protein binding of drugs associated with it. The protein binding of lidocaine is known to be high and primarily dependent on alpha-1-acid glycoprotein. What impact should a myocardial infarction have on this patient's pharmacologic response (assuming that the myocardial infarction had no effect on hepatic blood flow)?

Considerations

- Lidocaine is administered via a constant IV infusion.

- Lidocaine has a high extraction ratio.

- Lidocaine possesses high protein binding to alpha-1-acid glycoprotein.

Because lidocaine has a high extraction ratio and binds extensively to alpha-1-acid glycoprotein, $Cl_h = Q_h$.

$$C_{ss(total)} = \frac{K_0}{Cl_h} \text{ or } \frac{K_0}{Q_h}$$

Substituting for $C_{ss(total)}$

$$C_{ss(free)} = F_p \times C_{ss(total)} = F_p \times \frac{K_0}{Q_h}$$

Impact on $C_{ss(total)}$

Because K_0 and Q_h are unchanged, $C_{ss(total)}$ should remain unchanged.

Impact on $C_{ss(free)}$

Because K_0 and Q_h are unchanged and F_p is decreased, $C_{ss(free)}$ should decrease, which could result in a reduced pharmacologic response (**Figure 9-10**).

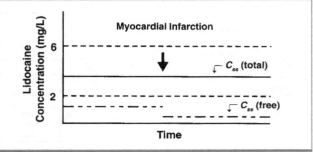

FIGURE 9-10.
Change in free steady-state plasma lidocaine concentrations due to myocardial infarction.

Consequence

Because only total (bound and unbound) lidocaine concentrations can be measured clinically, you should anticipate a reduced pharmacologic response despite similar steady-state total lidocaine concentrations. This reduced response may necessitate high total lidocaine concentrations and a higher dose to achieve the desired response.

Clinical Correlate

This reduced response is why lidocaine's dose is generally titrated to a clinical response based on electrocardiogram readings (i.e., decrease in arrhythmias) rather than dosed to a therapeutic concentration.

These three examples represent how the well-stirred model and knowledge of the pharmacokinetic characteristics of a drug can be used to predict the effect of changes in hepatic blood flow, protein binding, and intrinsic clearance. These same principles can be used to assess a wide variety of clinically relevant situations.

Renal Elimination

As stated previously, drug elimination refers to metabolism and excretion (**Figure 9-11**). Some drugs are primarily excreted unchanged; others are extensively metabolized before excretion. The fraction of drug metabolized is different for various agents. The overall elimination rate is the sum of all metabolism and excretion processes and is referred to as *total body elimination*.

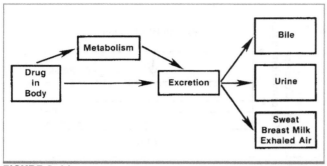

FIGURE 9-11.
Drug elimination.

Total body elimination = drug excreted unchanged + drug metabolized.

Excretion is the process that removes a drug from tissues and the circulation. A drug can be excreted through urine, bile, sweat, expired air, breast milk, or seminal fluid. The most important routes of excretion for many drugs and their metabolites are the urine and bile. For anesthetic gases, pulmonary excretion can play a significant role.

Excretion may occur for a biotransformed drug or for a drug that remains unchanged in the body. For example, penicillin G is primarily excreted unchanged in the urine. Elimination of this drug is thus dependent on renal function.

Renal excretion is the net effect of three distinct mechanisms within the kidneys:

1. Glomerular filtration

2. Tubular secretion

3. Tubular reabsorption

With glomerular filtration, blood flows into the capsule of the glomerulus, and there is a passive diffusion of fluids and solutes across the porous glomerular membrane (**Figure 9-12**). In a healthy adult, up to 130 mL of fluid may cross the glomeruli per minute (total of both kidneys).

Three factors influence glomerular filtration:

1. Molecular size

2. Protein binding

3. Glomerular integrity and total number of functioning nephrons

Drugs dissolved in the plasma may be filtered across the glomerulus; drugs that are protein bound or have a molecular weight greater than 60,000 dalton

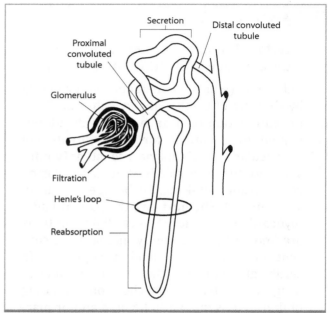

FIGURE 9-12.
Renal nephron.

are not filtered. Pathophysiologic changes in the kidneys may also alter glomerular filtration.

Some drugs are actively secreted from the blood into the proximal tubule, which contains urine. These drugs (primarily weak organic acids and some bases) are excreted by carrier-mediated active processes that may be subject to competition from other substances in the body due to broad specificity of the carriers. For example, probenecid and penicillin are both actively secreted. If given together, probenecid competes with penicillin for secretion, so penicillin is secreted less rapidly (it has a longer half-life). This particular relationship can be used in therapeutic situations to extend the duration of penicillin action.

Most drugs also undergo tubular reabsorption back into the blood. This process occurs passively in the distal tubules for drugs that are lipid soluble or not highly ionized. For other agents, it can occur as an active process and (as with tubular secretion) is subject to competition from other agents. An example of reabsorption is glucose, which normally undergoes 100% reabsorption in the distal tubules of the kidneys. With renal dysfunction, glucose often is not reabsorbed and may appear in the urine. Other examples of agents that are actively reabsorbed include endogenous substances such as vitamins, electrolytes, and amino acids.

Tubular reabsorption is dependent on the physical and chemical properties of the drug and the pH of the urine. Drugs that are highly ionized in the urine have less tubular reabsorption; they tend to stay in the urine and are excreted. Drugs must be uncharged to pass easily through biologic membranes. Tubular reabsorption of some compounds may also be dependent on urine flow rate. Urea, for example, has a high tubular reabsorption at low urine flow rates and a low tubular reabsorption at high urine flow rates. Because renal clearance is determined by filtration, active secretion, and reabsorption, it is fairly complicated.

Total renal clearance, Cl_r, can be determined from the following equation:

$$Cl_r = \text{amount excreted in urine}_{(t_1 \to t_2)} / \text{AUC}_{(t_1 \to t_2)}$$

where AUC is the area under the plasma concentration curve. However, because it is not easy to differentiate these processes when measuring the amount of drug in the urine, renal clearance is calculated from the ratio of the urine excretion rate to the drug concentration in plasma:

$$Cl_r = \frac{\text{drug excretion rate}}{\text{drug plasma concentration}}$$

There are several different methods to calculate renal drug clearance. In one method, the excretion rate of the drug is estimated by determining the drug concentration in a volume of urine collected over short time periods after drug administration. This excretion rate is then divided by the plasma concentration of drug entering the kidneys at the midpoint of the urine collection period.

To express this as an equation:

$$Cl_r = \frac{\text{amount of drug in urine from } t_1 \text{ to } t_2 / (t_2 - t_1)}{C_{\text{midpoint}}}$$

where t_1 and t_2 are the times of starting and stopping the collection, respectively, and C is the plasma concentration at the midpoint of t_1 and t_2. Therefore, overall renal clearance is calculated usually without differentiating among filtration, secretion, and reabsorption. This method is commonly used to calculate creatinine clearance when the "amount of drug" is the amount of creatinine that appears in the urine over 24 hours, $t_2 - t_1 = 24$ hours, and C_{midpoint} is the serum creatinine determined at the midpoint of the urine collection period.

Relationship between Renal Clearance and Glomerular Filtration Rate

If a drug is exclusively eliminated renally and the only renal process involved is glomerular filtration, the relationship between total body clearance and glomerular filtration rate (GFR) is as shown in **Figure 9-13**. Creatinine clearance is commonly used as a measure of GFR. Remember that creatinine undergoes some tubular secretion; therefore, GFR can sometimes be slightly overestimated. As GFR increases, clearance of drug increases. When GFR is zero, clearance is zero. Recall that the equation for the line is $Y = mX + b$. Then, the line in Figure 9-13 can be defined as follows:

$$\text{Clearance} = (\text{slope})\,(\text{GFR}) + 0$$

or

$$\text{Clearance} = (\text{slope})\,(\text{GFR})$$

However, if a drug is excreted by glomerular filtration as well as some other route (e.g., biliary excretion), the relationship illustrated in **Figure 9-14** could exist. As GFR increases, the clearance of drug increases; but when GFR is zero, clearance is still greater than zero. In this example, the equation for the line is as follows:

$$\text{Clearance} = \text{slope (GFR)} + y\text{-intercept}$$
$$Y = mX + b$$

and we see that when GFR is zero, clearance is the value of the y-intercept, which is nonrenal clearance.

This approach has been used to relate the aminoglycoside elimination rate constant (K) to creatinine clearance. When dosing these agents, we must consider the individual's GFR, as reflected by creatinine

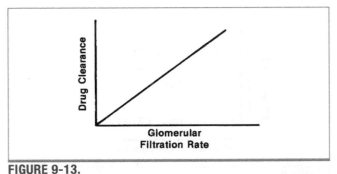

FIGURE 9-13.
Relationship between drug clearance and glomerular filtration rate for a drug that is exclusively eliminated by glomerular filtration.

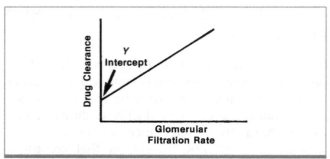

FIGURE 9-14.
Relationship between drug clearance and glomerular filtration rate for a drug that is eliminated by renal and nonrenal processes.

clearance. The relationship observed between K and creatinine clearance is shown in **Figure 9-15**.[1] Therefore, K can be predicted for aminoglycosides (such as gentamicin) based on an individual's creatinine clearance.

With the equation for a line, $Y = mX + b$:

$$K = 0.00293 \text{ hr}^{-1} \times \text{creatinine clearance (in mL/min)} + 0.014$$

Clinical Correlate

Note that drugs that are cleared almost solely by renal mechanisms will have a y-intercept of zero or very close to zero. Drugs that have extrarenal routes of elimination will have larger y-intercepts.

Determining patient-specific creatinine clearance can be accomplished by either direct measurement

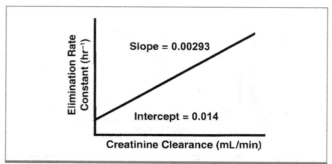

FIGURE 9-15.
Relationship between elimination rate constant and creatinine clearance for aminoglycosides.

of the amount of creatinine contained in a 24-hour urine sample or by estimating this parameter using standard mathematical equations. Direct measurement is the most accurate of these.

When using this method, creatinine clearance (CrCl) is determined as follows:

$$\text{CrCl} = \frac{UV}{P \times 1440}$$

where:

U = urinary creatinine concentration

V = volume of urine collected

P = plasma creatinine concentration (taken at midpoint of urine collection)

1440 = number of minutes in 24 hours

Although there are several formulas for estimating creatinine clearance, the Cockcroft–Gault equation is commonly used:

9-1
$$\text{CrCl}_{male} = \frac{(140 - age)\text{IBW}}{72 \times \text{SCr}}$$

or

$$\text{CrCl}_{female} = 0.85\frac{(140 - age)\text{IBW}}{72 \times \text{SCr}}$$

where:

CrCl = creatinine clearance (milliliters per minute)

age = patient's age (years)

IBW = ideal body weight (kilograms)

SCr = serum creatinine concentration (milligrams per deciliter [mg/dL])

Adjusting this equation for a patient's body surface area is not necessary clinically.

This formula also requires the following patient data:

- Ideal body weight (lean body weight) or adjusted body weight (AdjBW)
- Age
- Sex
- Steady-state serum creatinine concentration

IBW may be estimated as follows:

9-2 $\quad IBW_{males} = 50 \text{ kg} + 2.3 \text{ kg for each inch}$
$$\text{over 5 feet in height}$$

$$IBW_{females} = 45.5 \text{ kg} + 2.3 \text{ kg for each inch}$$
$$\text{over 5 feet in height}$$

In obese patients, the use of total body weight (TBW) overestimates whereas the use of IBW underestimates creatinine clearance.

In patients whose TBW is more than 20% over their IBW, adjusted body weight (AdjBW) should be used to estimate creatinine clearance:

9-3 $\quad AdjBW = IBW + 0.4(TBW - IBW)$

For a patient who weighs less than IBW, the actual body weight would be used.

It is important to note that the use of serum creatinine values less than 1 mg/dL will greatly elevate the calculated creatinine clearance value when using **Equation 9-1**. This is especially true in the elderly. In patients with serum creatinine values of less than 1 mg/dL, it has been recommended to either round the low serum creatinine value up to 1 mg/dL before calculating creatinine clearance, or round the final calculated creatinine clearance value down. Creatinine clearance, estimated creatinine clearance, and other GFR estimations, such as the modification of diet in renal disease (MDRD) equations, are more fully discussed in Lesson 12.

Reference

1. Matzke GR, Jameson JJ, Halstenson CE. Gentamicin distribution in young and elderly patients with various degrees of renal function. *J Clin Pharmacol.* 1987;27:216–20.

REVIEW QUESTIONS

9-1. The major organ(s) responsible for drug elimination is (are) _____.
A. Liver
B. Brain
C. Kidney
D. A and C

9-2 The body converts a drug to a less active substance by a process called _____.
A. Phosphorylation
B. Hydrogenation
C. Biotransformation
D. Distransformation

9-3. Biotransformation is also known as _____.
A. Absorption
B. Elimination
C. Renal excretion
D. Metabolism

9-4. Hepatic elimination encompasses the processes of _____.
A. Biotransformation and glucuronidation
B. Biotransformation and excretion
C. Glomerular filtration and oxidation
D. All of the above

9-5. Glucuronidation is _____.
A. Oxidation metabolism
B. Hydrolysis metabolism
C. Phase II biotransformation process
D. All of the above

9-6. Biotransformation may be dependent on factors such as age, _____.
A. Height, and gender
B. Gender, and weight
C. Disease, and genetics
D. Disease, and gender

9-7. Which of the following is not a Phase I reaction?
A. Glucuronidation
B. Oxidation
C. Hydrolysis
D. Reduction

9-8. The basic functional unit of the liver is the _____.
A. Renal lobule
B. Hepatocyte
C. Liver cell
D. Liver lobule

9-9. The liver receives its blood from the _____.
A. Portal artery and hepatic vein
B. Portal vein and hepatic artery
C. Portal artery and hepatic artery
D. Vena cava and aorta

9-10. A drug administered orally goes through the liver before it is available to the systemic circulation via which of the following?
A. Hepatic artery
B. Vena cava
C. Hepatic vein
D. Renal artery

9-11. Because the extraction ratio can maximally be 1, the maximum value that hepatic clearance can approach is that of _____.
A. Creatinine clearance
B. Glomerular filtration
C. Hepatic blood flow
D. Renal blood filtration

9-12. Intrinsic clearance is the maximal ability of the liver to eliminate drug in the absence of any blood flow limitations.
A. True
B. False

9-13. Smoking is known to increase the enzymes responsible for theophylline metabolism (a drug with a low hepatic extraction). Would a patient with a history of smoking likely require a higher, lower, or equivalent theophylline total daily dose compared to a nonsmoking patient?

    A. Lower

    B. Higher

    C. Equivalent

9-14. Heart failure reduces cardiac output and hepatic blood flow. Consequently, the total daily dose of lidocaine may need to be decreased in a patient with heart failure who has a myocardial infarction.

    A. True

    B. False

9-15. Which of the following types of metabolism do drugs with a high extraction ratio undergo to a significant extent?

    A. Zero-order

    B. First-pass

    C. Intraluminal

    D. Nonlinear

9-16. Significant first-pass metabolism means that much of the drug's metabolism occurs before its arrival at the _____.

    A. Hepatocyte

    B. Systemic circulation

    C. Portal blood

    D. Liver lobule

9-17. The liver receives blood supply from the GI tract via the _____.

    A. Portal vein

    B. Hepatic artery

    C. Hepatic vein

    D. Portal artery

9-18. For a drug that is totally absorbed without any presystemic metabolism and then undergoes hepatic extraction, which of the following is the correct equation for F?

    A. $F = 1 - K_a$

    B. $F = 1 - F_p$

    C. $F = 1 - E$

    D. $F = 1$ – the fraction of the drug absorbed

9-19. Route of administration, extraction ratio, and protein binding are all factors that should be considered when trying to assess the effect of disease states on plasma concentrations of drugs eliminated by the liver.

    A. True

    B. False

9-20. What impact will administration of a drug that inhibits the hepatic cytochrome P450 system have upon theophylline clearance?

    A. Increase

    B. Decrease

9-21. Disease states may increase or decrease drug protein binding.

    A. True

    B. False

9-22. Liver function is best assessed by _____.

    A. Serum transaminase concentrations

    B. Serum albumin concentrations

    C. Serum bilirubin concentrations

    D. No one test can adequately assess hepatic function

9-23. Which metabolic process is most affected by hepatic disease?

    A. Phase I reactions

    B. Phase II reactions

9-24. Drug elimination encompasses both _____.

    A. Metabolism and excretion

    B. Metabolism and biotransformation

    C. Absorption and metabolism

    D. Metabolism and distribution

9-25. Two important routes of drug excretion are _____.

    A. Hepatic and tubular secretion

    B. Biliary and metabolic

    C. Renal and biliary

    D. Renal and metabolic

9-26. Fluid is filtered across the glomerulus through active transport.

   A. True

   B. False

9-27. Tubular secretion most often occurs with weak organic acids.

   A. True

   B. False

9-28. Which of the following statements about tubular reabsorption is *false*?

   A. Tubular reabsorption depends on the pH of the urine.

   B. Highly ionized drugs tend to remain in the urine.

   C. Tubular reabsorption can only be an active transport process.

   D. A and C.

9-29. Renal clearance can be calculated from the ratio of which of the following rates to the drug's concentration in plasma?

   A. Tubular reabsorption rate

   B. Tubular secretion rate

   C. Glomerular filtration rate

   D. Excretion rate

9-30. For aminoglycoside doses, which of the following must be calculated to estimate an individual patient's drug elimination rate? An individual patient's _____.

   A. Pulmonary clearance

   B. Biliary clearance

   C. Creatinine clearance

   D. A and C

9-31. For aminoglycosides, the terminal elimination rate constant can be estimated from the creatinine clearance using which of the following equations?

   A. $K = 0.00293 \text{ hr}^{-1} \times$ (creatinine clearance in mL/min) + 1.4

   B. $K = 0.00293 \text{ hr}^{-1} \times$ (creatinine clearance in mL/min) + 0.014

   C. $K = 2.93 \text{ hr}^{-1} \times$ (creatinine clearance in mL/min)

   D. $K = 0.00293 \text{ hr}^{-1} +$ (creatinine clearance in mL/min)

ANSWERS

9-1. A,B,C. *Incorrect answers*

   D. CORRECT ANSWER

9-2 A, B, D. *Incorrect answers*

   C. CORRECT ANSWER

9-3. A, B, C. *Incorrect answers*

   D. CORRECT ANSWER

9-4. A. CORRECT ANSWER

   B, C, D. *Incorrect answers*

9-5. A, B, D. *Incorrect answers*. Oxidation and hydrolysis are Phase I reactions.

   C. CORRECT ANSWER

9-6. A, B, D. *Incorrect answers*

   C. CORRECT ANSWER

9-7. B, C, D. *Incorrect answers*

   A. CORRECT ANSWER

9-8. A, B, C. *Incorrect answers*

   D. CORRECT ANSWER

9-9. A, C, D. *Incorrect answers*

   B. CORRECT ANSWER

9-10. A, B, D. *Incorrect answers*

   C. CORRECT ANSWER

9-11. A, B, D. *Incorrect answers*

   C. CORRECT ANSWER

9-12. A. CORRECT ANSWER

   B. *Incorrect answer*

9-13. A, C. *Incorrect answers*

   B. CORRECT ANSWER. Smoking raises the concentrations of enzymes that also metabolize theophylline, so more theophylline would be metabolized, requiring a higher theophylline dose.

9-14. A. CORRECT ANSWER

   B. *Incorrect answer*

9-15. A. *Incorrect answer.* Zero-order processes are not determined by amount of hepatic extraction.

B. CORRECT ANSWER

C. *Incorrect answer.* Intraluminal metabolism is independent of hepatic extraction.

D. *Incorrect answer.* Nonlinear metabolism involves only saturation or induction of hepatic enzymes.

9-16. A, C, D. *Incorrect answers*

B. CORRECT ANSWER

9-17. A. CORRECT ANSWER

B, C, D. *Incorrect answers*

9-18. A, B, D. *Incorrect answers*

C. CORRECT ANSWER. *F* represents the fraction of drug that reaches the systemic circulation; *E* is the extraction ratio.

9-19. A. CORRECT ANSWER

B. *Incorrect answer*

9-20. A. *Incorrect answer*

B. CORRECT ANSWER. Theophylline is a low-extraction drug and its clearance is roughly equal to intrinsic hepatic clearance (Cl_i), so the effect of cytochrome P450 enzyme induction is likely to decrease intrinsic and overall clearance.

9-21. A. CORRECT ANSWER

C. *Incorrect answer*

9-22 A, B, C. *Incorrect answers*

D. CORRECT ANSWER. No single test can define hepatic function

9-23 A. CORRECT ANSWER

B. *Incorrect answer*

9-24. A. CORRECT ANSWER

B. *Incorrect answer.* Biotransformation is a type of metabolism.

C. *Incorrect answer.* Absorption is not an elimination process.

D. *Incorrect answer.* Distribution is not an elimination process.

9-25. A, B, D. *Incorrect answers*

C. CORRECT ANSWER

9-26. A. *Incorrect answer*

B. CORRECT ANSWER

9-27. A. CORRECT ANSWER

B. *Incorrect answer*

9-28. A. *Incorrect answer.* Urine pH does affect tubular reabsorption.

B. *Incorrect answer.* Highly ionized drugs do remain in the urine because ionized forms of drugs do not cross membranes well.

C. CORRECT ANSWER

D. *Incorrect answer*

9-29. A. *Incorrect answer.* Tubular reabsorption rate cannot be directly measured.

B. *Incorrect answer.* Tubular secretion rate cannot be directly measured.

C. *Incorrect answer.* Glomerular filtration rate does not account for tubular secretion or reabsorption.

D. CORRECT ANSWER

9-30. A, B, D. *Incorrect answers.* Aminoglycosides do not undergo hepatic or pulmonary clearance.

C. CORRECT ANSWER

9-31. A. *Incorrect answer.* The *y*-intercept is wrong. Aminoglycosides undergo little if any extrarenal elimination and, therefore, the *y*-intercept value should be close to zero.

B. CORRECT ANSWER

C. *Incorrect answer.* The answer should represent the approximate fraction of drug excreted per hour, and this value should be less than one.

D. *Incorrect answer.* The correct answer should be expressed as a product, not a sum (i.e., A × B, not A + B).

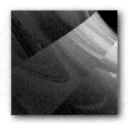

Discussion Points

D-1. Research the metabolism of primidone and discuss the clinical significance of its metabolites. Discuss the proper method to monitor a patient receiving primidone.

D-2. Select several drugs whose prescribing information indicates that the dose should be decreased with hepatic impairment. Describe the pharmacokinetics of these drugs and discuss why this drug's dose should be decreased. Finally, indicate specifically how you would go about decreasing this dose.

D-3. Research the pharmacokinetics of carbamazepine and discuss its metabolism when given alone and when given with other enzyme inhibitors or inducers. Specifically, how would you begin a patient on carbamazepine and how would you monitor and adjust its dose?

D-4. Research the various oral fluoroquinolones to determine which can affect the metabolism of theophylline and to what extent. Discuss why some of these drugs affect theophylline and others do not.

D-5. Describe several clinical situations in which a drug's ability to compete for renal secretion with another drug can be either useful or harmful.

D-6. Describe situations in which alteration of urine pH with urine acidifier or alkalinizing agents can be used to enhance the clinical response of other drugs.

D-7. Look up and compare the various equations that can be used to calculate the elimination rate constant for gentamicin, tobramycin, and amikacin. Are these equations the same or different? Try to explain why they are either the same or different.

Nonlinear Processes

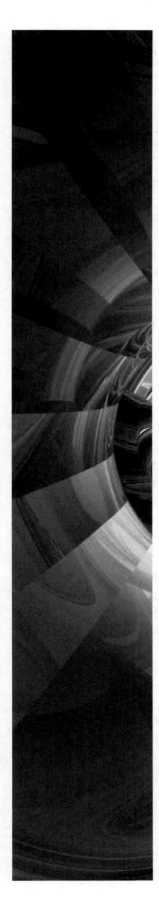

OBJECTIVES

After completing Lesson 10, you should be able to:

1. Describe the relationship of both drug concentration and area under the plasma drug concentration versus time curve (AUC) to the dose for a nonlinear, zero-order process.

2. Explain the various biopharmaceutic processes that can result in nonlinear pharmacokinetics.

3. Describe how hepatic enzyme saturation can result in nonlinear pharmacokinetics.

4. Use the Michaelis–Menten model for describing nonlinear pharmacokinetics.

5. Describe V_{max} and K_m.

6. Use the Michaelis–Menten model to predict plasma drug concentrations.

7. Use the $t_{90\%}$ equation to estimate the time required for 90% of the steady-state concentration to be reached.

Until now, we have used a major assumption in constructing models for drug pharmacokinetics: drug clearance remains constant with any size dose. This is the case only when drug elimination processes are first order (as described in previous lessons). With a first-order elimination process, as the dose of drug increases, the plasma concentrations observed and the AUC increase proportionally. That is, if the dose is doubled, the plasma concentration and AUC also double (**Figure 10-1**).

Because the increase in plasma concentration and AUC is linear with drug dose in first-order processes, this concept is referred to as *linear pharmacokinetics.* When these linear relationships are present, they are used to predict drug dosage. For example, if a 100-mg daily dose of a drug produces a steady-state peak plasma concentration of 10 mg/L, we know that a 200-mg daily dose will result in a steady-state plasma concentration of 20 mg/L. (Note: linear does not refer to the plot of natural log of plasma concentration versus time.)

With some drugs (e.g., phenytoin and aspirin), however, the relationships of drug dose to plasma concentrations and AUC are not linear. As the drug dose increases, the peak concentration and the resulting AUC do not increase proportionally (**Figure 10-2**). Therefore, such drugs are said to follow nonlinear, zero-order, or dose-dependent pharmacokinetics (i.e., the pharmacokinetics change with the dose given). Just as with drugs following linear pharmacokinetics, it is important to predict the plasma drug concentrations of drugs following zero-order

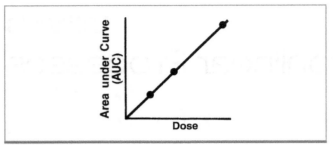

FIGURE 10-1.
Relationship of AUC to drug dose with first-order elimination, where clearance is not influenced by dose.

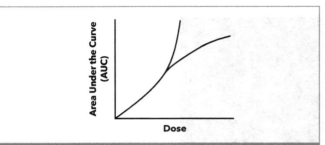

FIGURE 10-2.
Relationship of AUC to drug dose with dose-dependent pharmacokinetics.

pharmacokinetics. In this lesson, we discuss methods to characterize drugs that follow nonlinear pharmacokinetics.

Nonlinear pharmacokinetics may refer to an increase or decrease in several different processes, including absorption, distribution, and renal or hepatic elimination (**Table 10-1**). For example, with nonlinear absorption, the fraction of drug in the gastrointestinal (GI) tract that is absorbed per minute changes with the amount of drug present. Although absorption and distribution can be nonlinear, nonlinear pharmacokinetics usually refers to the processes of drug elimination.

When a drug exhibits nonlinear pharmacokinetics, usually the processes responsible for drug elimination are saturable at therapeutic concentrations. These elimination processes may include renal tubular secretion (as seen with penicillins) and hepatic enzyme metabolism (as seen with phenytoin). When an elimination process is saturated, any increase in drug dose results in a disproportionate increase in the plasma concentrations achieved because the amount of drug that can be eliminated over time cannot increase. This situation is contrary

to first-order linear processes, in which an increase in drug dosage results in an increase in the amount of drug eliminated over any given period.

Of course, most elimination processes are capable of being saturated if enough drug is administered. However, for most drugs, the doses administered do not cause the elimination processes to approach their limitations.

Clinical Correlate

Many drugs exhibit mixed-order pharmacokinetics, displaying first-order pharmacokinetics at low drug concentrations and zero-order pharmacokinetics at high concentrations. It is important to know the drug concentration at which a drug order switches from first to zero. Phenytoin is an example of a drug that switches order at therapeutic concentrations, whereas theophylline does not switch until concentrations reach the toxic range.

TABLE 10-1. Drugs Having Dose- or Time-Dependent Pharmacokinetics

Process	Agent	Mechanism
Absorption	Riboflavin, methotrexate, gabapentin	Saturable gut wall transport
	Penicillins	Saturable decomposition in GI tract
Distribution	Methotrexate	Saturable transport into and out of tissues
	Salicylates	Saturable protein binding
Renal elimination	Penicillin G	Active tubular secretion
	Ascorbic acid	Active reabsorption
Extrarenal elimination	Carbamazepine	Enzyme induction
	Theophylline, phenytoin	Saturable metabolism

GI = gastrointestinal.

For a typical drug having dose-dependent pharmacokinetics, with saturable elimination, the plasma drug concentration versus time plot after a dose may appear as shown in **Figure 10-3**.

After a large dose is administered, an initial slow elimination phase (clearance decreases with higher plasma concentration) is followed by a much more rapid elimination at lower concentrations (curve A). However, when a small dose is administered (curve B), the capacity of the elimination process is not reached, and the elimination rate remains constant. At high concentrations, the elimination rate approaches that of a zero-order process (i.e., the amount of drug eliminated over a given period remains constant, but the fraction eliminated changes). At low concentrations, the elimination rate approaches that of a first-order process (i.e., the amount of drug eliminated over a given time changes, but the fraction of drug eliminated remains constant).

A model that has been used extensively in biochemistry to describe the kinetics of saturable enzyme systems is known as *Michaelis–Menten kinetics* (for its developers). This system describes the relationship of an enzyme to the substrate (in this case, the drug molecule). In clinical pharmacokinetics, it allows prediction of plasma drug concentrations resulting from administration of drugs with saturable elimination (e.g., phenytoin).

The equation used to describe Michaelis–Menten pharmacokinetics is as follows:

$$\text{Drug elimination rate} = \frac{-dC}{dt} = \frac{V_{max}C}{K_m + C}$$

where $-dC/dt$ is the rate of drug concentration decline at time t and is determined by V_{max}, the theoretical maximum rate of the elimination process.

K_m is the drug concentration when the rate of elimination is half the maximum rate, and C is the total plasma drug concentration.

V_{max} is expressed in units of amount per unit of time (e.g., milligrams per day) and represents the maximum amount of drug that can be eliminated in the given time period. For drugs metabolized by the liver, V_{max} can be determined by the quantity or efficiency of metabolizing enzymes. This parameter will vary, depending on the drug and individual patient.

K_m, the Michaelis constant, is expressed in units of concentration (e.g., mg/L) and is the drug concentration at which the rate of elimination is half the maximum rate (V_{max}). In simplified terms, K_m is the concentration above which saturation of drug metabolism is likely.

V_{max} and K_m are related to the plasma drug concentration and the rate of drug elimination as shown in **Figure 10-4**. When the plasma drug concentration is less than K_m, the rate of drug elimination follows first-order pharmacokinetics. In other words, the amount of drug eliminated per hour directly increases with the plasma drug concentration. When the plasma drug concentration is much less than K_m, the first-order elimination rate constant (K) for drugs with nonlinear pharmacokinetics is approximated by V_{max}; therefore, as V_{max} increases (e.g., by hepatic enzyme induction), K increases.

With drugs having saturable elimination, as plasma drug concentrations increase, drug elimination approaches its maximum rate. When the plasma concentration is much greater than K_m, the rate of drug elimination is approximated by V_{max}, and elimination proceeds at close to a zero-order process.

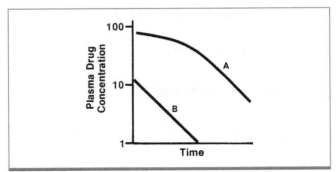

FIGURE 10-3.
Dose-dependent clearance of enzyme-saturable drugs.

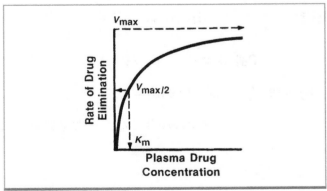

FIGURE 10-4.
Relationship of drug elimination rate to plasma drug concentration with saturable elimination.

Next, we consider how V_{max} and K_m can be calculated and how these determinations may be used to predict plasma drug concentrations in patients.

Calculation of V_{max}, K_m, and Plasma Concentration and Dose

For drugs that have saturable elimination at the plasma concentrations readily achieved with therapeutic doses (e.g., phenytoin), prediction of the plasma concentrations achieved by a given dose is important. For these predictions, it is necessary to estimate V_{max} and K_m. Therefore, we must apply the Michaelis–Menten equation presented earlier in this lesson:

$$\frac{-dC}{dt} = \frac{V_{max}C}{K_m + C}$$

The change in drug concentration over time is related to the Michaelis–Menten parameters V_{max}, K_m, and the plasma drug concentration (C). We know that at steady state (after multiple drug doses) the rate of drug loss from the body (milligrams removed per day) is equal to the amount of drug administered (daily dose). In the Michaelis–Menten equation, $-dC/dt$ indicates the rate of drug loss from the body; therefore, at steady state:

$$\frac{-dC}{dt} = \text{daily drug dose} = \frac{V_{max}C}{K_m + C}$$

Now we have an equation that relates V_{max}, K_m, plasma drug concentration, and daily dose (at steady state). To use this relationship, it is first helpful to transform the equation to a straight-line form:

10-1
$$\text{Daily dose} = \frac{V_{max}C}{K_m + C}$$

$$\text{Daily dose} (K_m + C) = V_{max}C$$

$$\text{Daily dose} (K_m) + \text{daily dose} (C) = V_{max}C$$

$$\text{Daily dose} (C) = V_{max}C - \text{daily dose} (K_m)$$

Then:

$$\text{Daily dose} = -K_m \left(\text{daily dose}/C\right) + V_{max}$$

$$Y = mX + b$$

where m is slope and b is the y-intercept.

So the relationship of the Michaelis–Menten parameters, C, and dose can be expressed as a straight line (**Figure 10-5**). If the straight line can be defined, then V_{max} and K_m can be determined; if V_{max} and K_m are known, then the plasma concentrations at steady state resulting from any given dose can be estimated.

To define the line, it is necessary to know the steady-state concentrations achieved at a minimum of two different doses. For example, a patient receiving 300 mg of phenytoin per day achieved a steady-state concentration (trough) of 9 mg/L; when the daily dose was increased to 400 mg/day, a steady-state concentration of 16 mg/L was achieved. The data for this patient can be plotted as shown in **Figure 10-6**. Then a line is drawn between the two points, intersecting the y-axis. The y-intercept equals V_{max} (observed to be 700 mg/day), and the slope of the line equals $-K_m$.

Calculating K_m

10-2
$$\text{Slope} = -K_m = \frac{\text{dose}_{initial} - \text{dose}_{increased}}{\text{dose}/C_{initial} - \text{dose}/C_{increased}}$$

$$= \frac{300 \text{ mg/day} - 400 \text{ mg/day}}{\left(\dfrac{300 \text{ mg/day}}{9 \text{ mg/L}} - \dfrac{400 \text{ mg/day}}{16 \text{ mg/L}}\right)}$$

$$= \frac{-100 \text{ mg/day}}{33.3 \text{ L/day} - 25 \text{ L/day}}$$

$$= -12.0 \text{ mg/L}$$

So K_m equals 12 mg/L.

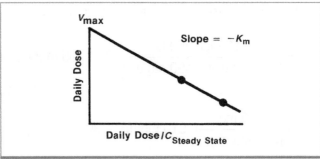

FIGURE 10-5.
Linear plot of the Michaelis–Menten equation.

Calculating Dose

Knowing V_{max} and K_m, we can then predict the dose necessary to achieve a given steady-state concentration or the concentration resulting from a given dose. If we wish to increase the steady-state plasma concentration to 20 mg/L, we can use the Michaelis–Menten equation to predict the necessary dose:

$$dose = \frac{V_{max}C}{K_m + C}$$

$$= \frac{(700 \text{ mg/day})(20 \text{ mg/L})}{12 \text{ mg/L} + 20 \text{ mg/L}}$$

$$= \frac{14,000 \text{ mg}^2/(\text{day} \times \text{L})}{32 \text{ mg/L}}$$

$$= 438 \text{ mg/day}$$

Note how units cancel out to yield mg/day.

Calculating Steady-State Concentration from This K_m and Dose

If we wish to predict the steady-state plasma concentration that would result if the dose is increased to 500 mg/day, we can rearrange the Michaelis–Menten equation and solve for C:

10-3
$$C = \frac{K_m(\text{daily dose})}{V_{max} - \text{daily dose}}$$

$$= \frac{12 \text{ mg/L } (500 \text{ mg/day})}{700 \text{ mg/day} - 500 \text{ mg/day}}$$

$$= \frac{12 \text{ mg/L } (500 \text{ mg/day})}{200 \text{ mg/day}}$$

$$= 30 \text{ mg/L}$$

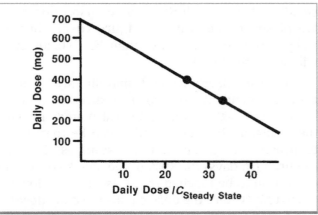

FIGURE 10-6.
Plot of patient data using two steady-state plasma phenytoin concentrations at two dose levels.

See Lesson 15 for examples of how these calculations are applied.

Clinical Correlate

When performing this calculation using sodium phenytoin or fosphenytoin, be sure to convert doses to their phenytoin free-acid equivalent before substituting these values into the equation. To convert, multiply the daily dose by 0.92 (92% free phenytoin). Fosphenytoin injection, although containing only 66% phenytoin free acid, is actually labeled in phenytoin sodium equivalents such that the 0.92 factor also applies to this product when drug dose is expressed as phenytoin equivalents.

The preceding example demonstrates how plasma drug concentrations and drug dose can be predicted. However, it also shows that for drugs like phenytoin, with saturable elimination, when plasma concentrations are above K_m, small dose increases can result in large increases in the steady-state plasma concentration.

When clearance changes with plasma concentration, there is no true half-life as with first-order elimination. As clearance changes, the elimination rate changes as does the time to reach steady state. With high doses and high plasma concentrations (and resulting lower clearance), the time to reach steady state is much longer than with low doses and low plasma concentrations (**Figure 10-7**). Theoretically, if the dose is greater than V_{max}, steady state will never be reached.

Because clearance and half-life are concentration-dependent factors, a traditional time to steady-state value cannot be calculated. Instead, the Michaelis–Menten equation can be rearranged to provide an equation that estimates the time required (in days) for 90% of the steady-state concentration to be reached ($t_{90\%}$), as shown below for phenytoin (where the dose equals the daily dose):

10-4 $\quad t_{90\%} = \dfrac{K_m(V)}{(V_{max} - \text{daily dose})^2}[2.3V_{max} - 0.9 \text{ dose}]$

From the previous example, when dose = 300 mg/day, V_{max} = 700 mg/day, and K_m = 12 mg/L, volume of distribution (V) can be estimated as 0.65 L/kg body weight, or (0.65 × 77 kg body weight) = 50 L.

$$t_{90\%} = \frac{12 \text{ mg/L } (50 \text{ L})}{(700 \text{ mg/day} - 300 \text{ mg/day})^2}[2.3(700 \text{ mg/day}) - 0.9(300 \text{ mg/day})]$$

$$= \frac{600 \text{ mg}}{(400 \text{ mg/day})^2}[1610 \text{ mg/day} - 270 \text{ mg/day}]$$

$$= (0.00375 \text{ day}^2/\text{mg})(1340 \text{ mg/day})$$

$$= 5.0 \text{ days}$$

When the dose is increased to 400 mg/day:

$$t_{90\%} = \frac{12 \text{ mg/L } (50 \text{ L})}{(700 \text{ mg/day} - 400 \text{ mg/day})^2}[2.3(700 \text{ mg/day}) - 0.9(400 \text{ mg/day})]$$

$$= \frac{600 \text{ mg}}{(300 \text{ mg/day})^2}[1610 \text{ mg/day} - 360 \text{ mg/day}]$$

$$= (0.0067 \text{ day}^2/\text{mg})(1250 \text{ mg/day})$$

$$= 8.38 \text{ days}$$

We can see that as the dose is increased, it takes a longer time to reach steady state, drug continues to accumulate, and the plasma drug concentration continues to rise. When this occurs with a drug such as phenytoin, toxic effects (e.g., ataxia and nystagmus) probably will be observed if the high dosage is given on a regular basis.

Clinical Correlate

The $t_{90\%}$ equation will provide only a rough estimate of when 90% of steady state has been reached, and its accuracy is dependent on the K_m value used. Other ways to check to see if a patient is at steady state are to examine two levels drawn approximately a week apart. If these levels are ±10% of each other, then you can assume steady state. Additionally, it is safe to wait at least 2 weeks (and preferably 4 weeks) after beginning or changing a dose before obtaining new steady-state levels.

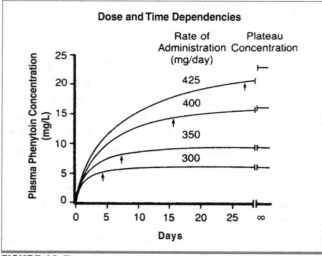

FIGURE 10-7.
Time to reach $t_{90\%}$ (represented by arrows) at different daily dosages.

REVIEW QUESTIONS

10-1. Which drug pairs demonstrate nonlinear pharmacokinetics?

   A. Theophylline and methotrexate
   B. Carbamazepine and phenytoin
   C. Acetaminophen and sulfonamides
   D. A and B

10-2. Nonlinear pharmacokinetics means that the plot of plasma drug concentration versus time after a dose is a straight line.

   A. True
   B. False

10-3. When hepatic metabolism becomes saturated, any increase in drug dose will lead to a disproportionate increase in the plasma concentration achieved.

   A. True
   B. False

10-4. When the rate of drug elimination proceeds at half the maximum rate, the drug concentration is known as _____.

   A. V_{max}
   B. K_m
   C. $\frac{1}{2}V_{max}$
   D. $(V_{max})(C)$

10-5. At very high concentrations—concentrations much higher than the drug's K_m—drugs are more likely to approach zero-order elimination.

   A. True
   B. False

10-6. Which of the equations below describes the form of the Michaelis–Menten equation that relates daily drug dose to V_{max}, K_m, and the steady-state plasma drug concentration?

   A. Daily dose = $-K_m$(daily dose/C)(V_{max})
   B. Daily dose = $-K_m$(daily dose/C) + V_{max}
   C. Daily dose = $-K_m$(daily dose × C) + V_{max}
   D. Daily dose = $-K_m$ – (daily dose/C) + V_{max}

The following information is for **Questions 10-7 to 10-11.** A patient, JH, is administered phenytoin free acid, 300 mg/day for 2 months (assume steady state is achieved), and a plasma concentration determined just before a dose is 10 mg/L. The phenytoin dose is then changed to 400 mg/day; 2 months after the dose change, the plasma concentration determined just before a dose is 18 mg/L. Assume that the volume of distribution of phenytoin is 45 L.

10-7. Calculate K_m for this patient.

   A. 12.9 mg/L
   B. 25 mg/L
   C. 37.5 mg/L
   D. 10 mg/L

10-8. For the same patient, JH, determine V_{max}.

   A. 123 mg/day
   B. 900 mg/day
   C. 500 mg/day
   D. 687 mg/day

10-9. For the case of JH above, plot both concentrations on a daily dose/C versus V_{max} plot and then determine this patient's V_{max}.

   A. Approximately 550 mg/day
   B. Approximately 400 mg/day
   C. Approximately 675 mg/day
   D. Approximately 800 mg/day

10-10. After the dose of 400 mg/day is begun, how long will it take to reach 90% of the steady-state plasma concentration?

   A. Approximately 14 days
   B. Approximately 9 days
   C. Approximately 30 days
   D. Approximately 90 days

10-11. If the patient, JH, misunderstood the dosage instructions and consumed 500 mg/day of phenytoin, what steady-state plasma concentration would result?

A. 29.4 mg/L

B. 34.5 mg/L

C. 27.2 mg/L

D. 19.6 mg/L

ANSWERS

10-1. D. CORRECT ANSWER (Both A, B agents demonstrate nonlinear pharmacokinetics)

A,B,C. *Incorrect answers*

10-2. A. *Incorrect answer*

B. CORRECT ANSWER. *Linear pharmacokinetics* means that the AUC and plasma concentrations achieved are directly related to the size of the dose administered. Drugs with linear pharmacokinetics may exhibit plasma concentrations versus time plots that are not straight lines, as with multicompartment drugs.

10-3. A. CORRECT ANSWER. There will be a disproportionate increase in the plasma concentration achieved because the amount of drug that can be eliminated over time cannot increase.

B. *Incorrect answer*

10-4. A. *Incorrect answer.* V_{max} is the maximum rate of hepatic metabolism.

B. CORRECT ANSWER

C. *Incorrect answer.* $\frac{1}{2}V_{max}$ is only one-half of the maximum hepatic metabolism and does not relate K_m to V_{max}.

D. *Incorrect answer.* $(V_{max})(C)$ is only the numerator of the Michaelis–Menten equation.

10-5. A. CORRECT ANSWER. At very low concentrations, drugs are more likely to exhibit first-order kinetics because hepatic enzymes are usually not yet saturated, whereas at higher concentrations, enzymes saturate, moving clearance toward zero-order kinetics.

B. *Incorrect answer.*

10-6. A, C, D. *Incorrect answers*

B. CORRECT ANSWER

10-7. A. CORRECT ANSWER. The K_m is calculated from the slope of the line above:

$$\text{slope} = -K_m = \frac{\text{dose}_1 - \text{dose}_2}{\text{dose}_1/C_1 - \text{dose}_2/C_2}$$

$$= \frac{300 \text{ mg/day} - 400 \text{ mg/day}}{\left(\dfrac{300 \text{ mg/day}}{10 \text{ mg/L}} - \dfrac{400 \text{ mg/day}}{18 \text{ mg/L}}\right)}$$

$$= \frac{-100 \text{ mg/day}}{30 \text{ L/day} - 22.22 \text{ L/day}}$$

$$= \frac{-100 \text{ mg/day}}{7.78 \text{ L/day}}$$

$$= -12.9 \text{ mg/L}$$

So K_m equals 12.9 mg/L.

B, C, D. *Incorrect answers.* Use dose pairs of 300 and 400 and concentration pairs of 10 and 18 to calculate K_m.

10-8. A, C. *Incorrect answers.* Try again; you probably made a math error.

B. *Incorrect answer.* Try again, and use either set of dose and concentration pairs (i.e., 300 and 10 or 400 and 18).

D. CORRECT ANSWER.

$$\text{Daily dose} = -K_m(\text{daily dose}/C) + V_{max}$$

$$400 = (-12.9 \text{ mg/L})\left(\frac{400 \text{ mg/day}}{18 \text{ mg/L}}\right) + V_{max}$$

$$400 = (-12.9 \text{ mg/L})(22.22 \text{ L/day}) + V_{max}$$

$$400 = -277.75 \text{ mg/day} + V_{max}$$

$$686.64 = V_{max}$$

10-9. A, B, D. *Incorrect answers*

C. CORRECT ANSWER. See the figure at the bottom of the page for an example plot of the daily dose versus daily dose/C.

10-10. A, C, D. *Incorrect answers*

B. CORRECT ANSWER. The time to reach steady state is calculated by:

$$t_{90\%} = \frac{K_m(V)}{(V_{max} - \text{dose})^2}\left[2.3V_{max} - 0.9\,\text{dose}\right]$$

$$= \frac{12.9\text{ mg/L }(45\text{ L})}{(687\text{ mg/day} - 400\text{ mg/day})^2}[2.3(678\text{ mg/day}) - 0.9(400\text{ mg/day})]$$

$$= \frac{580.5\text{ mg}}{278\text{ mg/day}}[1559\text{ mg/day} - 360\text{ mg/day}]$$

$$= (0.00705\text{ day}^2/\text{mg})(1199\text{ mg/day})$$

$$= 8.5\text{ days}$$

10-11. A. *Incorrect answer.* Perhaps you used a 400-mg dose instead of a 500-mg dose.

B. CORRECT ANSWER. The steady-state plasma concentration resulting from a daily dose of 500 mg would be estimated from the line equation as follows:

$$\text{Daily dose} = -K_m(\text{dose}/C) + V_{max}$$

$$500\text{ mg/day} = -12.9\text{ mg/L}\left(\frac{500\text{ mg/day}}{C}\right) + 687\text{ mg/day}$$

Rearranging gives:

$$\frac{-187\text{ mg/day}}{-12.9\text{ mg/L}} = \frac{500\text{ mg/day}}{C}$$

$$14.5\text{ L/day} = \frac{500\text{ mg/day}}{C}$$

$$\frac{14.5\text{ L/day}}{500\text{ mg/day}} = \frac{1}{C}$$

$$0.029\text{ L/mg} = \frac{1}{C}$$

$$C = 34.5\text{ mg/L}$$

C, D. *Incorrect answers.* You may have made a simple math error.

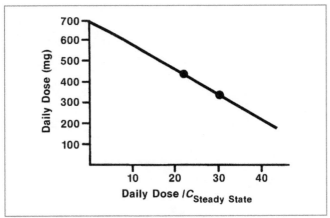

Daily dose versus daily dose divided by steady-state concentration.

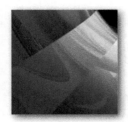 Discussion Points

D-1. When using the Michaelis–Menten equation, examine what happens when daily dose is much lower than V_{max}, and when it exceeds V_{max}.

D-2. When using the $t_{90\%}$ equation, examine what happens to $t_{90\%}$ when dose greatly exceeds V_{max}.

D-3. Using two steady-state plasma drug concentrations and two doses to solve for a new K_m, V_{max}, and dose using the Michaelis–Menten equation, examine the values of K_m and V_{max} obtained using this process. Are these values close to the actual patient population parameters?

D-4. Discuss several practical methods to determine when a nonlinear drug has reached steady state.

D-5. Examine the time to 90% equation and note the value of K_m that is used in this equation. Substitute several different phenytoin K_m values based on a range of population values (i.e., from approximately 1 to 15 mg/L) and describe the effect this has on your answer. Based on this observation, what value of K_m would you use when trying to approximate the $t_{90\%}$ for a newly begun dose of phenytoin?

D-6. Discuss the patient variables that can affect the pharmacokinetic calculation of a nonlinear drug when using two plasma drug concentrations obtained from two different doses.

D-7. Examine the package insert for Cerebyx® (fosphenytoin) and answer the following questions:

A. What salt is this product?

B. What percent phenytoin sodium is it?

C. What percent phenytoin free acid is it?

D. How many milligrams of Cerebyx® is equivalent to 100 mg of sodium phenytoin injection?

E. What therapeutic advantage does this product offer?

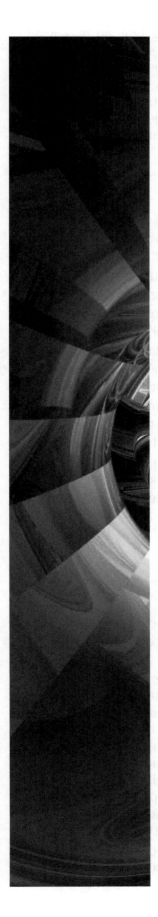

Pharmacokinetic Variation and Model-Independent Relationships

OBJECTIVES

After completing Lesson 11, you should be able to:

1. Identify the various sources of pharmacokinetic variation.

2. Explain how the various sources of pharmacokinetic variation affect pharmacokinetic parameters.

3. Describe how to apply pharmacokinetic variation in a clinical setting.

4. Name the potential sources of error in the collection and assay of drug samples.

5. Explain the clinical importance of correct sample collection, storage, and assay.

6. Describe ways to avoid or minimize errors in the collection and assay of drug samples.

7. Explain the basic concepts and calculations of the model-independent pharmacokinetic parameters of total body clearance, mean residence time (MRT), volume of distribution at steady state, and formation clearance.

Sources of Pharmacokinetic Variation

An important reason for pharmacokinetic drug monitoring is that a drug's effect may vary considerably among individuals given the same dose. These differences in drug effect are sometimes related to differences in pharmacokinetics. Some factors that may affect drug pharmacokinetics are discussed below. However, irrespective of pharmacokinetics, drug effects may vary among individuals because of differences in drug sensitivity.

Age

At extremes of age, major organ functions may be considerably reduced compared with those of healthy young adults. In neonates (particularly if premature) and the elderly, renal function and the capacity for renal drug excretion may be greatly reduced. Neonates and the elderly are also more likely to have reduced hepatic function. Renal function declines at a rate of approximately 1 mL/min/yr after the age of 40 years. In the neonate, renal function rapidly progresses in infancy to equal or exceed that of adults. Pediatric patients may have an increased rate of clearance because a child's drug metabolism rate is increased compared to adults. When dosing a drug for a child, the drug may need to be administered more frequently.

Other changes also occur with aging. Compared with adults, the neonate has a higher proportion of body mass made up of water and a lower proportion of body fat. The elderly are likely to have a lower proportion of body water and lean tissue (**Figure 11-1**). Both of these changes—organ function and body makeup—affect the disposition of drugs and how they are used. Reduced function of the organs of drug elimination generally requires that doses of drugs eliminated by the affected organ be given less frequently. With alterations in body water or fat content, the dose of drugs that distribute into those tissues must be altered. For drugs that distribute into body water, the neonatal dose may be larger per kilogram of body weight than in an adult.

Disease States

Drug disposition is altered in many disease states, but the most common examples involve the kidneys and liver, as they are the major organs of drug elimination. In patients with major organ dysfunction, drug clearance decreases and, subsequently, drug half-life lengthens. Some diseases, such as renal failure or cirrhosis, may even result in fluid retention and an increased volume of drug distribution.

Alterations in drug clearance and volume of distribution require adjustments in the dose administered and/or the dosing interval. For most drugs, when clearance is decreased but the volume of distribution is relatively unchanged, the dose administered may be similar to that in a healthy person although the dosing interval may need to be increased. Alternatively, smaller doses could be administered over a shorter dosing interval. When the volume of distribution is altered, the dosing interval can often remain the same but the dose administered should change in proportion to the change in volume of distribution.

Clinical Correlate

When adjusting a dose of a drug that follows first-order elimination, if you do not change the dosing interval, then the new dose can be calculated using various simple ratio and proportion techniques. For example, if gentamicin peak and trough serum drug concentrations (in a patient receiving 120 mg every 12 hours) were 9 and 2.3 mcg/mL, respectively, then a new dose can be calculated: "if 120 mg gives a peak of 9, then X mg will give a desired peak of 6," yielding an answer of 80 mg every 12 hours. Likewise, one can check to see if this trough would be acceptable with this new dose: "if 120 mg gives a trough of 2.3, then 80 mg will give a trough of X," yielding an answer of 1.5 mcg/mL.

EXAMPLE

Effect of Volume of Distribution and Impaired Renal/Hepatic Function on Drug Dose

A 23-year-old male experienced a major traumatic injury from a motor vehicle accident. On the third day after injury, his renal function is determined to be good (creatinine clearance = 120 mL/min), and his weight has increased from 63 kg on admission to 83 kg. Note that fluid accumulation (as evidenced by weight gain) is an expected result of traumatic injury. He is treated with gentamicin for gram-negative bacteremia.

An initial gentamicin dose of 100 mg is given over 1 hour, and a peak concentration

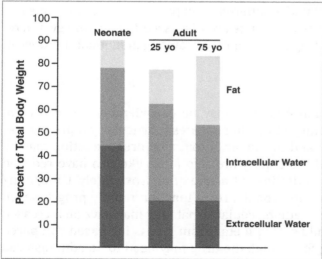

FIGURE 11-1.
Effect of age on body composition.

of 2.5 mg/L is determined. Four hours after the peak, the plasma concentration is determined to be 0.6 mg/L, and the elimination rate constant and the volume of distribution are determined to be 0.36 hr^{-1} and 33.6 L, respectively. This volume of 33.6 L equals 0.40 L/kg compared to a typical V of 0.2–0.3 L/kg. In this case, the patient's gentamicin elimination rate constant is similar to that found in people with normal renal function, but the volume of distribution is much greater. To maintain a peak plasma gentamicin concentration of 6–8 mg/L, a much larger dose would have to be administered at a dosing interval of 6 or 8 hours. Using the multiple-dose infusion equation from Lesson 5 (see **Equation 5-1**), we would find that a dose as high as 220 mg given every 6 hours would be necessary to achieve the desired plasma concentrations.

On the other hand, we would expect patients with impaired renal function to have a lower creatinine clearance and, therefore, a smaller elimination rate constant compared to patients with normal renal function. A smaller than normal elimination rate constant would produce a longer half-life and would require an increase in the dosage interval. In patients with both impaired renal function and abnormal volume of distribution values, the dose and dosing interval should be adjusted accordingly.

Just as renal dysfunction may alter the dosage requirement for drugs eliminated renally, hepatic dysfunction alters the dosage requirement for hepatically metabolized or excreted drugs. For example, the daily dose of theophylline must be reduced in patients with liver dysfunction. With this agent, however, a consistent plasma concentration (as opposed to a large difference in peak and trough plasma concentrations) is desired. Therefore, with liver dysfunction, smaller doses of theophylline than usual are generally administered but at the usual dosage intervals (two to four times daily). For a continuous intravenous (IV) infusion, the infusion rate must be reduced.

Genetic Factors, Pharmacogenetics, and Pharmacogenomics

Interpatient variability in drug response may result from genetically determined differences in metabolism, distribution, and target proteins of drugs. Pharmacogenetics is the study of genetic variations that lead to interpatient variations in drug response. This concept is often used interchangeably with pharmacogenomics. In the strictest sense, pharmacogenetics refers to monogenetic variants in drug response while pharmacogenomics refers to the entire spectrum of genes that interacts to determine drug safety and efficacy. The goals of these two areas of study are to optimize drug therapy and limit drug toxicity based on an individual's genetic profile. Information gained from studies in these areas will enable clinicians to use genetic tests to select a drug, drug dose, and treatment duration that will have the greatest likelihood for achieving therapeutic outcomes with the least potential for adverse effects in a given patient based on DNA profiles. Much work has already been done in the area of cancer treatment, and information is emerging in the areas of cardiology, neurology, and infectious diseases.

Genetic variations commonly occur either as rare defects or polymorphisms. Rare mutations occur in less than 1% of the population while polymorphisms occur in at least 1% of humans. To date, polymorphisms in drug-metabolizing enzymes are the most documented examples of genetic variants that result in altered drug response and toxicity. We will briefly discuss two examples of polymorphic metabolizing enzymes and corresponding drugs whose plasma concentrations and pharmacologic effect may be altered as a result of genetic variation: CYP2C9 and warfarin, and CYP2C19 and clopidogrel.

CYP2C9 is a polymorphic isoenzyme that metabolizes warfarin, phenytoin, and tolbutamide. The S-isomer of warfarin is metabolized by this isoenzyme, and genetic alterations can result in significant reductions in clearance necessitating substantial dose reductions. On the other hand, ultrarapid metabolizers of CYP2C9 require higher doses of warfarin.

Another factor to consider with warfarin metabolism is its target enzyme vitamin K oxidoreductase or VKOR. Warfarin inhibits VKOR, thereby preventing carboxylation of vitamin K–dependent clotting factors II, VII, IX, and X. Genetic alterations in VKOR can result in rare cases of warfarin resistance in which carriers of these mutations require extremely high warfarin doses, or actually may cause a lack of response to warfarin at any dose. Specifically, the VKORC1 genotype in combination with CYP2C9 genotype explains approximately 30% of the interpatient variability in warfarin doses commonly encountered in clinical practice.

Patients who are intermediate metabolizers or poor metabolizers of CYP2C19 may experience a reduced response to clopidogrel and potentially require higher doses or alternative antiplatelet therapy for adequate clinical outcomes. The reason is that clopidogrel is a prodrug that must undergo conversion via CYP2C19 to its active form.

There are many other examples of differences in response to drugs and adverse drug reactions due to variation in a patient's genetic sequence. These sequence variations can affect enzymes responsible for drug metabolism, drug targets, and drug transporters, all of which will lead to deviation in absorption, distribution, metabolism, and elimination. With isoniazid, for example, there are two distinct subsets of the population with differences in isoniazid elimination (**Figure 11-2**). The elimination of isoniazid is said to exhibit a bimodal pattern. This difference in clearance is caused by genetically controlled differences in hepatic microsomal enzyme production. Likewise, genetic differences in drug elimination also have been observed for hydralazine, warfarin, and phenylbutazone. Polymorphism has been observed in some patients associated with decreased expression of P-glycoprotein (a drug transporter in the duodenum). In these patients, the bioavailability of P-glycoprotein substrates, such as digoxin, is greatly increased; therefore, a decrease in dose may be required.[1]

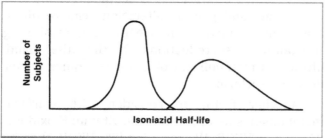

FIGURE 11-2.
Bimodal distribution for isoniazid half-life.

Many variants have also been observed in the cytochrome P450 enzyme system. These variations can cause different responses to drugs metabolized by the CYP450 enzyme system. For example, poor CYP2D6 metabolizers have been found to have elevated plasma concentrations, and poor CYP2C19 metabolizers were found to have an increased incidence of fluoxetine adverse effects.[2]

Pharmacogenomic research is still in progress. Many sequence variations have currently been observed, but there are countless polymorphisms left to be discovered. Currently, more than 100 drugs contain references (e.g., abacavir, carbamazepine, tramadol, and warfarin) to pharmacogenetic information in their approved labeling, and guidelines for the use of genetic information in drug prescribing are beginning to emerge, including those from the Clinical Pharmacogenetics Implementation Consortium. These guidelines are available through the Pharmacogenomics Knowledge Base website (www.PharmGKB.org).

Obesity

Obesity alters drug pharmacokinetics. Because obesity is common in our society, it is an important source of pharmacokinetic variation. With obesity, the ratio of body fat to lean tissue is greater than in nonobese patients. Fat tissue contains less water than lean tissue, so the amount of body water per kilogram of total body weight is less in the obese person than in the nonobese person.

For some drugs, alterations in body makeup that accompany obesity require changes in drug dosages. Drugs that are lipophilic (such as thiopental) and distribute well into fat tissues must often be given in larger doses to achieve the desired effects. Drugs that distribute primarily in extracellular fluids (such as the aminoglycosides) may be given in higher absolute doses to the obese person, but the overall milligram per kilogram dose will be lower. The morbidly obese person who is twice ideal body weight will have an aminoglycoside volume of distribution that is approximately 1.4 times greater than a person of ideal body weight.[3]

Other Factors

Many other factors may affect drug pharmacokinetics, including pregnancy and drug interactions. Specific changes in pharmacokinetics during pregnancy include increased renal drug clearance, alterations in volume of distribution, and changes in plasma protein binding. Another example of an effect on pharmacokinetics is the histamine-2 blocker, cimetidine, which inhibits the hepatic enzymes that metabolize theophylline, thereby decreasing theophylline clearance. When evaluating drug pharmacokinetics in an individual patient, the clinician must consider the many factors that may cause variations from the expected results.

Potential Sources of Error in the Collection and Assay of Biologic Samples

Pharmacokinetic calculations depend greatly on the validity of the reported drug concentration from a biologic sample (e.g., blood, serum, or plasma). Using incorrect concentration values to calculate dosages can result in subtherapeutic or supratherapeutic (i.e., toxic) drug concentrations. Inaccurate concentration values can result from incorrect drug sampling or assay procedures. To ensure that drug concentrations are valid, several factors should be considered:

- Proper laboratory sample collection and handling

- Physiochemical factors affecting assay accuracy

- Proper laboratory instrument calibration and controls check

- Proper drug administration and sample timing

Sample Collection and Handling

To measure drug concentrations, whole blood is usually collected in a blood collection tube called a *serum separator tube* (SST). The SST contains a gel barrier that separates the fluid portion of blood from the solid portion (**Figure 11-3**). After collection, the blood is first allowed to clot, which takes approximately 30 minutes, and is then centrifuged for at least 15 minutes to separate the solid components of the blood (blood cells, fibrin, fibrinogen, etc.) from the fluid component. This fluid component is called *serum*. If whole blood is centrifuged before it clots, then only the blood cells are separated from the fluid component, which is called *plasma*.

Most assays of therapeutically monitored drugs are performed on serum, hence the term *serum drug*

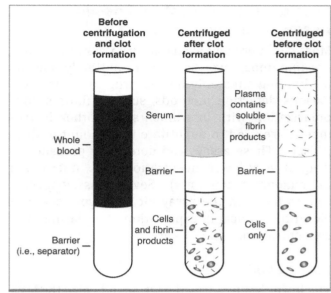

FIGURE 11-3.
Blood products.

concentration. However, the operations manual for specific assay instruments often indicate whether a particular drug may be tested using plasma or serum. Most instruments allow the use of either serum or plasma. The assay should be performed within 24 hours of sample collection. If this is not possible, refrigerate the sample (at 2–6°C) until the assay can be performed.

If plastic or glass SSTs are used, it is important to ensure that the drug to be assayed is not affected (i.e., absorbed or adsorbed) by the polymeric gel barrier used to separate the plasma from the cells. The composition of this barrier depends on the brand of SST used. The barriers are usually made of acrylic, silicon, or polyester polymers, and although they are generally chemically inert, they can absorb or adsorb the drug being tested.

The degree of absorption or adsorption depends on the hydrophilicity of the drug, the type of barrier used in the SST, the amount of contact time, and the volume of the plasma sample. For example, decreases ranging from 6% to 64% were reported in measured concentrations of phenytoin, phenobarbital, lidocaine, quinidine, and carbamazepine when plasma was stored in Vacutainer SST collection tubes.[4] Adsorption or absorption of drug by the SST barrier is of particular concern when small sample volumes are used (e.g., in pediatric patients) or prolonged storage times are required.

Physicochemical Factors Affecting Assay Accuracy

Most commercially available drug assay methods are immunoassays that use an antibody specific for binding sites only on the drug to be assayed. Various detection methods, such as fluorescence polarization with instruments and other instruments, are used to quantitate the amount of drug present. These assays can detect the presence of drug at very low concentrations (i.e., microgram or nanogram amounts). Several assay-specific factors listed in the assay kit package insert can aid in the clinical interpretation of a plasma drug concentration.

Lower Limit of Drug Detection

The lower limit of drug detection indicates the lowest drug concentration that the assay can reliably report. This is a function of the particular assay instrument and is called *assay sensitivity*, which is the lowest measurable drug concentration that can be distinguished from zero with 95% confidence. Plasma drug concentrations lower than this concentration should be reported as less than this value.

Clinical Correlate

Use caution when interpreting a serum drug concentration reported as <X (e.g., <0.5 mg/L). This is not the same value as X, but instead means that the sample has no detectable drug concentration above the assay's lower limit of sensitivity. Consequently, this value could be 0, and it could have been 0 for many hours. One cannot reliably use this value to calculate patient-specific *K* values.

Upper Limit of Drug Detection

The upper limit of drug detection indicates the highest drug concentration that can be accurately measured. Plasma drug concentrations above the upper limit will often be reported as higher than this value. If this occurs, assay parameters can be adjusted to increase the dilution volume of the plasma sample, thus allowing higher drug concentrations to be measured.

Assay Interference

Assay interferences are generally categorized as cross-reactivity and physiologic interferences. The degree of cross-reactivity with other structurally similar compounds is called *assay specificity*. Cross-reactivity is a function of the specificity of the antibody used to bind to the drug. Often, this antibody will also at least partially bind to other compounds that are structurally related to the desired analyte, such as metabolites and chemical analogues of the analyte.

For example, gentamicin assays cross-react with the seldom-used aminoglycoside netilmicin, and amikacin assays cross-react with kanamycin; however, gentamicin and tobramycin assays do not generally cross-react. In addition, patients with impaired renal function who are receiving vancomycin have been shown to accumulate a vancomycin metabolite called *vancomycin crystalline degradation product 1* (CDP-1). CDP-1 can cross-react with older assays for vancomycin; however, many newer assay methodologies have reduced this assay interference to an acceptable amount. Clinicians must still be aware of this potential for cross-reactivity. Physiologic substances in the patient's sample may also interfere with the assay. Examples include excess amounts of bilirubin, hemoglobin (i.e., hemolyzed sample), protein, and triglycerides. Plasma drug concentrations are usually not affected by such interferences.

Clinical Correlate

Ask your laboratory's clinical chemistry department for copies of the assay kit package inserts for all drugs that they assay in-house. These inserts will provide useful information, such as the upper and lower limits of assay sensitivity, as well as interfering and cross-reacting substances.

Instrument Calibration and Controls Check

Each drug assay should be calibrated to establish a linear relationship between drug concentration and the instrument's detection method. Calibration of the assay is an automatic process of measuring and plotting different known drug concentrations (i.e., calibrators) based on the instrument's method of detection and measurement. Most assay instruments use some type of spectrophotometric measurement unit, such as fluorescence polarization. **Figure 11-4** is a plot of drug concentration versus the instrument's detection measure (polarization), showing the linear relationship between concentration and polarization. Note that the calibration curve is not linear at very high and very low drug concentrations.

Once this calibration plot or curve is stored in the instrument's software, other unknown drug concentrations (i.e., patient samples) can be accurately determined from this plot. As a quality control check, at least two different known concentrations (control values) should be tested for each drug assay per working shift. If these control values are out of range, as defined per individual laboratory standards, then this assay should be recalibrated and measurement of the patient's plasma drug concentration repeated.

Drug Administration and Sample Timing

To accurately assess drug concentration data and make dosing recommendations, it is important to be aware of administration and sampling factors that may affect the reported drug concentrations. First, drug administration times should be documented, noting any deviations from the recommended dosing schedule. Second, sampling times should be carefully noted so that adjustments can be made in dosage calculations if necessary. Third, it is important to note any other medications the patient is receiving. Occasionally, a patient's sample will contain two drugs, one of which can inactivate the other, particularly if both drugs are infused concomitantly, the sample is taken while the interfering drug is infusing, or a sample containing both drugs is stored at room temperature for a prolonged period.

A good example is the in vitro inactivation of the aminoglycosides by penicillins. Cephalosporins have not been shown to inactivate aminoglycosides.[5] Penicillins and aminoglycosides form a chemical complex that is not detected by commercially available drug assays.[6] This in vitro inactivation results in a falsely low plasma drug concentration report, which can in turn result in an unnecessary dosage increase. Quantitatively, the aminoglycoside concentration can decline to less than 10% of its original concentration within 24 hours of the beginning of this reaction. These reactions are time and temperature dependent. Refrigerating the sample slows the inactivation process, and freezing the sample stops it completely. To avoid the inactivation process, it is important to adjust the administration times to avoid concomitant infusions of aminoglycosides and penicillins. Drawing a plasma aminoglycoside concentration during infusion of the penicillin should be avoided as well.

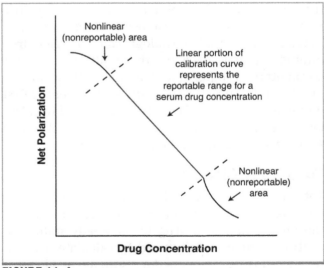

FIGURE 11-4.
Drug concentration versus net polarization.

Clinical Correlate

When assaying the concentration of an aminoglycoside from a patient who is concomitantly receiving a penicillin, the laboratory must perform the assay immediately or freeze the sample. Freezing the sample instantly stops the in vitro inactivation of the aminoglycoside by the penicillin, whereas refrigerating the sample only slows down this degradation reaction. If the assay is not performed immediately, the aminoglycoside concentration from the assay will be lower than the patient's actual serum aminoglycoside concentration.

Model-Independent Relationships

Until now, we have used a major assumption in constructing models for drug pharmacokinetics: that drug clearance remains constant with any size dose. Drug clearance remains constant for small or large doses when drug elimination processes are first order (as described in previous lessons). With a first-order elimination process, as the dose of drug increases, the plasma concentrations observed and the area under the plasma drug concentration versus time curve (AUC) increase proportionally. That is, if the dose is doubled, the plasma concentration and AUC also double.

Throughout this self-instructional course, we have emphasized the mathematical relationships of specific pharmacokinetic compartmental models (e.g., one- or two-compartment model after an IV bolus or oral dose administration). This lesson reviews several pharmacokinetic parameters that are derived without the assumption of a specific model.

The primary purpose of rigorous pharmacokinetic data analysis, compartmental or model-independent, is to determine the pharmacokinetic parameters useful in dosing drugs for patients. Consequently, multiple plasma drug concentrations are obtained at specific time points in healthy and diseased persons to assess a drug's population pharmacokinetic parameters. In clinical practice, it may be difficult to obtain multiple plasma samples after the first dose to determine a patient's pharmacokinetic parameters. Consequently, clinicians use population parameters from the literature to make individual patient dosage calculations.

Model-independent pharmacokinetic data analysis provides the opportunity to obtain pharmacokinetic values that do not depend on a compartmental model. Total body clearance, mean residence time (MRT), volume of distribution at steady state, and formation clearance are four of the most frequently used model-independent parameters and are the focus of this section.

The use of model-independent data analysis techniques to generate model-independent parameters offers several advantages over traditional compartmental approaches. First, it is not necessary to assume a compartmental model. Many drugs possess complex distribution patterns requiring two, three, or more exponential terms to describe their elimination. As the number of exponential terms increases, a compartmental analysis requires more intensive blood sampling and rigorous data calculations. Second, several drugs (e.g., gentamicin) can be described by one, two, or more distribution compartments, depending on the characteristics of the patients evaluated or the aggressiveness of the blood sampling. Therefore, a compartmental approach would require that pharmacokinetic parameters be obtained for each distribution pattern, making it difficult to compare one data set to another. Third, calculations are generally easier with model-independent relationships and do not require a computer with sophisticated software.

One drawback of using model-independent parameters is the inability to visualize or predict plasma concentration versus time profiles. This may result in the loss of specific information that provides important insight regarding drug disposition.

Like compartmental pharmacokinetic data analysis, the main purpose of assessing plasma concentration versus time data with model-independent relationships is to determine useful pharmacokinetic parameters. These parameters are usually, but not always, obtained from serial plasma concentration determinations after a single IV bolus or oral dose of a drug.

In practice, total body clearance and apparent volume of distribution are the two most important pharmacokinetic parameters because they facilitate the calculation of maintenance and loading dose regimens, respectively. Understanding the effect that disease, altered physiologic state, or drug–drug interaction may have on these pharmacokinetic parameters is important in applying these principles to clinical practice. AUC and area under the first moment curve (AUMC) are two tools used to calculate most model-independent parameters. AUC and AUMC are discussed in the next section.

Total Body Clearance

Total body clearance (Cl_t) is the most important pharmacokinetic parameter because it relates the dosing rate of a drug to its steady-state concentration. It is usually used to calculate a maintenance-dosing regimen. An estimate of Cl_t for a drug is usually obtained after a single IV bolus dose (**Figure 11-5**).

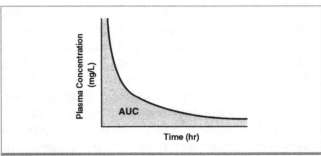

FIGURE 11-5.
Concentration versus time profile after a single intravenous dose. AUC = area under the plasma drug concentration versus time curve.

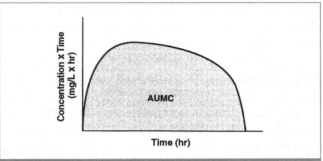

FIGURE 11-6.
Concentration × time versus time curve. AUMC = area under the first moment curve.

Total body clearance is calculated with the following equation:

$$Cl_t = \frac{X_0}{AUC_{0 \to \infty}}$$

(See **Equation 3-5**.)

where:

X_0 = drug dose

$AUC_{0 \to \infty}$ = area under the concentration versus time curve from time zero to infinity

This is a model-independent relationship because calculations do not depend on a specific compartmental model. In other words, we only need the dose and the $AUC_{0 \to \infty}$ to calculate total body clearance. Because the dose is known, a determination of the $AUC_{0 \to \infty}$ is all that is needed.

As you can see from **Figures 11-6** and **11-7**, the trapezoidal rule applies only to drugs whose clearance is constant with respect to dose (linear) and does not apply to drugs whose clearance is nonlinear. Remember, the trapezoidal rule is a model-independent approach used to directly calculate the AUC of the drug from time zero to the time point that coincides with the last measured plasma concentration value (t_{last}). However, because AUC must include all of the area from zero to infinity after a single IV bolus dose, an estimate of the area between t_{last} and infinity is needed.

This terminal area can be easily obtained by the following equation:

$$\text{Terminal area} = \frac{C_{last}}{\lambda}$$

where:

C_{last} = last measured plasma concentration

λ = terminal elimination rate constant

Two key assumptions in estimating this terminal AUC are that you have a reliable estimate of the terminal elimination rate constant (i.e., slope) and that this value remains constant between t_{last} and infinity. To determine several model-independent relationships, such as MRT and volume of distribution at steady state, it is important to understand how to calculate the AUMC. The AUMC is the area under the drug concentration versus time versus time curve. The AUMC is generated with the AUC data from the concentration versus time profile for a single IV bolus dose (see Figure 11-5). To calculate AUMC after a single IV bolus dose of a drug, it is necessary to collect serial drug plasma concentrations

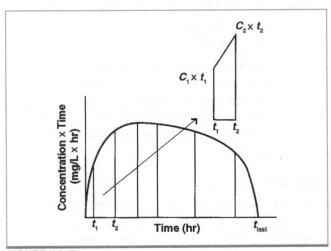

FIGURE 11-7.
Concentration × time versus time curve with trapezoids.

over time, determine concentration × time for each plasma concentration, and plot these values versus time on graph paper (see Figure 11-6).

As you can see from Figure 11-6, the shape of the [concentration × time] versus time curve is very different from the drug plasma concentration (C) versus time (t) plot used to calculate AUC. The trapezoidal rule can be used to calculate AUMC. Following a plot as in Figure 11-6, a series of straight lines can be drawn from the concentration × time point to its accompanying time value on the x-axis, forming individual trapezoids (**Figure 11-7**).

The area of each trapezoid is calculated with the following equation:

$$\text{Area of trapezoid} = \frac{(C_2 \times t_2) + (C_1 \times t_1)}{2}(t_2 - t_1)$$

The sum of all of the trapezoidal areas yields an estimate of the AUMC from time zero to the last observed time point. As in calculating AUC, it is important to obtain AUMC from time zero to infinity. Consequently, the terminal area, which includes the portion of the curve from t_{last} to infinity, must be estimated.

Assuming the terminal elimination slope remains constant over this time period, the terminal area is calculated with the following equation:

$$\text{Terminal area} = \frac{(C_{\text{last}} \times t_{\text{last}})}{\lambda} + \frac{C_{\text{last}}}{\lambda^2}$$

where:

C_{last} = last observed plasma concentration

t_{last} = time of the last observed plasma concentration

λ = terminal elimination rate constant from the concentration versus time curve. λ is used here (instead of K) to indicate that this represents elimination in a model-independent or noncompartmental analysis

Mean Residence Time

MRT is the average time intact drug molecules transit or reside in the body. For a population of drug molecules, individual molecules spend different times within the body. Following the principles of statistical probability, specific drug molecules may be eliminated quickly, whereas others may remain in the body much longer. Consequently, a distribution of transit times can be characterized by a mean value. In other words, elimination of a drug can be thought of as a random process. Residence time reflects how long a particular drug molecule remains or resides in the body. The MRT reflects the overall behavior of a large number of drug molecules. This parameter is not used frequently in clinical practice to monitor patients. However, it is useful when comparing the effect of disease, altered physiologic state, or drug–drug interaction on the pharmacokinetics of a specific drug.

MRT can be calculated with the following equation:

$$\text{MRT} = \frac{\text{AUMC}_{0\to\infty}}{\text{AUC}_{0\to\infty}}$$

Volume of Distribution at Steady State

Volume of distribution at steady state (V_{ss}) is a parameter that relates total amount of drug in the body to a particular plasma concentration after a single dose. This parameter is not affected by changes in drug elimination or clearance, making it a useful tool in assessing the effect disease, altered physiologic state, or drug–drug interaction may have on the volume of distribution of a drug. V_{ss} was calculated previously but was only applicable to a drug fitting a two-compartment model. The following equation for V_{ss} does not depend on the model used to describe drug distribution or elimination from the body:

$$V_{ss} = \text{MRT} \times \text{Cl}_t$$

And since:

$$\text{MRT} = \frac{\text{AUMC}_{0\to\infty}}{\text{AUC}_{0\to\infty}} \text{ and Cl}_t = \frac{X_0}{\text{AUC}_{0\to\infty}}$$

then:

$$V_{ss} = \frac{X_0 \times \text{AUMC}_{0\to\infty}}{(\text{AUC}_{0\to\infty})^2}$$

Formation Clearance

Formation clearance ($\text{Cl}_{P\to mX}$) is a model-independent parameter that provides a meaningful estimate of the portion of the total body clearance that is accounted for by production of a specific metabolite.

Formation clearance is analogous to systemic and renal clearance of a drug and refers to the formation of metabolites in the course of drug elimination. This parameter is not used to individualize a patient's drug dosing regimen, but is useful when assessing the impact that a specific drug treatment, disease, or altered physiologic state may have on a specific metabolic pathway of a drug.

The following equations are used to calculate the formation clearance of a drug:

$$Cl_{P \to m1} = F_{m1} Cl_t$$

where:

$Cl_{P \to m1}$ = fractional clearance of the parent drug (P) to form metabolite 1 (m_1)

F_{m1} = fraction of metabolite m_1 formed from a single dose of the parent drug

Cl_t = total body clearance

Or:

$$Cl_{P \to m1} = \left(\frac{m_{1,u}}{X_0} \right) \left(\frac{X_0}{AUC_{0 \to \infty}} \right)$$

$$= \frac{m_{1,u}}{AUC_{0 \to \infty}}$$

where:

$m_{1,u}$ = amount of metabolite m_1 excreted in the urine

For example, if a drug is metabolized by three separate enzyme systems, each producing a unique metabolite, what effect would the addition of a known hepatic enzyme inducer have on the individual metabolic pathways? **Figure 11-8** provides a visual perspective of this situation.

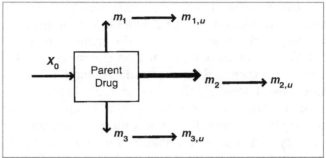

FIGURE 11-8.
Metabolic pathways for a parent drug, where m_1 = metabolite 1, $m_{1,u}$ = amount of m_1 excreted in the urine, m_2 = metabolite 2, $m_{2,u}$ = amount of m_2 excreted in the urine, m_3 = metabolite 3, and $m_{3,u}$ = amount of m_3 excreted in the urine.

To simplify this example, we will assume that systemic clearance equals hepatic clearance, these three metabolic pathways account for 100% of the hepatic clearance of the drug, the metabolite is rapidly secreted unchanged in the urine, and the dose is equal to 100 mg. **Table 11-1** shows the effect of an enzyme inducer on each metabolic pathway portrayed in Figure 11-8 as shown by changes in the percentage of drug dose excreted in the urine for each metabolite and formation clearance.

As Table 11-1 shows, the administration of an enzyme inducer substantially increased the systemic clearance of this drug, from 25 to 75 mL/min. However, the change in the percentage of the dose excreted as a specific metabolite does not exactly reflect the change in formation clearance values. The percentage of dose excreted in the urine for m_1 was reduced threefold, but no change in the formation clearance was observed. This means that the enzyme inducer had no effect on the enzyme responsible for producing m_1.

TABLE 11-1. Changes in Formation Clearance of Three Metabolites as a Result of Enzyme Induction

	Metabolite	Percentage of Dose Excreted in Urine	Formation Clearance (mL/min)
Control (Cl_t = 25 mL/min)	m_1	20	5
	m_2	50	12.5
	m_3	30	7.5
Enzyme induction (Cl_t = 75 mL/min)	m_1	6.7	5
	m_2	63.3	47.5
	m_3	30	22.5

On the other hand, treatment with the enzyme inducer produced only a 1.3-fold increase in the percentage of the dose excreted in the urine for m_2 but a fourfold increase in its formation clearance. Finally, the percentage of dose excreted in urine for m_3 was unchanged despite a threefold increase in its formation clearance. Because the formation clearance of a drug to a metabolite reflects more accurately the activity of that specific enzyme, the data would suggest that the enzyme(s) responsible for the formation of m_2 and m_3 was significantly increased by the enzyme inducer, whereas the enzyme(s) responsible for the formation of m_1 was unaffected. The preceding example demonstrates the value of formation clearance versus the more traditional approach of calculating the percentage of a drug dose excreted as a specific metabolite.

References

1. Evans WE, McLeod HL. Pharmacogenomics—Drug disposition, drug targets, and side effects. *N Engl J Med.* 2003;348(6):538–47.

2. Mancana D, Kerewin RW. Role of pharmacogenomics in individualizing treatment with SSRIs. *CNS Drugs.* 2003;17(3):143–51.

3. Bauer LA, Blouin RA, Griffin WO, et al. Amikacin pharmacokinetics in morbidly obese patients. *Am J Hosp Pharm.* 1980;37:519–22.

4. Dasgupta A, Dean R, Saldana S, et al. Absorption of therapeutic drugs by barrier gels in serum separator blood collection devices. *Am J Clin Pathol.* 1994;101:456–61.

5. Spruill WJ, McCall CY, Francisco GE. In vitro inactivation of tobramycin by cephalosporins. *Am J Hosp Pharm.* 1985;42:2506–9.

6. Riff LF, Jackson GG. Laboratory and clinical conditions for gentamicin inactivation by carbenicillin. *Arch Intern Med.* 1972;130:887–91.

REVIEW QUESTIONS

11-1. The proportion of total body weight that is water is highest in _____.

   A. Healthy adults

   B. Neonates

   C. Elderly

   D. Teenagers

11-2. With dysfunction of the major organs of drug elimination (kidneys and liver), which of the following may be affected?

   A. Drug clearance

   B. Volume of distribution

   C. Drug plasma protein binding

   D. All of the above may be affected

11-3. For drugs that distribute primarily in extra-cellular fluid, a dose for an obese person should be calculated using total body weight.

   A. True

   B. False

11-4. The fluid portion of a sample of whole blood centrifuged before it clots is called _____.

   A. Serum

   B. Plasma

   C. Serous fluid

   D. Citrated blood

11-5. The fluid portion of whole blood centrifuged after clot formation is called _____.

   A. Serum

   B. Plasma

   C. Serous fluid

   D. Citrated blood

11-6. Assay cross-reactivity refers to diminished assay performance caused by _____.

   A. Physiologic substances found in some patients' plasma that directly affect the assay itself

   B. Structurally related drug compounds or metabolites for which the assay method measures as if they were the desired assay compound

   C. An in vitro inactivation of one drug by another drug that is also present in the patient's plasma

   D. None of the above

Indicate *Yes* or *No* for **Questions 11-7 through 11-10**:

   Yes = the accuracy of the drug concentrations is of concern and should be redrawn.

   No = the accuracy of the drug concentrations is not of particular concern.

11-7. A gentamicin concentration from a sample stored at controlled room temperature and assayed 24 hours after it was collected from a patient receiving both ampicillin and gentamicin.

   A. Yes

   B. No

11-8. A plasma tobramycin concentration from a sample stored at controlled room temperature and assayed 24 hours after it was collected from a patient receiving both tobramycin and ceftazidime.

   A. Yes

   B. No

11-9. A plasma gentamicin concentration from a sample stored in a freezer until assayed 12 hours after it was collected from a patient receiving both ampicillin and gentamicin.

A. Yes

B. No

11-10. A plasma gentamicin concentration from a sample assayed immediately after it was collected from a patient receiving both piperacillin and gentamicin.

A. Yes

B. No

11-11. The trapezoidal rule can be used to calculate AUC for model-independent relationships.

A. True

B. False

11-12. The ratio of $AUMC_{\to\infty}$ to $AUC_{\to\infty}$ is called _____.

A. Trapezoidal rule

B. Total body clearance

C. Mean residence time

D. Formation clearance

11-13. Which statement(s) is/are *true* about the calculation of formation clearance ($Cl_{P\to mX}$)? Formation clearance can be used to calculate the _____.

A. Clearance rate of individual metabolites of a drug

B. Mean residence time

C. Total body clearance of a drug that has multiple metabolites

D. A and C

ANSWERS

11-1. A, C, D. *Incorrect answers*

B. CORRECT ANSWER. The proportion of the body that is water is greatest in the neonate and lowest in the elderly.

11-2. A, B, C. *Incorrect answers* as individual responses because all can be affected.

D. CORRECT ANSWER. Major organ dysfunction can affect most pharmacokinetic parameters.

11-3. A. *Incorrect answer*

B. CORRECT ANSWER. The proportion of fat tissue that is extracellular fluid is less than in lean tissue, but the drug will still distribute somewhat in the adipose extracellular fluid.

11-4. A. *Incorrect answer.* Serum is produced when centrifugation occurs after sample is allowed to clot

B. CORRECT ANSWER. Plasma contains clotting factors.

C. *Incorrect answer.* Serous fluid is a natural body fluid and is not centrifuged to remove cellular components.

D. *Incorrect answer.* Citrated blood contains citrate additives that keep the blood from clotting.

11-5. A. CORRECT ANSWER.

B. *Incorrect answer.* Plasma also contains clotting factors.

C. *Incorrect answer.* Serous fluid is a natural body fluid and is not centrifuged to remove cellular components.

D. *Incorrect answer.* Citrated blood contains citrate additives that keep the blood from clotting.

11-6. A. *Incorrect answer.* This is assay interference.

B. CORRECT ANSWER

C. *Incorrect answer.* Assay cross-reactivity does not involve assay measurement of inactivated products that result from some physiochemical process.

D. *Incorrect answer*

11-7. A. CORRECT ANSWER. Ampicillin will inactivate gentamicin in vitro.

   B. *Incorrect answer*

11-8. A. *Incorrect answer*

   B. CORRECT ANSWER. Aminoglycosides are not inactivated by cephalosporin agents, just penicillin products.

11-9. A. *Incorrect answer*

   B. CORRECT ANSWER. Freezing this sample will stop inactivation from occurring.

11-10. A. *Incorrect answer*

   B. CORRECT ANSWER. Inactivation does not have time to occur if you assay the sample immediately.

11-11. A. CORRECT ANSWER. The trapezoidal rule is a model-independent method for AUC calculation.

   B. *Incorrect answer*

11-12. A. *Incorrect answer*. Trapezoidal rule is a method to calculate AUC.

   B. *Incorrect answer*. Total body clearance is $X_0/AUC_{0\rightarrow\infty}$.

   C. CORRECT ANSWER

   D. *Incorrect answer*. Formation clearance is a calculation of metabolite clearance.

11-13. A, B, C. *Incorrect answers*. MRT is calculated using AUC and AUMC

   D. CORRECT ANSWER.

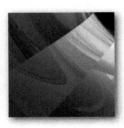

Discussion Points

D-1. Write a pharmacy protocol to ensure proper serum drug concentration collection and assay.

D-2. Try to get a package insert from your laboratory on any therapeutically monitored drug. Describe the type of information found. Specifically, how are the issues of assay sensitivity, specificity, and cross-reactivity noted?

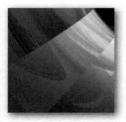

Definitions of symbols and key equations are as follows:

   AUC = area under plasma concentration versus time curve

   F = fraction of drug reaching systemic circulation

   Cl_t = total drug clearance from body = dose/AUC

   K_a = absorption rate constant

The following applies to **Questions PS3-1 to PS3-4**. The relative bioavailabilities of two dosage forms (a sustained-release tablet and an oral solution) of oral omeprazole are compared. The following plasma drug concentrations were obtained after 20 mg of each was administered:

Time after Dose (hr)	Concentration (ng/mL)	
	Sustained-Release Tablet	Oral Solution
0	0	0
0.5	2.98	9.03
1	6.11	23.99
1.5	8.09	27.64
2	9.76	24.80
3	12.34	16.06
4	13.18	13.28
5	12.52	11.16
6	11.25	8.79
8	7.63	5.62
12	2.78	1.63

Before proceeding to the questions below, on linear graph paper, plot the plasma drug concentration versus time data for the two formulations.

QUESTIONS

PS3-1. What is the $AUC_{0-12\,hr}$ for the oral tablet formulation (using the trapezoidal method)?

   A. 52.16 (ng/L) × hour

   B. 67.89 (ng/L) × hour

   C. 99.23 (ng/L) × hour

   D. 126.62 (ng/L) × hour

PS3-2. What is the $AUC_{0-12\,hr}$ for the oral solution formulation (using the trapezoidal method)?

   A. 60.52 (ng/L) × hour

   B. 79.43 (ng/L) × hour

   C. 122.75 (ng/L) × hour

   D. 143.18 (ng/L) × hour

PS3-3. What are the peak plasma drug concentrations for the oral tablet and oral suspension, respectively?

   A. 13.18 and 27.64 ng/L

   B. 13.28 and 6.11 ng/L

   C. 28.22 and 13.24 ng/L

   D. 3.87 and 9.47 ng/L

PS3-4. Which product has greater bioavailability?

   A. Oral solution

   B. Oral tablet

The following applies to **Question PS3-5**. A single oral dose (500 mg) of a sustained-release procainamide tablet was given, and the following plasma drug concentrations were determined:

Time after Dose (hr)	Plasma Drug Concentration (mg/L)
0	0
0.25	0.28
0.5	0.76
0.75	1.85
1	2.57
1.5	6.23
2	7.44
4	1.73
6	1.51
10	0.31

PS3-5. What is the absorption rate constant (K_a) of this formulation (using the method of residuals)?

A. 2.4 hr^{-1}

B. 3.1 hr^{-1}

C. 0.23 hr^{-1}

D. 1.5 hr^{-1}

ANSWERS

PS3-1. A, B, D. *Incorrect answers*

    C. CORRECT ANSWER. Using the equation found in Figure 3-10,

$$\frac{(2.98+0)(0.5-0)}{2} = 0.75$$

$$\frac{(2.98+6.11)(1-0.5)}{2} = 2.27$$

$$\frac{(6.11+8.09)(1.5-1)}{2} = 3.55$$

$$\frac{(8.09+9.76)(2-1.5)}{2} = 4.46$$

$$\frac{(9.76+12.34)(3-2)}{2} = 11.05$$

$$\frac{(12.34+13.18)(4-3)}{2} = 12.76$$

$$\frac{(13.18+12.52)(5-4)}{2} = 12.85$$

$$\frac{(12.52+11.25)(6-5)}{2} = 11.89$$

$$\frac{(11.25+7.63)(8-6)}{2} = 18.88$$

$$\frac{(7.63+2.78)(12-8)}{2} = 20.82$$

$$+ \underline{\hspace{2em}}$$

$$= 99.28 \text{ (ng/L)} \times \text{hr}$$

PS3-2. A, C, D. *Incorrect answers*

    B. CORRECT ANSWER. Using the equation found in Figure 3-10,

$$\frac{(0+9.03)(0.5-0)}{2} = 2.26$$

$$\frac{(9.03+23.99)(1-0.5)}{2} = 8.26$$

$$\frac{(23.99+27.64)(1.5-1)}{2} = 12.91$$

$$\frac{(27.63+24.8)(2-1.5)}{2} = 13.11$$

$$\frac{(24.8+16.06)(3-2)}{2} = 20.43$$

$$\frac{(16.06+13.28)(4-3)}{2} = 14.67$$

$$\frac{(13.28+11.16)(5-4)}{2} = 12.22$$

$$\frac{(11.16+8.79)(6-5)}{2} = 9.98$$

$$\frac{(8.79+5.62)(8-6)}{2} = 14.41$$

$$\frac{(5.62+1.63)(12-8)}{2} = 14.5$$

$$+ \underline{\hspace{2em}}$$

$$= 122.75 \text{ (ng/L)} \times \text{hr}$$

PS3-3. A. CORRECT ANSWER. Observe peak concentration from AUC plot.

B, C, D. *Incorrect answers*

PS3-4. A. CORRECT ANSWER. The oral tablet has a smaller AUC and, therefore, has a lower bioavailability than the oral solution.

B. *Incorrect answer*

PS3-5. A, B, C. *Incorrect answers*

D. CORRECT ANSWER. First, the data points at 4, 8, and 12 hours are on the straight-line terminal portion of the plot and, therefore, are not used to calculate the residual line. Next, the terminal, straight-line portion of the graph is back-extrapolated to the y-axis. For each time at which a concentration was actually determined, the concentration corresponding to the back-extrapolated line is noted (extrapolated concentration). The residual is the remainder of the actual concentration subtracted from the extrapolated concentration. The K_a is the negative slope of the natural log of the residual concentration versus time curve. We can choose any two residual points to determine the slope, but it is usually best to select the points most widely separated by time. Therefore,

$$K_a = -\left(\frac{\Delta y}{\Delta x}\right) = \frac{\ln 4.62 - \ln 1.53}{0.25 \text{ hr} - 1 \text{ hr}}$$

$$= -\left(\frac{1.53 - .43}{-0.75 \text{ hr}}\right)$$

$$= 1.47 \text{ hr}^{-1}$$

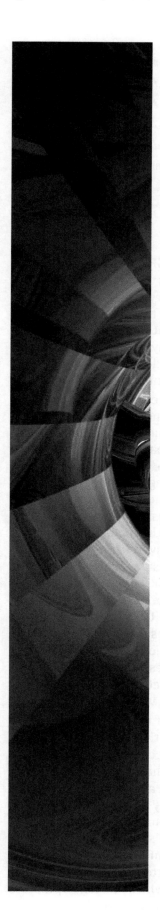

Aminoglycosides

Assessment of a patient's current renal function is an important component of ensuring correct drug dosing and achievement of desired therapeutic effect. This lesson reviews the various renal function assessment equations followed by cases on the appropriate dosing of aminoglycosides. The principles outlined are applicable to the pharmacokinetic modeling of most drugs exhibiting first order elimination.

Renal Function Assessment

The National Kidney Foundation (NKF) classifies chronic kidney disease (CKD) into five stages based on glomerular filtration rate (GFR) reported in units of mL/min/1.73 m^2 body surface area (BSA) as shown in **Table 12-1**. Recently, the NKF has recommended the use of the modified diet in renal disease (MDRD) equation (MDRDEQ) to estimate a patient's GFR as a screening tool for early detection of CKD (http://www.kidney.org/professionals/KDOQI/gfr.cfm).

GFR has historically been measured by renal clearance of substances that are 100% excreted via glomerular filtration with no renal tubular reabsorption or secretion, such as inulin clearance, and by renal clearance of radio-labeled ^{125}I-iothalamate, which has become the gold standard for GFR measurements. However, actual GFR measurements are not commonly done in clinical practice. Instead, clinicians rely on more easily performed estimations of GFR, such as measured creatinine clearance (CrCl), estimated CrCl, and now estimated GFR via the MDRD equation(s). It is important to understand the different methods for estimating renal function, their limitations, and place in practice so that evaluation of renal function and the drug dose adjustments can be made with the best clinical judgment.

CrCl measurement requires a 24-hour collection of urine as shown in the formula below:

$$\text{CrCl (mL/min)} = \frac{UV}{P \times 1440}$$

where:

U = urinary creatinine concentration (mg/dL)

V = volume of urine collected (mL)

P = plasma creatinine concentration (taken at midpoint of urine collection; mg/dL)

1440 = number of minutes in 24 hours

TABLE 12-1. Stages of Chronic Kidney Disease

Stage 1	Kidney damage with normal or increased GFR	>90 mL/min/1.73 m^2
Stage 2	Kidney damage with mildly decreased GFR	60–89 mL/min/1.73 m^2
Stage 3a	Moderately decreased GFR	45–59 mL/min/1.73 m^2
Stage 3b	Moderately decreased GFR	30–44 mL/min/1.73 m^2
Stage 4	Severely decreased GFR	15–29 mL/min/1.73 m^2
Stage 5	Kidney failure	<15 mL/min/1.73 m^2

GFR = glomerular filtration rate.

Due to the cumbersome nature of direct measurements of either GFR or CrCl, renal function is most commonly estimated with either the Cockcroft–Gault creatinine clearance equation (CGEQ) or the MDRD4$_{revised}$ estimated GFR equation. Both equations have limitations and different applicability to certain populations and have been studied to varying degrees for use in drug dosing adjustments. Cockcroft–Gault has historically been the most commonly used in drug development studies for drug dosing adjustment recommendations, but its accuracy in some patient populations has been debated. The various versions of the MDRDEQ were intended for use in estimating GFR to stage level of kidney disease and were developed in a sample that consisted primarily of patients with some degree of CKD. Thus, the MDRD equations may more accurately assess renal function in the CKD population but as such may not accurately assess renal function in non-CKD patients.[1] Because the equations account for different variables in their formulas, calculated values may differ between the two by up to 10% to 40%.[1,2] Thus, it is important to understand the intended/appropriate use of each of these equations and how to interpret them for drug dosing. **Table 12-2** shows several versions of both of these equations, including the most commonly used CGEQ using ideal body weight (IBW) or adjusted body weight (AdjBW).

Controversy continues to exist as to which equation, CGEQ or MDRDEQ, is best to use for renal adjustments of drug doses. Complicating this issue is the conversion to new global serum creatinine (SCr) assay standards that result in a more accurate measurement of creatinine (yielding a value 10% to 20% lower than older assays).[3] Newer measurements report two places past the decimal (i.e., 1.68 mg/dL). The MDRD4$_{revised}$ equation is the recommended version of the MDRD equation for use with these new assay standards for rapid GFR estimates while the CKD-EPI is recommended as the value to be reported by laboratories on chemistry panels. Further complicating the comparison is the potential for SCr to be falsely lowered in patients with reduced muscle mass which could affect any SCr dependent calculation. There is interest in developing estimates of renal function less dependent upon SCr.[4]

Much research has been done to determine which equation is the best; however, it appears that these equations are so dissimilar in their formulation that meaningful comparisons are difficult to perform and are subject to various patient demographic biases, especially age and obesity.[4,5,9-11] In addition the equations are often used to estimate renal function for drug dosing in specific patient populations that were not the focus of the original studies. The CGEQ was derived from a simple general linear multiple regression analysis such that each factor (age, weight, SCr value) in the equation is linearly expressed for the entire tested range of values. Conversely, the MDRDEQs were correlated using log transformed values and then re-expressed as a multiplicative linear model that now contains exponents for the variables of age and SCr and, therefore, produces a geometric relationship across the range of values for each variable tested.

Figure 12-1 is a plot of the age component for both equations, showing that the MDRDEQ calculates a much smaller decline in GFR from age 40 to 80 years than does the CGEQ. Therefore, the MDRDEQ may not predict age-related declines in renal function in the elderly as well as the CGEQ.[4,5] A recent study which evaluated GFR estimates in patients with renal disease suggests that the CGEQ using AdjBW performs similar to non-normalized CKD-EPI.[7] Despite many attempts to compare the equations the question of which strategy optimizes clinical outcomes remains unanswered.

TABLE 12-2. Equations Used to Estimate Creatinine Clearance (CrCl) or Glomerular Filtration Rate (GFR)

Cockcroft–Gault estimation of CrCl (mL/min/1.73 m²)

Original form used total weight with no BSA adjustment	$TBW(0.85 \text{ if female})(140 - age)/(72 \times SCr)$
Cockcroft–Gault equation most commonly recommended, using IBW or AdjBW*	$(IBW \text{ or } AdjBW^*)(0.85 \text{ if female})(140 - age)/(72 \times SCr)$

Modified diet in renal disease (MDRD) equations (mL/min/1.73 m²)

MDRD 6 variable equation with UUN	$198 (Cr^{-0.858} \times age^{-0.167}) \times BUN^{-0.293} \times UUN^{-0.249}$ [× 1.178 if black and × 0.822 if female]
MDRD 6 variable equation with albumin	$170 (Cr^{-0.999} \times age^{-0.176}) \times BUN^{-0.170} \times albumin^{-0.318}$ [× 1.178 if black and × 0.822 if female]
MDRD original 4 variable equation	$186 (Cr^{-1.154} \times age^{-0.203})$ [× 1.212 if black and × 0.742 if female]
MDRD revised 4 variable equation with new creatinine assay standards	$175 (Cr^{-1.154} \times age^{-0.203})$ [× 1.212 if black and × 0.742 if female]
CKD-EPI	$141 \times \min(SCr/\kappa, 1)^{\alpha} \times \max(SCr/\kappa, 1)^{-1.209} \times 0.993^{Age}$ [× 1.018 if female × 1.159 if black]
	where SCr (standardized SCr) = mg/dL
	κ = 0.7 (females) or 0.9 (males)
	α = −0.329 (females) or −0.411 (males)
	min = indicates the minimum of SCr/κ or 1
	max = indicates the maximum of SCr/κ or 1
	age = years
CKD-EPI Cystatin C	$133 \times \min(S_{cys}/0.8, 1)^{-0.499} \times \max(S_{cys}/0.8, 1)^{-1.328} \times 0.996^{Age} \times 0.932$ [if female]
	eGFR (estimated glomerular filtration rate) = mL/min/1.73 m²
	S_{cys} (standardized serum cystatin C) = mg/L
	min = indicates the minimum of $S_{cys}/0.8$ or 1
	max = indicates the maximum of $S_{cys}/0.8$ or 1
	age = years

AdjBW, adjusted body weight; BSA, body surface area; BUN, blood urea nitrogen; Cr, creatinine; IBW, ideal body weight; TBW, total body weight; UUN, urine urea nitrogen.

*AdjBW = IBW + 0.4(TBW − IBW); IBW(male) = 50 kg + 2.3 kg for each inch over 5 feet; IBW(female) = 45.5 kg + 2.3 kg for each inch over 5 feet.

In the absence of a trial evaluating outcomes resulting from use of the varying equations, it is reasonable to use the CGEQ to adjust drug dosing according to manufacturers' dosing tables because they were developed using this same CGEQ. By extension, most pharmacokinetic population values for the elimination rate constant (*K*) were also developed from regression analyses of drug clearance versus CrCl via the CGEQ, and thus more closely match existing drug dosing tables. Comparison of the use CGEQ versus MDRD and other GFR equations for drug dosing have also shown that CGEQ is the better method to use in most cases.[5] Practitioners should always refer to the package insert to verify which formula should be utilized to estimate need for drug dose adjustment.

The CGEQ estimation is influenced by age, body weight and SCr. A recent studies supports using an adjusted body weight to improve accuracy of the CGEQ. Rounding SCr values up to 1 mg/dL is controversial and not universally accepted as the best practice when estimating CrCl values. This controversy exists because the SCr is in the denominator of the equation, which results in overestimated SCr values.

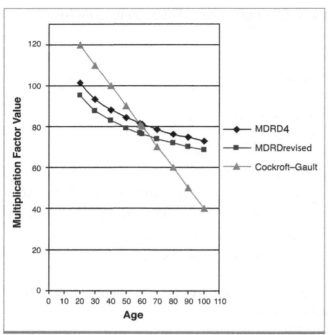

FIGURE 12-1.

A plot of age components of modified diet in renal disease (MDRD) equation and Cockcroft–Gault equation, showing that the MDRD calculates a much smaller decline in GFR from age 40 to 80 years than does the Cockcroft–Gault.

Source: Adapted from Spruill WJ, Wade WE, Cobb III HH. Estimating glomerular filtration rate with a modification of diet in renal disease equation: implications for pharmacy. *Am J Health-Syst Pharm.* 2007;64(6):652–60.

Clinical Correlate

Considerations when using the Cockcroft–Gault equation to adjust drug doses in declining renal function:

1. Use either actual IBW or an AdjBW in the formula and do not make any further BSA adjustments as this formula contains a body size factor of weight/72, which is sufficient to adjust the result for the patient's body size or BSA. Value, in units of mL/min, can now be assumed to approximate a patient's GFR expressed in units of mL/min/1.73 m^2.

2. Most drug manufacturers address dosing adjustments in patients with renal impairment by providing tables showing CrCl versus drug dose, with instructions to adjust dose based on patients' estimated CrCl calculated using the CGEQ.

3. If your laboratory is reporting SCr values that are calibrated to the IDMS-traceable creatinine assay, be aware that these newer SCr assays will report values to two places past the decimal and will produce values that are lower by as much as 10% to 20% (i.e., ~0.3 mg/dL) compared with older assay methods. This, in turn, will result in a CGEQ estimation of CrCl that is slightly higher than that using the older creatinine calibration techniques. Consequently, a clinical adjustment may be needed when applying a manufacturer's dosing adjustment data based on older creatinine assays to this newer reported creatinine value.

4. No recommendations can be made regarding rounding of the SCr value due to a lack of published studies; therefore, the potential ramifications of choosing to do so should be carefully considered.

Considerations when using MDRD equations to adjust doses:

1. Note that the MDRD equations are predictors of GFR and not CrCl, and, therefore, their use as replacements of CGEQ estimates for CrCl for drug dosing adjustments will require an individualized assessment of many dosing situations as GFR calculated from MDRD is not interchangeable with CrCl calculated by CGEQ. A reasonable approach would be to use the equation that was used to provide drug dosing recommendations by the manufacturer and then use the corresponding equation in practice while applying clinical judgment to assess the appropriate drug dosing adjustments especially in scenarios where the CGEQ and MDRD equation yield values that are significantly different.

2. The MDRD equations were initially validated in patients with chronic kidney disease and may not be as easily

generalized to other subsets of patients, including those without CKD or the elderly. The more commonly used CGEQ also has limitations in some populations that differ from the one in whom it was originally studied, but has shown in many comparison studies versus MDRD (GFR) to be the better choice for making drug dosing adjustments (mostly because it is the most consistent with manufacturer-labeling based dosing recommendations).

3. The MDRD equation may or may not actually be more "accurate" than the CGEQ for estimating GFR in patients with CKD; however, it can be calculated and reported using routine clinical chemistry analyzer software, as it does not require the patient's weight or height.

4. There is **no** useful conversion factor to convert MDRD GFR to the equivalent CGEQ value because of the differences in the regression models used. Sometimes the MDRD value will be higher and sometimes the CGEQ values will be higher and often they will be significantly different from one another for the same patient. It is likely that clinical studies will begin to include drug dosing adjustments based on the newer (non-CGEQ) estimates of glomerular filtration. It is important to verify prescribing information to discern which estimate of renal function was used prior to recommending dose adjustments.

Aminoglycoside Dosing

Individualization of aminoglycoside dosing regimens is important to optimize efficacy while minimizing potential toxicity. **Cases 1–4** outline traditional dosing methods of individualized dosing, and **Cases 5–7** focus on the extended interval administration of aminoglycosides.

Because the currently available IV aminoglycosides (gentamicin, tobramycin, and amikacin) exhibit similar pharmacokinetics, case discussions

of one aminoglycoside can be extrapolated to any other. Although amikacin has the same pharmacokinetic profile as other aminoglycosides, it requires doses and target concentrations approximately two to four times as high as the other aminoglycosides.

Several key points should be reviewed before beginning these cases. Aminoglycosides are excreted unchanged by renal glomerular filtration. The elimination, therefore, is proportional to a patient's GFR, which can be estimated by determining CrCl.

Estimation of Elimination Rate Constant (K) and Volume of Distribution (V) for All Aminoglycosides

Calculate Estimated Creatinine Clearance

Sometimes it is impractical or impossible to collect a 24-hour urine specimen; CrCl must then be estimated from SCr. Although there are several formulas for estimating CrCl, we use the Cockcroft–Gault equation[10]:

$$CrCl_{male} \ mL/min = \frac{(140 - age)BW}{72 \times SCr}$$

(See **Equation 9-1**.)

or

$$CrCl_{female} \ mL/min = \frac{(0.85)(140 - age)BW}{72 \times SCr}$$

where:

CrCl = creatinine clearance (mL/min per 1.73 m^2 BSA)

age = patient's age (years)

BW = ideal body weight (kilograms) or adjusted body weight (AdjBW) in obese patients

SCr = serum creatinine concentration (milligrams per deciliter [mg/dL])

Calculate Ideal Body Weight or Adjusted Body Weight

Because creatinine is produced by muscle metabolism (and not by fat), we must use the patient's total body weight (actual) IBW or AdjBW when estimating creatinine clearance. IBW should be used to calculate CrCl for patients of normal weight (BMI 19–24.5) or overweight (BMI 25–30). Patients who are overweight (BMI >30) are by definition >20% normal weight (BMI 30/20) = 1.2). In this population, an AdjBW should be used. If a patient's total body weight is less than their IBW, then TBW should be used to avoid overestimation of CrCl.

The IBW for adult males can be estimated as follows:

IBW = 50 kg + 2.3 kg for each inch over 5 feet in height   (See **Equation 9-2**.)

The IBW for adult females is as follows:

IBW = 45.5 kg + 2.3 kg for each inch over 5 feet in height   (See **Equation 9-2**.)

In obese patients, the use of total body weight in the CGEQ overestimates creatinine clearance calculations, and the use of IBW underestimates calculation of this variable. Consequently, an AdjBW likely represents a more accurate estimate of creatinine clearance in these patients and should be used. If a patient's actual body weight is >20% above his or her IBW then the AdjBW must be used to calculate CrCl[9,12]:

AdjBW = IBW + 0.4(TBW − IBW)   (See **Equation 9-3**.)

For a patient who weighs less than IBW (or BMI <19), the total body (actual) weight provides a more accurate estimate and should be used in the CGEQ to calculate CrCl.[7]

Clinical Correlate

Close examination of the Cockcroft–Gault equation reveals that SCr values less than 1 mg/dL could greatly elevate the calculated CrCl value. This is especially true for elderly patients (or those with conditions associated with lower muscle mass such as bedbound or paralyzed patients) for whom unrealistically high CrCl values may be calculated using this equation. The elderly often have reduced muscle mass as a fraction of TBW, and so may generate less creatinine than a younger patient of similar weight. In these patients, the SCr value may not be an appropriate indicator of the patient's true renal function. Some authors have suggested to round SCr values up to 1 mg/dL or round final CrCl down to 100 mL/min, but this is not universally accepted as the most accurate practice. Although these recommended adjustments may yield a more accurate estimation in some cases, they still add error to the original CrCl calculation and may not be necessary for all patients with SCr <1.0 (who are otherwise healthy and ambulatory) as some studies have shown that actual SCr values used in the calculation (even when below 1.0) produce more accurate results compared to a 24-hour urine creatinine collection calculation than rounding the value up to 1.0 mg/dL.[5,12]

Calculate Estimated Elimination Rate and Volume of Distribution

To calculate an initial maintenance dose and dosing interval using traditional dosing methods, we must use population estimates for the elimination rate constant (K) and the volume of distribution (V). Population estimates of K are derived from small studies that correlate an aminoglycoside's clearance (and hence K) to the patient's CrCl (**Figure 12-2**). Creatinine clearance and aminoglycoside clearance are not equal; some amount of aminoglycoside is eliminated by organs other than the kidneys. When creatinine clearance is zero, the aminoglycoside clearance is still approximately 0.014 mL/min, reflecting this nonrenal clearance and, perhaps, some active tubular secretion.

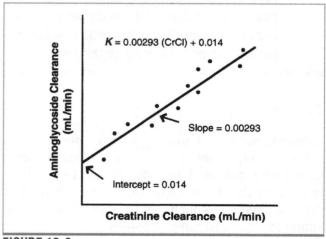

FIGURE 12-2.
Aminoglycoside clearance versus creatinine clearance.

The equation for the line of best fit through these points can be used to estimate an elimination rate constant (K) for this sample of patients, as shown here:

$$Y = mX + b$$

Or, for example, one commonly used regression equation is as follows:

$$\text{slope}(K) = 0.00293 \,(\text{CrCl}) + 0.014$$

where K is the elimination rate constant for aminoglycosides (population estimate). This equation will be used throughout the lesson for all aminoglycosides. The volume of distribution for gentamicin and tobramycin ranges between approximately 0.2–0.4 L/kg[15]. These estimates also involve the appropriate calculations of CrCl and IBW (or AdjBW). For obese patients AdjBW should be used in estimation of CrCl and aminoglycoside volume of distribution estimates. Because many small-sample studies have been done to estimate K and V, there are many different estimates for both.

To estimate K and V, we shall use the following:

 12-1 $K = 0.00293(\text{CrCl}) + 0.014$

12-2 $V = 0.24 \,\text{L/kg} \,(\text{IBW or AdjBW})$

Clinical Correlate

Consideration in the selection of a correct adjusted weight to be used in aminoglycoside calculations is critical. Use of an incorrect weight in calculations may under or overestimate volume leading to incorrect estimation of empiric doses. Although aminoglycoside penetration into adipose tissue is considered to be limited, studies suggest that a dosing weight should be utilized to account for the water content in adipose tissue.[13,14]

When calculating aminoglycoside volume of distribution, one can use either actual (if less than ideal) IBW or an AdjBW$_{AG}$ (if greater than 30% above IBW) formula that the uptake of drug in adipose tissue as well as the increased blood volume due to adipose tissue.

 12-3 $\text{AdjBW}_{AG} = \text{IBW} + 0.4\,(\text{TBW} - \text{IBW})$

Note that this AdjBW$_{AG}$ is same as that for use in the creatinine clearance formula. In clinical practice, the AdjBW is commonly used for aminoglycoside calculations. Also note that the AdjBW used for dose calculations may vary for each medication.

Clinical Correlate

The values for K and V represent population estimates of the elimination rate constant and volume of distribution, respectively, based on statistical averages with relatively large standard deviations. For this reason, it is important to obtain peaks and troughs after the initial dosing regimen is established to properly adjust the dosage and dosing interval based on the individual patient's specific pharmacokinetic data.

Clinical Correlate

Some clinicians would use the above K and V equations as initial population estimates for all aminoglycosides; however, other clinicians may use equations with slightly different numbers based on regression equations derived from similar studies. Additionally, most clinicians will use the same estimates for all aminoglycosides; however, some will use slightly different equations for each aminoglycoside. We will use the above equation for all aminoglycosides as they are all excreted renally via the exact same mechanism.

Desired Aminoglycoside Plasma Concentrations

The traditional ranges for desired aminoglycoside plasma concentrations for gentamicin and tobramycin are a peak of 4–10 mg/L and a trough of

1–2 mg/L. For amikacin, a peak of 15–30 mg/L and a trough of 5–10 mg/L is recommended.[12] Attainment of adequate peak concentrations is related to the efficacy in treating some infections (to ensure appropriate C_{max}:MIC ratio for these concentration-dependent drugs), and a low trough concentration may minimize the risk of nephrotoxicity and ototoxicity.

CASE 1

A 66-year-old white female, SG, is hospitalized for pyelonephritis with bacteremia secondary to a previously untreated urinary tract infection. The medical resident orders a pharmacy dosing consult to begin this patient on an aminoglycoside. Other pertinent patient data include height, 5'6"; weight, 58 kg; and SCr, 1.12 mg/dL.

Problem 1A. Calculate an appropriate aminoglycoside maintenance dose and loading dose, including the most appropriate dosing interval, for patient SG. Assume a desired C_{peak} of 6 mg/L and a C_{trough} of 1 mg/L.

Population values of K and V for the aminoglycosides should be used to estimate maintenance doses. A patient usually will receive a loading dose over 1 hour when therapy is initiated because a loading dose quickly brings aminoglycoside plasma concentration close to the desired therapeutic concentration. If a loading dose is not given, the patient's aminoglycoside concentration will not reach the desired concentration until steady state is achieved—in three (87.5% of steady state) to five (96.9% of steady state) drug half-lives.

Lessons 4 and 5 describe the mathematical models used for various multiple-dose IV drug dosing situations. For aminoglycosides, which are usually given intravenously over 30–60 minutes at regular (i.e., intermittent) intervals, Lesson 5 describes the appropriate dosing equation. A quick review of Lessons 4 and 5 may help you understand the derivation of these equations. Briefly, this equation is arrived at by taking the equation from Lesson 4 for

a single IV bolus dose and adding the appropriate factors for the following:

- Multiple doses
- Simultaneous drug administration and drug elimination
- Drug administration over 30–60 minutes instead of an intravenous bolus
- Attainment of steady state (for simplicity, 1 hour is assumed for the drug administration time)

The equation is as follows:

$$C_{ss\,peak} = \frac{K_0(1-e^{-Kt})}{VK(1-e^{-K\tau})}$$

(See **Equation 5-1.**)
where:

$C_{ss\,peak}$ = desired peak concentration at steady state (milligrams per liter)

K_0 = drug infusion rate (also maintenance dose you are trying to calculate, in milligrams per hour)

V = volume of distribution (population estimate for aminoglycosides, in liters)

K = elimination rate constant (population estimate for aminoglycosides, in reciprocal hours)

t = infusion time (hours)

τ = desired or most appropriate dosing interval (hours)

To solve this equation, we must perform the following:

1. Determine creatinine clearance (CrCl).

2. Insert population estimates for V and K.

3. Choose a desired C_{peak}, based on clinical and microbiologic data.

4. Determine our infusion time in hours.

5. Calculate an appropriate dosing interval (τ), as shown below.

6. Determine K_0 (maintenance dose, in milligrams per hour).

To calculate an initial maintenance dose and dosing interval, we use the population estimates of K and V calculated from **Equations 12-1** and **12-2**:

$$K = 0.00293 \text{ hr}^{-1} \times \text{CrCl (in mL/min)} + 0.014$$

$$V = 0.24 \text{ L/kg} \times \text{IBW}$$

For patient SG, we can calculate the IBW:

$$\text{IBW} = 45.5 + 2.3 \text{ kg per inch over 60 inches}$$

$$= 45.5 + 2.3(6) = 59.3 \text{ kg}$$

However, because SG's actual body weight of 58 kg is less than her IBW (59.3 kg), we should use her actual body weight in the calculation of CrCl and in the estimation of her volume of distribution (V).

Estimated CrCl (via the Cockcroft–Gault equation) is as follows:

$$\text{CrCl}_{\text{female}} \text{ mL/min} = \frac{(\text{BW}^*)(140 - \text{age})0.85}{72 \times \text{SCr}}$$

$$= \frac{(58)(140 - 66)0.85}{72 \times 1.12}$$

$$= 45.24 \text{ mL/min}$$

Note: Select between actual (if less than ideal) IBW or an AdjBW$_{\text{AG}}$ (if greater than 30% above IBW) formula that reflects this 10% of distribution into adipose tissue as follows:

$$\text{estimated } K = 0.00293 \text{ (CrCl)} + 0.014$$

$$= 0.00293 \text{ (45)} + 0.014$$

$$= 0.146 \text{ hr}^{-1}$$

$$\text{estimated } T\tfrac{1}{2} = 0.693/K \quad \text{(See Equation 3-3.)}$$

$$= 0.693/0.146 \text{ hr}^{-1}$$

$$= 4.75 \text{ hr}^{-1}$$

$$\text{estimated } V = 0.24 \text{ L/kg (weight)}$$

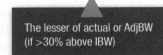

The lesser of actual or AdjBW (if >30% above IBW)

$$V = (0.24 \text{ L/kg})(58 \text{ kg}) = 13.92 \text{ L}$$

$$C_{\text{peak desired}} = 6 \text{ mg/dL}$$

$$C_{\text{trough desired}} = 1 \text{ mg/dL}$$

Estimation of Best Dosing Interval (τ)

The choice of dosing interval influences the C_{peak} and C_{trough} eventually obtained as well as the magnitude of the fluctuations in C_{peak} and C_{trough}. The equation below is used to determine the most appropriate dosing interval (τ) that will yield the desired C_{peak} and C_{trough}. As can be seen, this calculation is driven by the patient's elimination rate constant (K) and the C_{peak} and C_{trough} desired:

12-4 $$\tau = \frac{1}{-K}(\ln C_{\text{trough (desired)}} - \ln C_{\text{peak (desired)}}) + t$$

where t is the duration of the infusion in hours. This equation can be used to evaluate several different C_{peak} and C_{trough} combinations to find an appropriate dosing interval.

Derivation of Above Dosing Interval Equation

The above dosing interval equation comes from a simple rearrangement of the equation for K as shown below. For a concentration versus time curve (following first-order elimination), the terminal slope equals $-K$ and:

$$-K = \frac{Y_2 - Y_1}{X_2 - X_1} = \frac{\ln C_{\text{trough}} - \ln C_{\text{peak}}}{\tau - t}$$

This equation can be rearranged to easily calculate τ as shown below:

Step 1. Rearrange **Equation 12-4** and then solve for:

$$(-K)(\tau - t) = \ln C_{\text{trough}} - \ln C_{\text{peak}}$$

Step 2. Divide both sides by $-K$:

$$\tau - t = \frac{\ln C_{\text{trough}} - \ln C_{\text{peak}}}{-K}$$

Step 3. Transpose t to the right-hand side of the equation:

$$\tau = \frac{\ln C_{\text{trough}} - \ln C_{\text{peak}}}{-K} + t$$

Step 4. Rearrange:

$$\tau = \frac{1}{-K}(\ln C_{\text{trough}} - \ln C_{\text{peak}}) + t$$

Step 5. Further rearrange **Step 4** by considering the rule of logarithms:

$$\log a - \log b = \log (a/b)$$

Therefore:

$$\tau - \frac{1}{-K} \ln \left[\frac{\text{trough}}{\text{peak}} \right] + t$$

The equation in either **Steps 4** or **5** can be used to calculate the dosing interval (τ). You may find the equation in **Step 5** easier to enter into a hand-held calculator. Calculating the dosing interval with both equations (**Steps 4** and **5**) will serve as an added arithmetic check, because both methods should give the same answer.

Calculation of Best Dosing Interval (τ) for Patient SG

For patient SG, the calculation of the dosing interval (τ, in hours) proceeds as follows if we want a C_{peak} of 6 mg/L and a C_{trough} of 1 mg/L:

$$\tau = \frac{1}{-K} (\ln C_{\text{trough (desired)}} - C_{\text{peak (desired)}}) + t$$

$$= \frac{1}{-0.146} (\ln 1 \text{ mg/L} - \ln 6 \text{ mg/L}) + 1 \text{ hr}$$

$$= (-6.85)(0 - 1.79) + 1 \text{ hr}$$

$$= (-6.85)(-1.79) + 1 \text{ hr}$$

$$= 13.26 \text{ hours}$$

At this point, we know that the best dosing interval to obtain our desired C_{peak} and C_{trough} concentrations is 13.26 hours. In practice, this number would be rounded down to 12 hours.

Calculation of Maintenance Dose for SG

Next, we must determine the maintenance dose to be given at our desired interval of 12 hours. Note that in this example we are calculating the maintenance dose first, and will use it to calculate the proper loading dose.

Once K and V have been estimated, the desired C_{peak} and C_{trough} concentrations 'determined, and τ calculated, these values can be substituted in our general equation and solved for K_0 (maintenance dose):

$$C_{ss\,\text{peak}} = \frac{K_0(1 - e^{-Kt})}{VK(1 - e^{-K\tau})}$$

(See **Equation 5-1**.)

where:

$C_{ss\,\text{peak}}$ = desired peak drug concentration at steady state (milligrams per liter)

K_0 = drug infusion rate (also maintenance dose you are trying to calculate, in milligrams per hour)

V = volume of distribution (population estimate for aminoglycosides, in liters)

K = elimination rate constant (population estimate for aminoglycosides, in reciprocal hours)

t = duration of infusion (hours)

τ = desired or most appropriate dosing interval (hours)

Then:

$$6 \text{ mg/L} = \frac{K_0(1 - e^{-(0.146 \text{ hr}^{-1})(1 \text{ hr})})}{0.146 \text{ hr}^{-1}(13.9 \text{ } L)(1 - e^{-0.146 \text{ hr}^{-1}(12 \text{ hr})})}$$

$$= \frac{K_0(0.1358)}{(2.03)(0.8265)}$$

$$10.1 = K_0(0.1358)$$

$$74.13 \text{ mg} = K_0$$

which would be given over 1 hour for an infusion rate (K_0) of 74.13 mg/hr.

Therefore, patient SG should receive 74.13 mg every 12 hours. In practice, the dose would be rounded to either 70 or 80 mg every 12 hours. This amount is the initial estimated maintenance dose that would be given until C_{peak} and C_{trough} results are obtained. Because we rounded the dose up from the calculated value of 74.13 to 80 mg, the actual

$C_{ss\ peak}$ is slightly higher than our desired value of 6 mg/L. This actual $C_{ss\ peak}$ can be determined via a simple ratio:

$$\text{desired level} \times \frac{\text{actual (rounded) dose}}{\text{calculated dose}} = \text{actual peak}$$

For this patient, the actual $C_{ss\ peak}$ is calculated as follows:

$$6\ \text{mg/L} \times \frac{80\ \text{mg}}{74.13\ \text{mg}} = 6.47\ \text{mg/L}$$

Problem 1B. Calculate the C_{trough} concentration expected from the dose of 80 mg every 12 hours for patient SG.

The answer to this problem requires the use of another equation:

$$C = C_0 e^{-Kt} \quad \text{(See **Equation 3-2**.)}$$

where:

> C = drug concentration at time t
>
> C_0 = drug concentration at time zero or some earlier time
>
> e^{-Kt} = fraction of original or previous concentration remaining at time t

This general equation can be rewritten to show the calculation of patient SG's C_{trough} concentration after she receives her dose of 80 mg every 12 hours:

$$C_{ss\ trough} = C_{ss\ peak} e^{-Kt'}$$

(See **Equation 3-2**.)

where $t' = \tau -$ time of infusion (t), or the change in time from the first concentration to the second.

In this case, we are saying that C_{trough} equals C_{peak} multiplied by the fraction of C_{peak} remaining (as described by $e^{-Kt'}$) after elimination has occurred for t hours (i.e., 11 hours). As shown in **Figure 12-3**, because the peak concentration occurs at the end of the 1-hour infusion, t' in this equation is always τ (dosing interval) minus t (duration of infusion).

You should understand how t, τ, and t' differ.

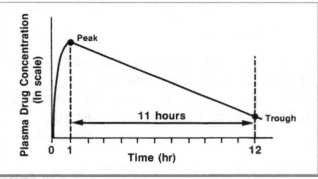

FIGURE 12-3.
Hours of elimination after drug peaks.

In patient SG's case, the estimated C_{trough} would be:

$$
\begin{aligned}
C_{ss\ trough} &= C_{ss\ peak} e^{-Kt'} \\
&= (6.47\ \text{mg/L}) e^{-(0.146\ \text{hr}^{-1})(12\ \text{hr}-1\ \text{hr})} \\
&= (6.47\ \text{mg/L}) e^{-(0.146\ \text{hr}^{-1})(11\ \text{hr})} \\
&= (6.47\ \text{mg/L}) e^{-1.606} \\
&= (6.47\ \text{mg/L})(0.200) \\
&= 1.29\ \text{mg/L; round to 1.3 mg/L}
\end{aligned}
$$

This calculation tells us that 80 mg every 12 hours will give an estimated C_{peak} of 6.47 mg/L and an estimated C_{trough} of 1.3 mg/L. Remember that we actually picked a desired C_{trough} of 1 mg/L, but we also shortened the desired dosing interval from 13.2 to 12 hours, making the estimated C_{trough} higher than the initial desired C_{trough}. If, based on clinical judgment, a lower C_{trough} is desired, the dose can be recalculated with a longer dosing interval, such as 18 hours or choose to round the dose down to 70 mg every 12 hours. In most clinical situations, every 12-hour dosing would likely be preferred.

In patient SG's case, if a C_{trough} close to 2 mg/L had been attained, it would have been because we chose a dosing interval shorter than that recommended by our dosing interval calculation. Therefore, we would need to reexamine the rounding of our dosing interval and would probably round it up from 13.2 to 18 hours.

CASE 2

In Case 1, we showed how to calculate an appropriate maintenance dose and dosing interval. For this case, we use the data presented in Case 1 and continue treating patient SG.

Problem 2A. Calculate an appropriate loading dose to approximate a plasma concentration of 6 mg/L.

There are several methods to calculate a loading dose, and two are presented. Because one method requires estimation of the maintenance dose first, the loading dose is determined after the maintenance dose and dosing interval are calculated. In clinical practice, the loading and maintenance doses would be calculated at the same time.

Like all drugs given at the same maintenance dose via intermittent administration, aminoglycosides will not reach the desired steady-state therapeutic concentration for three to five drug half-lives. Therefore, subtherapeutic concentrations may exist for 1–2 days of therapy in patients with longer half-lives. **Figure 12-4-A** shows a plasma drug concentration versus time simulation for an aminoglycoside given at the same dose six times.

In Lesson 3, we learned that a patient's drug half-life is dependent on the elimination rate

constant (K). Mathematically, $T\frac{1}{2}$ equals $0.693/K$ and, vice versa, K equals $0.693/T\frac{1}{2}$. Thus, time to reach steady state is dependent on the elimination rate constant (K) for a given patient.

Clinical Correlate

This is an interesting and conflicting concept. Reaching a steady-state drug concentration depends only on the patient's elimination rate (K). Steady state occurs in three to five drug half-lives. The time to steady state cannot be shortened with a loading dose infusion. However, a loading dose infusion can produce a plasma drug concentration approximately equal to the eventual steady-state concentration (see **Figure 12-4B**). That is, a loading dose infusion will quickly bring the patient's drug concentration to a concentration that approximates the concentration at steady state. In addition, any time the dose or dosing interval is changed, it will take another three to five half-lives to reach a new steady-state concentration. After changing a dosing regimen, remember to allow enough time to reach a new steady-state concentration before repeating plasma drug concentrations.

Calculating a Loading Dose

The loading dose infusion can be calculated from the formula for an intermittent infusion not at steady state as shown in Lesson 5:

$$C_{ss\,peak} = \frac{K_0}{VK}(1 - e^{-Kt})$$

where:

$C_{ss\,peak}$ = desired peak drug concentration at steady state

K_0 = loading dose (in mg) to be infused ÷ duration of infusion (in hours)

V = volume of distribution (population estimate, in liters)

K = elimination rate constant (population estimate, in reciprocal hours)

t = duration of infusion (1 hour)

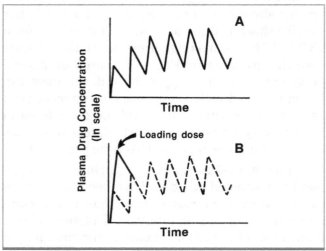

FIGURE 12-4A.
Drug accumulation to steady state without a loading dose.
FIGURE 12-4B.
Concentration versus time simulation for the same aminoglycoside dose preceded by a loading dose.

Clinical Correlate

In Lesson 5, we calculated the loading dose of a drug administered by IV push, $X_0 = C_{0(desired)}V$. This equation assumes a rapid infusion of a drug. Because aminoglycosides are infused over 30 minutes to an hour, the equation below must be used to calculate a loading dose to account for the amount of drug eliminated over the infusion period. The term $(1 - e^{-Kt})$ represents the fraction remaining after (t), the time of infusion.

This equation can be rearranged to isolate K_0 on one side of the equation:

$$K_0 = \frac{C_{ss\,peak}(VK)}{(1 - e^{-Kt})}$$

Patient SG's loading dose infusion can then be calculated:

> 6 mg/L (desired peak) can be used instead of actual peak (6.3 mg/L)

$$\text{Loading Dose} = \frac{(6\ mg/L)(13.9)(0.146\ hr^{-1})}{(1 - e^{-(0.146)(1\ hr)})}$$

$$= \frac{12.2\ mg/hr}{0.136}$$

$$= 89.6\ mg/hr$$

By this method, the loading dose infusion can be determined *before* the maintenance dose is calculated, but only with a complicated equation.

Another, easier loading dose formula that requires calculation of the maintenance dose first is shown below:

> maintenance dose

$$\text{loading dose} = \frac{K_0}{(1 - e^{-K\tau})}$$

where:

K_0 = estimated maintenance dose expressed as mg/hr

$1/(1 - e^{-K\tau})$ = accumulation factor at steady state (see **Equation 4-2**)

τ = dosing interval at which estimated maintenance dose is given

With this loading dose formula you are, in essence, multiplying the desired maintenance dose by a factor (the accumulation factor) representing the sum of the fraction of doses that have accumulated at steady state. This factor describes how much the concentration will be increased at steady state.

These two formulas are derivations of each other, as shown below. Begin with our general formula and rearrange it to solve for K_0:

$$C_{ss\,peak} = \frac{K_0(1 - e^{-Kt})}{VK(1 - e^{-K\tau})}$$

$$K_0 = \frac{C_{ss\,peak}(VK)}{(1 - e^{-Kt})}$$

> This corresponds to the circled portion of the next equation.

The first numerator/denominator combination in the above equation is also found in the equation for the loading dose:

$$\text{loading dose} = \left(\frac{C_{ss\,peak}(VK)}{(1 - e^{-Kt})}\right)$$

Therefore, the right-hand term of this loading dose equation can be substituted into the general equation for K_0 (**Step 1** below) and then rearranged (**Step 2** below) to then yield our other loading dose formula:

Step 1: $K_0 = (\text{loading dose})(1 - e^{-K\tau})$

Step 2: $(\text{loading dose}) = \dfrac{K_0}{(1 - e^{-K\tau})}$

For patient SG, the loading dose should be as follows:

$$\text{loading dose} = \frac{K_0}{(1 - e^{-K\tau})}$$

$$= \frac{74.3 \text{ mg/hr}}{1 - e^{(-146 \text{ hr}^{-1})(12 \text{ hr})}}$$

$$= \frac{74.3 \text{ mg/hr}}{1 - 0.173}$$

$$= \frac{74.3 \text{ mg/hr}}{0.827}$$

$$= 89.8 \text{ mg}$$

Both loading dose formulas will give approximately the same number. However, some prefer the loading dose equation that requires the maintenance dose to be calculated first because it is simple. Patient SG should receive a loading dose of 90 mg (rounded) followed by a maintenance dose of 80 mg every 12 hours beginning 12 hours after the loading dose. The 90-mg loading dose should give an approximate C_p of 6.47 mg/L. Based on the estimated parameters, steady state should be attained in three to five half-lives (3 × 4.75 = 14.25 hours; 5 × 4.75 = 23.75 hours). (See **Equation 3-3**.)

CASE 3

To continue with patient SG from Cases 1 and 2, blood was drawn for drug concentration assessment around the fourth dose (i.e., approximately 5 minutes before dose was due and immediately after the 1-hour dose infusion). C_{peak} and C_{trough} were determined as follows:

- 7:55 AM C_{trough} was 0.2 mg/L (before fourth dose)
- 8–9 AM   80-mg dose was infused over 1 hour
- 9 AM C_{peak} was 4.2 mg/L (after fourth dose)

In this example, the trough level was taken just before the fourth dose was given, and the peak level was obtained just after the fourth dose was given. This procedure is normal and appropriate if the concentrations are at steady state. **Figure 12-5** illustrates that, at steady state, C_{trough} from a trough and peak is equal to the C_{trough} from a peak and trough because all C_{trough} and all C_{peak} values are the same. We know that if we measured a C_{trough} after the C_{peak}, it would equal the C_{trough} before the C_{peak}. This is not true before steady state is reached. In this case, therefore, when a peak and trough is ordered, the literal interpretation would be as follows:

1. Give the infusion from 8:00 to 9:00 AM.

2. Draw a sample to determine C_{peak} at approximately 9:00 AM.

3. Wait until the end of SG's 12-hour dosing interval (approximately 7:55 PM) to draw a sample prior to the next dose to determine C_{trough}.

In practice, this method is too cumbersome for pharmacy, nursing, and laboratory staff, so usually a trough and peak is drawn once steady state has been attained.

It is recommended that C_{peak} be measured either at the end of a 1-hour infusion, 30 minutes after the end of a 30-minute infusion, or 1 hour after an intramuscular injection. Infusing aminoglycosides over 1 hour allows simpler pharmacokinetic calculations in that the duration of infusion (t) is 1 hour and the infusion rate (K_0) is simply the dose given. Remember that K_0 is expressed as milligrams per hour. So, if the drug is infused over 30 minutes (0.5 hour), then K_0 = dose (mg)/0.5 (hour).

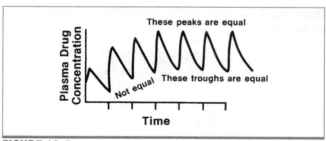

FIGURE 12-5.
Peak and trough concentrations at steady state.

Clinical Correlate

An actual peak and trough, as opposed to a trough and peak, is sometimes ordered on the first (i.e., not at steady state) dose of a drug to estimate volume of distribution and K in a patient whose drug half-life is quite long. (See Lesson 13, Vancomycin, Case Two, for a case on this.) This is possible because, if you remember, K can be calculated at any time point if we have two drug concentration values and the amount of time between them.

Problem 3A. Are patient SG's concentrations of 4.2 mg/L (peak) and 0.2 mg/L (trough) at steady state?

Patient SG's concentrations were determined around the fourth dose, meaning 36 hours after her first dose. To determine whether these serum values are steady-state concentrations, we must use C_{peak} and C_{trough} to calculate SG's actual K and $T\frac{1}{2}$. These calculations are done in Problem 3C, and the results are 0.277 hr^{-1} for K and 2.5 hours for $T\frac{1}{2}$. Five half-lives would equal 12.5 hours (2.5 × 5), which is less than the 36 hours elapsed. Therefore, these concentrations are considered to be at steady state. If the drug is not at steady state, the predose C_{trough} would be less than the postdose C_{trough} and would overestimate K. If the K is larger (indicating more rapid elimination) verification that C_{peak} and C_{trough} were drawn at correct times to ensure values are appropriate to use for estimating patient specific pharmacokinetic parameters.

Problem 3B. How can you determine when to order drug concentration samples so they are likely to be at steady state?

You want to determine C_{peak} and C_{trough} after the patient is at steady state. Therefore, you must draw blood samples three to five drug half-lives after the first dose. You must estimate the patient's K and $T\frac{1}{2}$ using population estimates as in Case 1 and then multiply the $T\frac{1}{2}$ by three to five. As shown in Lesson 4, after three half-lives, concentrations are 87.5% of steady state, whereas after five half-lives, they are 96.9% of steady state. Use judgment when choosing

three, four, or five half-lives to calculate time to steady state. Plasma concentration sampling should be scheduled to follow the dose that achieves steady state.

For patient SG, the estimated K and $T\frac{1}{2}$ (from Case 1, Problem 1A) were 0.146 hr^{-1} and 4.75 hours, respectively. Therefore, steady state would be reached in 23.6 (5 × 4.75) hours. You could then schedule C_{peak} and C_{trough} determinations at the next dose after 24 hours have elapsed.

Clinical Correlate

By calculating the patient's actual elimination rate (K) and volume of distribution (V), pharmacists can more accurately predict patient-specific pharmacokinetic data, thereby optimizing patient care. Once patient-specific parameters are known, it is important not to continue to use population estimates to adjust dosages or dosage intervals.

Problem 3C. Adjust patient SG's dosing regimen, based on C_{peak} and C_{trough} concentrations, to obtain the desired C_{peak} of 6 mg/L and C_{trough} of 1 mg/L.

Adjustment of patient SG's dose involves using the measured drug concentrations to calculate an actual K and V and then substituting these new values for our initial estimates of K and V, in **Equations 3-2, 5-1, and 12-4**, used in Case 1. The formula for K below comes from a rearrangement of the general equation used to calculate the slope of the natural log of plasma drug concentration versus time line as described in Case 1. Remember that because concentration decreases with time, the slope (and hence, $-K$) is a negative number.

Calculation of SG's Actual Elimination Rate (K)

To calculate K, the equation is as follows:

$$K = -\left(\frac{\ln C_{trough} - \ln C_{peak}}{\tau - t} \right)$$

(See **Equation 3-1.**)

where:

K = elimination rate constant (in reciprocal hours)

C_{trough} = measured trough concentration (0.2 mg/L)

C_{peak} = measured peak concentration (4.2 mg/L)

τ = dosing interval at the time concentrations are obtained (12 hours)

t = duration of infusion (1 hour)

Again, remembering a rule of logarithms:

$$\ln a - \ln b = \ln (a/b)$$

we can simplify this equation for hand-held calculators:

$$K = -\frac{\ln\left(\dfrac{C_{trough}}{C_{peak}}\right)}{\tau - t}$$

This equation version is more calculator-friendly

Either form of this equation may be used to calculate K, as follows:

$$K = -\frac{\ln 0.2 \text{ mg/L} - \ln 4.2 \text{ mg/L}}{12 \text{ hr} - 1 \text{ hr}}$$

$$= -\frac{-1.61 - 1.44}{11}$$

$$= -\frac{-3.05}{11}$$

$$= 0.277$$

Therefore, $K = 0.277 \text{ hr}^{-1}$, compared to 0.146 hr^{-1}, which was our estimate, or:

$$K = -\frac{\ln\left(\dfrac{0.2 \text{ mg/L}}{4.2 \text{ mg/L}}\right)}{12 \text{ hr} - 1 \text{ hr}}$$

$$= -\frac{\ln(0.48)}{11 \text{ hr}}$$

$$= -\frac{-3.04}{11 \text{ hr}}$$

$$= -0.277 \text{ hr}^{-1}$$

Patient SG's actual K of 0.277 hr^{-1} is greater than the estimated value of 0.146 hr^{-1}, so her elimination probably was greater than estimated. Her actual drug half-life ($T\frac{1}{2}$) is 2.5 hours, shorter than the population-estimated $T\frac{1}{2}$ of 4.75 hours:

$$T\tfrac{1}{2} = 0.693/K \quad \text{(See Equation 3-3.)}$$

$$= 0.693/0.277 \text{ hr}^{-1}$$

$$= 2.5 \text{ hours}$$

The formula for K above can also be used to calculate the slope, $-K$, for any two points on the natural log of plasma drug concentration versus time line. For instance, suppose that instead of a C_{peak}, patient SG had a concentration measured at 11:00 AM (2 hours after C_{peak}). This concentration was 2.41 mg/L. You can still calculate her K value as follows (**Figure 12-6**):

$$K = -\frac{\ln 0.2 \text{ mg/L} - \ln 2.41 \text{ mg/L}}{12 \text{ hr} - 1 \text{ hr} - 2 \text{ hr}}$$

$$= -\frac{-1.61 - 0.883}{9}$$

$$= -\frac{-2.493}{9}$$

$$= 0.277$$

Note that this K value is the same as the one calculated with the measured C_{peak} and C_{trough} concentrations.

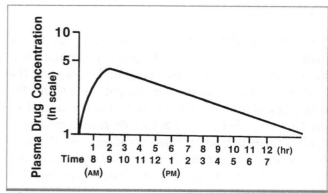

FIGURE 12-6.
K from any two points.

Calculation of SG's Actual Volume of Distribution (V)

Patient SG's actual volume of distribution (V) is calculated with the equation from Case 1. Use the actual C_{peak} and C_{trough} values, dose, and dosing interval.

$$C_{ss\,peak} = \frac{K_0(1-e^{-Kt})}{VK(1-e^{-K\tau})}$$

This equation can also be rearranged to isolate V on one side of the equation if the reader so prefers, although it is not normally necessary.

$$V = \frac{K_0(1-e^{-Kt})}{C_{ss\,peak}K(1-e^{-K\tau})}$$

(See **Equation 5-1**.)

where:

t = the duration of the infusion

τ = dosing interval at the time concentrations are obtained

In this case, some of the variables substituted in this equation are different from those used when initially estimating a dose. The changes from Case 1 are shown here in **bold** type:

$C_{ss\,peak} = C_{peak}$ measured at steady state

K_0 = **maintenance dose infused at time C_{peak} and C_{trough} were measured**

V = **patient's actual volume of distribution that you are trying to determine based on C_{peak} and C_{trough} values**

K = **actual elimination rate constant calculated from patient's C_{peak} and C_{trough} values**

t = duration of infusion (hours)

τ = **patient's dosing interval at time C_{peak} and C_{trough} were measured**

In patient SG's case, she received a maintenance dose of 80 mg every 12 hours, with subsequent C_{peak} and C_{trough} concentrations of 4.2 and 0.2 mg/L, respectively. Her K value from these concentrations was 0.277 hr^{-1}.

If we substitute these values into the previous equation, we can solve for patient SG's actual V:

$$4.2\ mg/L = \frac{(80\ mg/hr)(1-e^{-(0.277\ hr^{-1})(1\ hr)})}{(V)(0.277\ hr^{-1})(1-e^{-(0.277\ hr^{-1})(12\ hr)})}$$

$$4.2\ mg/L = \frac{(80)(0.242)}{(V)(0.277)(0.964)}$$

$$1.122\,(V) = 19.36$$

$$V = 17.3\ L$$

Patient SG's V value of 17.3 L (which equals 0.298 L/kg IBW) is larger than estimated and would make her actual C_{peak} and C_{trough} lower than what was estimated using the smaller Vd.

Now that we have calculated the patient's actual K and V, we need to recalculate the dose and dosing interval. We must first calculate the new dosing interval (τ) and then calculate the new dose

$$\tau = \frac{1}{-K}(\ln C_{trough\,(desired)} - \ln C_{peak\,(desired)}) + t$$

where t is the duration of infusion in hours and K is the actual elimination rate calculated from patient's peak and trough values, and *not* the estimated value of 0.147 hr^{-1}. It is important to note that when we calculate our new dosing interval, the values we insert into the equation are our desired levels and not the levels reported by the laboratory on the dose of 80 mg every 12 hours. Then:

$$\tau = \frac{1}{-0.277\ hr^{-1}}(\ln 1\ mg/L - \ln 6\ mg/L) + 1\ hr$$

$$= (-3.61)(0-1.79) + 1\ hr$$

$$= (-3.61)(-1.79) + 1\ hr$$

$$= 6.46\ hr + 1\ hr = 7.46\ hours, \text{ rounded to every 8 hours}$$

(See **Equation 12-4**.)

This adjusted τ should be compared with our initial τ estimate of 13.18 hours from Case 1, Problem 1A. Because our real τ is shorter than previously estimated, C_{peak} and C_{trough} values less than those predicted also would be expected. In other words, we initially administered a dose every 12 hours when, in actuality, the patient needed a dose every 7.5 hours.

This calculated dosing interval of 7.5 hours may be rounded up to 8 hours for ease in scheduling.

Problem 3D. How is patient SG's adjusted maintenance dose now calculated?

Once again, we shall use the general equation from Case 1 and solve for K_0. This time, we shall replace the estimates of K and V with the calculated (actual) values and use the adjusted τ value of 8 hours:

$$C_{ss\,peak} = \frac{K_0(1-e^{-Kt})}{VK(1-e^{-K\tau})}$$

(See **Equation 5-1.**)
where:

$C_{ss\,peak}$ = desired steady-state C_{peak} (6 mg/L)

K_0 = drug infusion rate (also adjusted maintenance dose you are trying to calculate, in milligrams per hour)

V = actual volume of distribution determined from patient's measured C_{peak} and C_{trough} values, in liters

K = actual elimination rate constant calculated from patient's measured C_{peak} and C_{trough} values, in reciprocal hours

t = infusion time, in hours

τ = adjusted dosing interval rounded to a practical number

The following equation shows the calculation of the new maintenance dose:

$$6\ mg/L = \frac{K_0}{(17.25\ L)(0.277\ hr^{-1})}\left[\frac{(1-e^{-0.277\ hr^{-1}(1\ hr)})}{(1-e^{-0.277\ hr^{-1}(8\ hr)})}\right]$$

$$6\ mg/L = \frac{K_0}{(4.78)}\frac{0.242}{0.891}$$

$$25.5 = K_0\ 0.242$$

$$K_0 = 105.6\ mg,\ rounded\ to\ 100\ mg$$

If 105.6 mg gives a peak of 6 mg/L, then our rounded dose of 100 mg will give a peak of 5.7 mg/L.

$$\frac{100\ mg}{105.6\ mg} = \frac{X}{6\ mg/L}$$

$$X = 5.68\ mg/L$$

Problem 3E. If we give 100 mg every 8 hours, what will be our steady-state C_{trough}?

If we give 105.6 mg exactly every 7.5 hours, our C_{trough} would be precisely as desired: 1 mg/L. But because we rounded our dosing interval and adjusted the maintenance dose down to practical numbers, we must calculate the steady-state C_{trough} that will result. Our roundings could change our actual $C_{trough\ values}$.

This C_{trough} calculation is performed similarly to the one in Case 1, Problem 1B:

$$C_{ss\,trough} = C_{ss\,peak}e^{-Kt'}$$

(See **Equation 3-2.**)

$$= 5.68\ mg/L\ [e^{-(0.277hr^{-1})(\tau-1\ hour)}]$$

$$= 5.68\ mg/L\ [e^{-(0.277)(7)}]$$

$$= 5.68\ (e^{-1.939})$$

$$= 5.68\ (0.144)$$

$$= 0.82\ mg/L$$

So, in this case, a dose of 100 mg every 8 hours will give a steady-state C_{trough} of 0.82 mg/L, which is still well below the usual maximum acceptable trough concentration of 2 mg/L.

CASE 4

Four days later, another set of peak and trough concentrations are obtained. Patient SG has been receiving 100 mg every 8 hours. However, her renal function has declined, as seen by an increase in SCr from 1.12 mg/dL at baseline to 1.91 mg/dL today. C_{peak} and C_{trough} were determined as follows:

- 7:55 AM C_{trough} was 2.8 mg/L.
- 8:00 to 9:00 AM   A 100-mg dose was infused over 1 hour.
- 9:00 AM C_{peak} was 9.6 mg/L.

A new adjusted K, τ, V, and maintenance dose (K_0) were calculated using the methods described in

Case 3. These values are shown below; see if you obtain the same numbers:

new $K = 0.176$ hr^{-1}

new $T\frac{1}{2} = 3.94$ hours

new $V = 12.6$ L

new $\tau = 11.2$ (rounded to 12 hours)

new maintenance dose (K_0) = 70 mg every 12 hours (72.7 mg rounded down to 70

new trough concentration = 0.834 mg/L (using the expected peak of 5.78 from the rounded down dose of 70 mg rather than the 6 mg/L peak we used to calculate the 72.7 mg dose)

Problem 4A. Because patient SG's C_{trough} on 100 mg every 8 hours is now too high (2.8 mg/L), how long would you wait before beginning the new dose of 70 mg every 12 hours?

Before switching, you must wait for the patient's C_{trough} to decrease to approximately 1 mg/L. Therefore, the dose should be held for some time before you begin a new lower dose. The formula for calculating the number of hours to hold the dose is as follows:

$$C_{ss \text{ trough (desired)}} = C_{ss \text{ trough}}e^{-Kt'}$$

(See **Equation 3-2.**)

where t' is the amount of time to hold the dose after the end of the 8-hour dosing interval.

This formula is an application of the general formula described in Case 1:

$$C = C_0e^{-Kt} \quad \text{(See Equation 3-2.)}$$

which means:

concentration at a time = previous concentration
$\times$ fraction of dose remaining

In patient SG's case:

$$1 \text{ mg/L} = (2.8 \text{ mg/L}) \, e^{-0.176 \text{ hr}^{-1}(t')}$$

$$0.357 \text{ mg/L} = e^{-0.176(t')}$$

Next, take the natural log of both sides:

$$\ln 0.357 = \ln (e^{-0.176(t')})$$

$$-1.03 = -0.176(t')$$

$$t' = 5.85 \text{ hours}$$

Thus, we should hold patient SG's dose for an additional 5.9 (round to 6) hours after the next C_{trough} time and then begin her new dose. The next C_{trough} time for this patient would be 3:45 PM, 7.75 hours after her last dose (8:00 AM). The C_{trough} at this time, at steady state, would also be expected to be approximately 2.8 mg/L. We would need to hold the regularly scheduled 4:00 PM dose for 6 hours, until 10:00 PM, at which time we would then begin her new dose of 70 mg every 12 hours.

The calculation of the time to hold a dose can be illustrated (**Figure 12-7**) by plotting patient SG's C_{peak} and C_{trough} values on semilog graph paper and then extending the line connecting them until it reaches our desired C_{trough} of 1 mg/L. You can then count the hours needed to reach this 1-mg/L concentration and hold the dose accordingly.

Another, and often more practical, way to estimate the time to hold a patient's dose is by examining the half-life. By definition, the drug concentration decreases by one-half over each half-life. In the following paragraph, we can then estimate how many drug half-lives to wait for the concentration to approach our desired 1 mg/L.

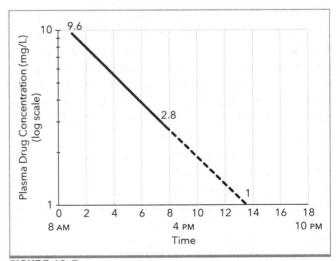

FIGURE 12-7.
Calculation of the time to hold a dose by plotting levels on semilog paper.

For patient SG (trough of 2.8 mg/L and $T\frac{1}{2}$ of 3.94 hours), the concentration will drop to 1.4 mg/L (half of 2.8) in one half-life of approximately 4 hours (3.94 hours to be exact) and then drop to 0.7 mg/L (half of 1.4) in another 4 hours. Therefore, we could hold patient SG's doses for approximately two half-lives (4 × 2 = 8 hours) before beginning our new dose. This would certainly put us below the desired level of 1 mg/L (which is where we wanted to be to restart the new dose in the above calculation, but allows us to use more simplified math with half-lives rather than longer, more specific formulas to determine when the level will be exactly 1 mg/L for restarting therapy.

In patient SG's case, another dose was given from 8:00 to 9:00 AM, after the C_{trough} of 2.8 was obtained at 7:55 AM. Therefore, her next C_{trough} will occur at approximately 3:45 PM (shortly before the next scheduled dose). We need to hold this dose for an additional 8 hours from the time of the last time point when the concentration would be 2.8 mg/L and then begin our new regimen of 70 mg every 12 hours. (i.e., 8 hours, and approximately two half-lives) after the last dose, the concentration would be 0.7 mg/L and we could begin our new dose. In this scenario, that would be 12 midnight.

Extended-Interval Aminoglycoside Dosing

An alternative method to conventional dosing of aminoglycosides is extended-interval dosing, which is administering large doses over extended intervals (24, 36, or 48 hours) based on the patient's renal function. The theory behind this approach is that administering large doses produces higher peak serum concentrations than achieved with conventional dosing and, thus, increases the peak serum concentration to bacterial minimum inhibitory concentration (MIC) ratio (Peak/MIC).

Additionally, administering drug at an extended-interval creates an aminoglycoside-free period that reduces accumulation of aminoglycoside in tissues such as the inner ear and kidney, resulting in decreased drug-related toxicity. It is known that uptake of aminoglycosides by tissues is a saturable process. Administering smaller doses at a more frequent interval does not saturate this process and ultimately leads to higher tissue concentrations than those achieved with extended-interval dosing.

Thus, this latter dosing method may actually result in less toxicity to the patient. This drug-free interval may also decrease the development of adaptive resistance.

Several characteristics of aminoglycosides as a class enable these drugs to be administered by the extended-interval method. Aminoglycosides demonstrate concentration-dependent bactericidal action such that as the concentration of the drug in the serum increases, the rate and extent of bacterial killing increases. Because of this property, it is suggested that the optimal serum peak aminoglycoside concentration to bacterial MIC ratio is >10:1. It appears that bactericidal activity occurs in a biphasic fashion; initially, bacteria are killed at a very rapid rate in a concentration-dependent manner. After a time frame of approximately 2 hours, the rate of bacterial killing declines, which may be due to bacterial adaptive resistance.

Aminoglycosides also exhibit a long postantibiotic effect (PAE) of approximately 4–6 hours. Postantibiotic effect is defined as the amount of time that drug concentration falls below the MIC before regrowth of the bacteria resumes.[17-20] PAE is generally thought to increase with high peak concentrations of aminoglycosides.

A third characteristic of aminoglycosides that support extended-interval dosing is a decrease in the development of adaptive resistance. Adaptive resistance results in decreased efficacy of an antibiotic and the emergence of resistant organisms. It is a reversible process if a sufficient drug-free interval between doses is allowed.[20] Administering doses every 24–48 hours rather than every 8 hours would allow for more drug-free time over the course of a day and potentially allow bacteria to return closer to baseline susceptibility for these agents.

Situations in which extended-interval aminoglycoside dosing probably should *not* be used include pregnancy, ascites, or significant third spacing, hemodynamic instability, unstable or poor renal function (CrCl <20 mL/min), and burns >20%. Numerous methods have been proposed for extended-interval aminoglycoside dosing and monitoring. Several of these methods are presented here.

Method 1

The Sanford Guide to Antimicrobial Therapy 2017 recommends that for gentamicin and tobramycin, the dose in patients with a CrCl >80 mL/min is 5.1 mg/kg (7 mg/kg for seriously ill patients) every 24 hours, and for amikacin, 15 mg/kg every 24 hours.[16,21] A patient's IBW is used in these calculations unless actual weight exceeds ideal weight by ≥30%. In this case, an AdjBW is used [**Equation 9-3:** AdjBW = IBW + (0.4 × (TBW − IBW).] Goal serum peak concentrations from these doses are 16–24 mcg/mL and 56–64 mcg/mL for gentamicin/tobramycin and amikacin, respectively. Expected trough levels for all three drugs are <1 mcg/mL. **Table 12-3** lists recommended doses in patients with a reduced CrCl.[16]

Method 2

A second method of extended-interval aminoglycoside dosing consists of administering a dose of 7 mg/kg of gentamicin or tobramycin at an interval based on the patient's CrCl ≥60 mL/min, every 24 hours; 40–59 mL/min, every 36 hours; 20–39 mL/min, every 48 hours. For patients with a CrCl <20 mL/min, it is recommended to monitor serial serum concentrations and administer a subsequent dose once the serum level is <1 mcg/mL. With the first dose, a 6- to 14-hour (often 8- to -12 hour) postinfusion serum level is measured and plotted on a once-daily aminoglycoside nomogram (**Figure 12-8**) to determine if the dosage interval should be altered for future doses.[19]

TABLE 12-3. Recommended Extended-Interval Dosing in Patients with Declining Renal Function[21]

Creatinine Clearance	Gentamicin/ Tobramycin	Amikacin
80–60 mL/min	4 mg/kg q 24 hr	12 mg/kg q 24 hr
60–40 mL/min	3.5 mg/kg q 24 hr	7.5 mg/kg q 24 hr
40–30 mL/min	2.5 mg/kg q 24 hr	4 mg/kg q 24 hr
30–20 mL/min	4 mg/kg q 48 hr	7.5 mg/kg q 48 hr
20–10 mL/min	3 mg/kg q 48 hr	4 mg/kg q 48 hr
<10 mL/min	2 mg/kg q 72 hr*	3 mg/kg q 72 hr*

*For patients receiving dialysis, these doses should be administered after dialysis.

Source: The Sanford Guide to Antimicrobial Therapy. 47th ed. Sperryville, VA: Antimicrobial Therapy, Inc.; 2017:217.

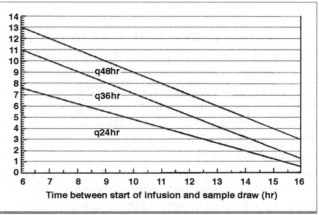

FIGURE 12-8.
Once-daily aminoglycoside adjustment nomogram (gentamicin or tobramycin, 7 mg/kg).

Source: Reproduced with permission from Nicolau DP, Freeman CD, Belliveau PP, et al. Experience with a once-daily aminoglycoside program administered to 2,184 adult patients. *Antimicrob Agents Chemother.* 1995;39(3):650–5.

Method 3

A third method consists of administering an initial gentamicin or tobramycin dose of 7 mg/kg, or 5 mg/kg for urinary tract infections, or 15 mg/kg amikacin followed by measuring a serum concentration 6–14 hours after the start of the infusion.[22] This measured value is then plotted on a once-daily aminoglycoside nomogram, and the dosing interval is determined. Because this nomogram is based on a dose of 7 mg/kg, if a smaller dose is administered, the measured serum level should be multiplied by a factor equal to 7 divided by the mg/kg dose given. For example, if a patient is treated with the 5 mg/kg dose, 7 divided by 5 equals 1.4, which is then multiplied by the measured serum concentration. This product is plotted on a once-daily aminoglycoside nomogram. For amikacin serum concentrations, plot one half the measured concentration on the nomogram. In situations in which the measured, or adjusted, value falls on one of the three lines, choose the longer interval for administering future doses. Body weight used for these dosage calculations is the patient's actual weight. In cases in which the patient's actual weight is >30% over their IBW, the AdjBW should be calculated and used in determining the dose. Initial dosing intervals are as follows: for CrCl >60 mL/min, every 24 hours; for CrCl 40–59 mL/min, every 36 hours; and for CrCl 20–39 mL/min, every 48 hours. If estimated CrCl is <20 mL/min, do not use extended-interval aminoglycoside dosing.

Method 4

An alternative method to those described above consists of using traditional or conventional dosing equations for calculating extended-interval doses. Goal serum peak and trough concentrations utilized should be 20–30 mcg/mL and <1 mcg/mL, respectively, for gentamicin and tobramycin. A minimum dosing interval of 24 hours is selected; increases in this value should be used in cases of declining renal function. The same equations for estimating K, V, dosing interval, and calculating the maintenance dose as used in traditional dosing methods are then applied.

Method 5

A fifth method is one that may be used in the treatment of patients with cystic fibrosis.[22] An initial dose of 10 mg/kg tobramycin or 20 mg/kg amikacin is administered over a 1-hour interval. Dosing weight is as described for Method 4. Serum levels are drawn 1 and 5 hours after the end of the infusion. From these two levels, one may calculate the patient's elimination rate and half-life. For patients with a half-life between 2 and 4 hours, administer the drug every 24 hours; for serum half-lives >4–6 hours, administer every 36 hours; for half-lives >6–8 hours, give every 48 hours. If calculated half-life is >8 hours, convert the patient to traditional dosing. If the calculated half-life is <2 hours, consider changing the patient to tobramycin 7 mg/kg every 12 hours, or amikacin 15 mg/kg every 12 hours. For these latter two regimens, consider monitoring half-life from serum levels to verify that the patient's half-life remains <2 hours.

CASE 5

JK is a 50-year-old female nursing home resident with a history of recurrent pneumonia and multiple courses of antibiotics over the last few months who is admitted to the hospital for exacerbation of chronic obstructive pulmonary disease. The patient has thick green sputum, low oxygen saturations, and a chest x-ray demonstrates bilateral lower lobe infiltration. Based on her past history, she is suspected of having *Pseudomonas aeruginosa* pneumonia. She is 5'5" tall and weighs 135 lb. Her admission SCr is 1 mg/dL.

Problem 5A. Calculate an extended-interval dose of tobramycin for this patient according to *The Sanford Guide to Antimicrobial Therapy 2017*.

The first step in solving this problem is to determine JK's creatinine clearance. Using the Cockcroft–Gault equation, we can determine this to be 61 mL/min.

$$CrCl_{female} \; mL/min = \frac{(140 - age)(BW)(0.85)}{72 \times SCr}$$

$$= \frac{(140 - 50)(57)(0.85)}{72 \times 1}$$

$$= 61 \, mL/min$$

Because *Pseudomonas aeruginosa* pneumonia is a serious infection, according to the *The Sanford Guide to Antimicrobial Therapy 2017*, we should administer 7 mg/kg tobramycin times her IBW of 57 kg every 24 hours. This results in a dose of 399 mg (round off to 400 mg) every 24 hours.

Problem 5B. According to the *The Sanford Guide to Antimicrobial Therapy 2017* in critically ill patients, a peak serum concentration should be drawn on the first dose of the aminoglycoside. The laboratory reports that JK has a peak serum tobramycin level of 23.2 mcg/mL. A serum trough level is also drawn and is reported as 0.8 mcg/mL. Based on these peak and trough levels, should JK's tobramycin dose be changed?

The Sanford Guide to Antimicrobial Therapy 2017 states that serum peak tobramycin levels should be between 16 and 24 mcg/mL, and trough levels should be <1 mcg/mL. JK's values are within these ranges; therefore, no changes in her dose are necessary at this time.

CASE 6

AM is a 32-year-old male with pyelonephritis due to *Klebsiella*, which is resistant to most antibiotics tested but susceptible to aminoglycosides. The physician orders gentamicin therapy with pharmacy to dose. He is 6 feet tall and weighs 175 lb. His current SCr is 0.85 mg/dL.

Problem 6A. Calculate an extended interval gentamicin dose for AM using the Hartford nomogram method (method 2 above).

Using the Cockcroft–Gault equation we can determine that AM's creatinine clearance is 137 mL/min. Note that for this patient IBW is the correct weight to use.

$$CrCl_{male} \ mL/min = \frac{(140 - age)(BW)}{72 \times SCr}$$

$$= \frac{(140 - 32)(77.6)}{72 \times 0.85}$$

$$= 137 \ mL/min$$

According to the Hartford nomogram method, he should receive 7 mg/kg every 24 hours. As stated previously an adjusted body weight is used if the patient is more than 30% above IBW. In this case the patient is not, so actual weight is used for empiric dose calculation:

$$IBW = 50 \ kg + 2.3 \ kg \ for \ each \ inch \ over \ 5 \ feet \ in \ height$$

$$IBW = 50 \ kg + 2.3(12) = 77.6 \ kg$$

$$Actual \ weight = \frac{175 \ lb}{2.2 \ lb/kg} = 79.5 \ kg$$

$$Percent \ above \ IBW = \frac{(ABW - IBW)(100)}{IBW}$$

$$= \frac{(79.5 - 77.6)(100)}{77.6} = 2.4\%$$

$$7 \ mg/kg \times 77.6 \ kg = 543 \ mg \ (round \ to \ 540 \ mg)$$

Clinical judgment should be used when performing these calculations in practice.

Problem 6B. Eleven hours after the beginning of AM's therapy, a serum gentamicin level is drawn and reported as 2.5 mcg/mL. Should AM's gentamicin therapy be adjusted?

Because an 11-hour postdose level of 2.5 mcg/mL falls within the range for 24-hour dosing, AM's gentamicin therapy does not require adjustment at this time.

Problem 6C. Calculate an extended-interval gentamicin dose for this patient using conventional or traditional dosing equations.

Step 1. Round the CrCl of 116 mL/min to 100 mL/min. Note, the practice of rounding CrCl values above 100 mL/min down to 100 mL/min is controversial and not universally agreed on by all practitioners; therefore, clinical judgment should be used.

Step 2. Estimate the patient's elimination rate constant.

$$K = 0.00293 \times CrCl + 0.014$$

$$= 0.00293 \ (100 \ mL/min) + 0.014$$

$$= 0.307 \ hr^{-1}$$

Step 3. Estimate the patient's volume of distribution.

$$V = 0.24 \ L/kg \ IBW$$

$$= 0.24 \ L/kg \times 77.6 \ kg$$

$$= 18.6 \ L$$

Step 4. Choose a desired steady-state peak serum concentration.
- The recommended range is 20–30 mcg/mL.
- For illustration purposes, we will choose 25 mcg/mL.

Step 5. Choose a desired steady-state trough serum concentration.
- The recommended value is <1 mcg/mL.
- For illustration purposes, we will choose 0.9 mcg/mL.

Step 6. Calculate a desired dosing interval.
- Because this method of dosing is extended interval, a minimum dosing interval of 24 hours should be used. This step is to determine if a patient should receive a dose at a 36- or 48-hour interval.

$$\tau = -1/K \ \times \ (\ln \ trough - \ln \ peak) + t$$

$$= -1/0.307 \times (\ln 0.9 - \ln 25) + 1$$

$$= 11.8 \ hours, \ which \ we \ will \ round \ up \ to \ 24 \ hours$$

Step 7. Calculate a maintenance dose to give the desired peak and trough concentrations.

$$C_{ss\,peak} = \frac{K_0(1-e^{-kt})}{VK(1-e^{-k\tau})}$$

$$25 \text{ mcg/mL} = \frac{K_0(1-e^{-0.307(1)})}{18.6L \times 0.307^{-1}(1-e^{-0.307(24)})}$$

$$K_0 = 540.4 \text{ mg q 24 hr (round to 540 mg)}$$

CASE 7

A 67-year-old female, AC, is involved in a motor vehicle accident resulting in multiple injuries. She undergoes surgical correction of her injuries and postoperatively is admitted to the intensive care unit requiring mechanical ventilation. On hospital day 7, her chest x-ray worsens, and sputum cultures isolate *E. coli* sensitive to amikacin. Renal function has remained stable with a SCr of 0.67 mg/dL. She is 5'4" and weighs 140 lb.

Problem 7A. This case represents an example of a hospital-acquired, or nosocomial, infection. Calculate an appropriate dose of amikacin for AC using dosing recommendations suggested in method 3.

The first step in solving this problem is to calculate her CrCl:

$$CrCl_{female} \text{ mL/min} = \frac{(140 - age)(BW)(0.85)}{72 \times SCr}$$

$$\frac{(140 - 67)(54.7)(0.85)}{72 \times 1}$$

$$= 47 \text{ mL/min}$$

> Notice that the SCr of <1 (i.e., 0.67) is rounded up to 1.00 for calculation purposes

According to the recommendations in method 3, she should receive 15 mg/kg as a single dose with a random serum level drawn 6–12 hours after this dose. The patient's actual weight is greater than ideal but is less than 20% above ideal body weight so ideal weight will be used in dose calculations.

$$IBW = 45.5 \text{ kg} + 2.3 \text{ kg for each inch over 5 feet in height}$$

$$IBW = 45.5 \text{ kg} + 2.3(4) = 54.7 \text{ kg}$$

$$Actual \text{ weight} = \frac{140 \text{ lb}}{2.2 \text{ lb/kg}} = 63.6 \text{ kg}$$

$$Percent \text{ above IBW} = \frac{(ABW - IBW)(100)}{IBW}$$

$$16.3\% = \frac{(63.6 - 54.7)(100)}{54.7}$$

She receives an initial dose of 15 mg/kg × 54.7 kg = 819 mg (rounded to 820.5 mg).

Note: Rounding SCr values up to 1 mg/dL is controversial and not universally accepted as the best practice when estimating CrCl values. It was done in this case to use as an example, but some literature suggests that using actual creatinine values (even in elderly patients) yields more accurate values than rounding up to 1 mg/dL.[6] Clinical judgment should be used when performing these calculations in practice.

Problem 7B. Ten hours after receiving her initial dose, a random amikacin level is 17 mcg/mL. Calculate an appropriate amikacin dosing interval for this patient.

Amikacin levels from an extended-interval dose are to be interpreted using an established once-daily aminoglycoside dosing nomogram. If we use the nomogram in Figure 12-8, it is necessary to divide the reported amikacin level by 2, and this number is then plotted on the nomogram (17 mcg/mL divided by 2 = 8.5 mcg/mL). Plotting this value on a once-daily aminoglycoside dosing nomogram demonstrates a dosing interval of every 48 hours. Therefore, this patient should receive amikacin 820 mg every 48 hours.

References

1. Levey AS, Bosch JP, Lewis JB, et al. A more accurate method to estimate glomerular filtration rate from serum creatinine: a new prediction equation. Modification of Diet in Renal Disease Study Group. *Ann Intern Med.* 1999;130(6):461–70.

2. Alagiakrishnan K, Senthilselvan A. Low agreement between the modified diet and renal disease formula and the Cockcroft–Gault formula for assessing chronic kidney disease in cognitively impaired elderly outpatients. *Postgraduate Medicine.* 2010;122(6):41–5.

3. Myers GL, Miller WG, Coresh J, et al. Recommendations for improving serum creatinine measurement: a report from the laboratory working group of the national kidney disease education program. *Clin Chem.* 2006;52(1):5–18.

4. Inker LA, Schmid CH, Tighiouart H, et al. Estimating glomerular filtration rate from serum creatinine and cystatin C. *N Engl J Med.* 2012;367(1):20–9.

5. Spruill WJ, Wade WE, Cobb HH. Estimating glomerular filtration rate with a modification of diet in renal disease equation: implications for pharmacy. *Am J Health-Syst Pharm.* 2007;64(6):652–60.

6. Dowling TC, Wang E, Ferrucci L, Sorkin JD. Glomerular filtration rate equations overestimate creatinine clearance in older individuals enrolled in the Baltimore longitudinal study on aging: impact on renal drug dosing. *Pharmacotherapy.* 2013;33(9):912–21.

7. Cartet-Farnier E, Goutelle-Audibert LG, Maire P, et al. Implications of using the MDRD or CKD-EPI equation for estimating renal function and drug dosage adjustment in elderly patients. *Fundam Clin Pharmacol.* 2017;31(1):110–19.

8. Khanal A, Peterson GM, Jose MD, Castelino RL. Comparison of equations for dosing of medications in renal impairment. *Nephrology.* 2017;22(6):470–7.

9. Higdon EA, Kimmons LA, Duhart Jr BT, Hudson JQ. Disagreement in estimates of kidney function for drug dosing in obese patients. *J Pharm Pract.* 2017;Jan 1:897190017737895.

10. Delanaye P, Guerber F, Scheen A, et al. Discrepancies between the Cockcroft-Gault and chronic kidney disease epidemiology (CKD-EPI) equations: implications for refining drug dose adjustment strategies. *Clin Pharmacokinet.* 2017;56(2):193–205.

11. Cockcroft DW, Gault MH. Prediction of creatinine clearance from serum creatinine. *Nephron.* 1976;16(1):31–41.

12. Winter MA, Guhr KN, Berg GM. Impact of various body weights and serum creatinine concentrations on the bias and accuracy of the Cockcroft-Gault equation. *Pharmacotherapy.* 2012;32(7):604–12.

13. Traynor AM, Nafziger AN, Bertino JS. Aminoglycoside dosing weight correction factors for patients of various body sizes. *Antimicrob Agents Chemother.* 1995;39(2):545–8.

14. Wurst R, Itokazu G, Rodvold K. Antimicrobial dosing in obese patients. *Clin Infect Dis.* 1997;25(1):112–8.

15. Dager WE. Aminoglycoside pharmacokinetics: volume of distribution in specific adult patient subgroups. *Ann Pharmacother.* 1994; 28(7–8):944–51.

16. Aminoglycoside once-daily and multiple daily dosing regimens. In: Gilbert DN, Eliopoulos GM, Chambers HF, et al., eds. *The Sanford Guide to Antimicrobial Therapy.* 47rd ed. Sperryville, VA: Antimicrobial Therapy, Inc.; 2017:117.

17. Maglio D, Nightingale CH, Nicolau DP, et al. Extended interval aminoglycoside dosing: from concept to clinic. *Int J Antimicrob Agents.* 2002;19(4):341–8.

18. Freeman CD, Nicolau DP, Belliveau PP, et al. Once-daily dosing of aminoglycosides: review and recommendations for clinical practice. *J Antimicrob Chemother.* 1997;39(6):677–86.

19. Nicolau DP, Freeman CD, Belliveau PP, et al. Experience with a once-daily aminoglycoside program administered to 2,184 adult patients. *Antimicrob Agents Chemother.* 1995;39(3):650–5.

20. Barclay ML, Begg EJ. Aminoglycoside adaptive resistance: importance for effective dosage regimens. *Drugs.* 2001;61(6):713–21.

21. Dosage of antimicrobial drugs in adult patients with renal impairment. In: Gilbert DN, Eliopoulos GM, Chambers HF, et al., eds. *The Sanford Guide to Antimicrobial Therapy*. 47rd ed. Sperryville, VA: Antimicrobial Therapy, Inc.; 2017:217.

22. The Nebraska Medical Center. Pharmacokinetic Training Packet for Pharmacists (2012). https://www.nebraskamed.com/sites/default/files/documents/for-providers/asp/pk_training packet_2012.pdf. Accessed January 29, 2018.

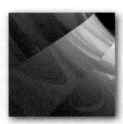

Discussion Points

D-1. In Case 1, Problem 1A, suppose SG was admitted to the hospital with gram-negative pneumonia. How would your maintenance dose differ in this patient to achieve a C_{peak} of 8 mg/L and a C_{trough} of 1 mg/L?

D-2. How would your loading dose differ for patient SG in Discussion Point 1 to achieve an approximate peak plasma concentration of 8 mg/L?

D-3. Steady-state peak and trough serum concentrations achieved with the maintenance dose you calculated in Discussion Point 1 were reported by the laboratory as peak = 6.8 mg/L, and trough = 1.8 mg/L. Calculate a new maintenance dose that will give you the desired peak and trough concentrations of 8 mg/L and 1 mg/L, respectively.

D-4. Calculate an extended-interval aminoglycoside dose for SG for a diagnosis of gram-negative pneumonia.

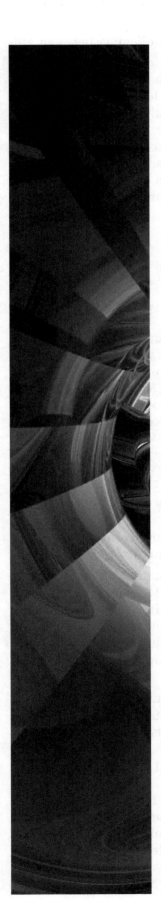

Vancomycin

In this lesson, Cases 1–4 focus on pharmacokinetic calculations for the antibiotic vancomycin. Before beginning, however, a few key points about vancomycin should be reviewed. Vancomycin is a drug most commonly used for methicillin-resistant *Staphylococcus aureus* (MRSA) and enterococci (group D *Streptococcus*) infections. For systemic infections, vancomycin is given by the intravenous (IV) route and is usually administered by intermittent infusion; only the IV route is considered in this lesson. Oral vancomycin is used for treatment of *Clostridium difficile* infection, but dose calculations and pharmacokinetic monitoring are not required when given by the oral route for this indication. To prevent an infusion-related adverse reaction called *red man syndrome*, an important consideration with IV vancomycin is the rate of infusion. Recommended infusion times are at least 1 hour and longer for larger doses (e.g., 1.5 or 2 g). Specific recommendations are given in "Therapeutic Monitoring of Vancomycin in Adult Patients: A Consensus Review of the American Society of Health-System Pharmacists, the Infectious Diseases Society of America, and the Society of Infectious Diseases Pharmacists."[1]

Pharmacokinetically, vancomycin is an example of a two-compartment model, a concept that is discussed in Lesson 6. After IV administration, vancomycin displays a pronounced distribution phase (α phase) (**Figure 13-1**) while the drug equilibrates between plasma and tissues. During this initial distribution phase (1–3 hours), plasma drug concentrations are quite high. As the drug distributes throughout the body, the plasma drug concentration declines rapidly over a short period. This biexponential elimination curve for vancomycin is an important consideration especially when evaluating peak plasma vancomycin concentration determinations. It is important not to obtain plasma drug concentrations during this initial distribution phase, as inaccurate pharmacokinetic calculations may result.

Because of vancomycin's initial distribution phase, there is some confusion about the therapeutic values for peak and trough concentrations. Older data that suggested peak concentrations of 30–40 mg/L are wrong because they were sampled during this initially high distribution phase. Appropriately sampled peak concentrations were then suggested to be approximately 18–26 mg/L, whereas trough concentrations were suggested to be between 5 and 10 mg/L, except for enterococci, for which vancomycin is only bacteriostatic and required a trough of between 10 and 15 mg/L. We now know that vancomycin troughs <10 mg/L should not be recommended for either MRSA or enterococci as they promote the development of resistance.[1]

In 2009, a consensus review of vancomycin, entitled "Therapeutic Monitoring of Vancomycin in Adult Patients: A Consensus Review of the American Society of Health-System Pharmacists, the Infectious Diseases Society of America,

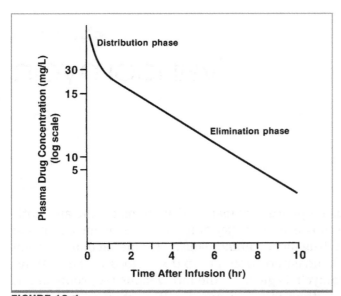

FIGURE 13-1.
Typical plasma concentration versus time curve for vancomycin, demonstrating distribution and elimination phases.

and the Society of Infectious Diseases Pharmacists" has presented the evidence for vancomycin toxicity and monitoring.[1] They concluded that vancomycin efficacy is best modeled as the total area under the drug concentration-time curve (i.e., concentration-independent killing) versus older methods of using peak and trough concentrations to predict efficacy. The ratio of the area under the serum drug concentration versus time curve to minimum inhibitory concentration (AUC/MIC) is a common research laboratory value used to predict efficacy. Unfortunately, most institutions cannot measure AUC/MIC for all pathogens so we instead use vancomycin trough concentrations that are approximated from AUC/MIC ratio measurements to both ensure adequate drug dosing and to decrease development of resistance. Recommended trough goal ranges may vary slightly based on the MIC of the infecting pathogen in each case and site of infection. MIC <1 mg/L requires a vancomycin trough of 10–20 mg/L (never <10 mg/L); an MIC of 1 mg/L requires a trough of 15–20 mg/L. Trough concentrations of 15–20 mg/L are also recommended for complicated infections such as pneumonia, endocarditis, meningitis, and osteomyelitis (or other serious or deep-seated infections). Unfortunately, this consensus paper also presents evidence for increasing nephrotoxicity associated with vancomycin trough concentrations >15 mg/L (and especially

>20 mg/L, thus creating a dilemma between efficacy and toxicity.

Although traditional monitoring of both vancomycin peak and trough levels is often not necessary, measuring both values may be useful to determine patient specific kinetic values in certain patient populations such as hemodynamically unstable patients with significantly decreased or changing renal function, in the elderly, and in those patients receiving concomitant nephrotoxic drugs.

Population Estimates for Vancomycin Volume of Distribution (*V*) and Elimination Rate Constant (*K*)

Similar to the aminoglycoside cases in Lesson 12, there are two commonly used population parameters to estimate volume of distribution (*V*) and elimination rate constant (*K*) that can be used to determine an initial vancomycin dose. The volume of distribution for vancomycin can vary based on patient population mix. We have chosen to use the following *V* based on a review of our patient population.

13-1   0.9 L/kg total body weight (TBW)

(Note that, unlike the aminoglycosides, it is recommended that TBW be used to calculate $V^{1,2}$.)

Vancomycin is eliminated almost entirely by glomerular filtration. Therefore, a reduction in renal function results in a decreased vancomycin clearance and an increased half-life. The average vancomycin half-life for a patient with normal renal function is approximately 6 hours ($K = 0.116$ hr^{-1}).

One method of determining population estimates for the elimination rate constant (*K*) based on creatinine clearance (CrCl) is as follows:

13-2 $K = 0.00083$ hr^{-1}[CrCl (in mL/min)] $+ 0.0044$

This equation, developed by Gary Matzke from regression analysis of vancomycin clearance versus creatinine clearance, has units of reciprocal hours, not milliliters per minute. In this type of equation, units are not supposed to cancel out; rather, they assume the units of the correlated value, *K*.

CASE 1

BW, a 51-year-old woman, 5'8" tall, weighing 150 lb, is admitted to the hospital for suspected severe postinfluenza community-acquired pneumonia. She has normal renal function with a serum creatinine (SCr) concentration of 1 mg/dL measured on the day of admission. Initially, she is treated with ceftriaxone and azithromycin, but on hospital day 3 a sputum culture reveals MRSA with a vancomycin MIC <1 mg/L. Pharmacy is then consulted for vancomycin dosing for BW.

Problem 1A. Determine an appropriate dosing regimen of vancomycin to achieve the desired steady-state plasma concentrations of 30 mg/L for the peak (drawn 2 hours after the end of a 2-hour infusion) and approximately 18 mg/L for the trough. How many doses are required to reach steady state?

Several approaches are available for the calculation of vancomycin dosages; one relatively simple method is presented here. With this method, we assume that the plasma concentrations during the elimination phase are more valuable for therapeutic drug monitoring than the relatively high, transient vancomycin concentrations of the distribution phase (the first 1–2 hours after the infusion). With this assumption, a one-compartment model can be used to estimate vancomycin dosage or plasma concentrations (**Figure 13-2**). We ignore the distribution phase.

To calculate an initial vancomycin dose, given the desired plasma concentrations, we use population estimates for CrCl, K, and V to solve first for

dosing interval and then dose, in a similar fashion to that done for the aminoglycosides, using the following first-order, one-compartment model equation:

$$CrCl = \frac{(140 - age)(Wt)}{72 \times SCr}$$

$$= \frac{(140 - 51)(63.9 \text{ kg}^*)}{72 \times 1}(0.85)$$

$$= \frac{(5687)}{72}(0.85)$$

$$= 67.1 \text{ mL/min}$$

Note: IBW used since actual weight is greater than IBW but is less than 30% greater than IBW.

$$K = 0.00083 \text{ hr}^{-1} \text{ CrCl (in mL/min)} + 0.0044$$

$$= 0.00083(67.1) + 0.0044$$

$$= 0.06 \text{ hr}^{-1}$$

$$T\frac{1}{2} = 0.693/0.061 \text{ hr}^{-1}$$

$$= 11.36 \text{ hours}$$

$$V = 0.9 \text{ L/kg} \times \text{Total body weight (TBW)}$$

$$= (0.9)(68.2 \text{ kg})$$

$$= 61.38 \text{ L}$$

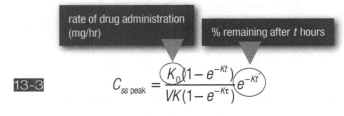

13-3
$$C_{ss\,peak} = \frac{K_0(1 - e^{-Kt})}{VK(1 - e^{-K\tau})}(e^{-Kt'})$$

τ = desired dosing interval, determined as follows:

13-4

$$\tau = \frac{1}{-K}\left(\ln C_{trough(desired)} - \ln C_{peak(desired)}\right) + t + t'$$

$$\tau = \frac{1}{-0.06}(\ln 18 \text{ mg/mL} - \ln 30 \text{ mg/L}) + 2 \text{ hr} + 2 \text{ hr}$$

$$= -16.67\,[-0.510] + 4$$

$$= 8.49 + 4$$

$$= 12.49 \text{ hr, rounded down to 12 hr}$$

Note: Additional 2 hr = extra time from end of infusion until level is drawn. Compare to **Equation 12-4.**

(See **Equation 5-1** and **Equation 12-4.**)

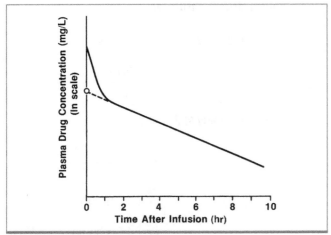

FIGURE 13-2.
Plasma concentration versus time curve for vancomycin, showing simplification with one-compartment model (dashed line).

where:

$C_{ss\,peak}$ = desired peak concentration 2 hours after infusion

K_0 = drug infusion rate (dose/infusion time)

t = duration of infusion (2-hour infusion for this case)

K = estimated elimination rate constant ($0.061\ hr^{-1}$)

V = volume of distribution (population estimate of 0.9 L/kg × 68.2 kg = 61.38 L)

t' = time between end of infusion and collection of blood sample (2 hours; inclusion of t' is different from the calculation for aminoglycosides [see Lesson 12] because sampling time for vancomycin is actually at least 4 hours after the beginning of the infusion)

τ = desired dosing interval

These values are then put into the equation:

$$C_{ss\,peak} = \frac{K_0(1 - e^{-0.06\,hr^{-1}(2\,hr)})}{(61.4\ L)(0.06\ hr^{-1})(1 - e^{-0.06\,hr^{-1}(12\,hr)})}e^{-0.06\,hr^{-1}(2\,hr)}$$

$$30\ mg/L = \frac{K_0(0.113)}{(61.4\ L)(0.06\ hr^{-1})(0.513)}(0.887)$$

$$K_0 = \frac{(30\ mg/L)(61.4\ L)(0.06^{-1})(0.513)}{(0.113)(0.887)}$$

$$=\sim 566.4\ mg\ vancomycin\ per\ 1\ hour$$
(to be infused over 2 hours)

Because vancomycin is infused over 2 hours,

Total dose = (566.4 mg/hr)(2 hr)

= 1132.8 mg vancomycin over 2 hours

Because vancomycin doses are usually rounded to the nearest 250 mg, our decision is whether to round up to 1250 mg or down to 1000 mg every 12 hours for this patient. Because of the severity of the pneumonia and concern for getting enough drug to the site of infection (alveoli of the lungs), the pharmacist decides to start BW on 1250 mg every 12 hours and draw peak and trough levels as soon as the patient is at steady state.

Because we rounded our maintenance dose to 1250 mg, we will need to calculate the predicted peak associated with the slightly higher dose than was calculated to achieve a peak of 30 mg/L. The peak change will be proportional to dose change and can be calculated as follows:

$$\frac{1132.8\ mg}{30\ mg/L} = \frac{1250\ mg}{X}$$

$$X = 33.1\ mg/L$$

With this regimen, we can then predict the vancomycin plasma concentration at the end of the dosing interval (trough):

13-5
$$C_{trough} = C_{ss\,peak}e^{-Kt''}$$

where $t'' = \tau - t - t'$

(See **Equation 3-2**.)

where t'' is the difference in time between the two plasma concentrations. In this case, t'' equals τ (12 hours) – t (2 hours) – t' (2 hours), or 8 hours.

$$C_{trough} = 33.1\ mg/L\ e^{(-0.06\,hr^{-1})(8\,hr)}$$

$$= 33.1\ mg/L\ e^{(-0.48)}$$

$$= 20.48\ mg/L$$

So the regimen should result in the desired plasma concentrations of 33.1 mg/L and approximately 20.48 mg/L.

The number of doses required to attain steady state can be calculated from the estimated half-life and the dosing interval. Steady state is attained in three to five half-lives. In patient BW's case, we will use three half-lives and our estimated K of 0.06 hr^{-1} in our calculations as follows:

Time to steady state = $3 \times T\frac{1}{2}$

$$T\frac{1}{2} = \frac{0.693}{K}$$

Time to steady state = $3 \times T\frac{1}{2}$

$$= 3 \times \frac{0.693}{0.06\ hr^{-1}}$$

$$= 3(11.55\ hr)$$

$$= 34.65\ hours$$

Range (34.65–57.75 hours) for 3–5 half lives. If doses are given every 12 hours, then steady state should be achieved by administration of the fourth dose (by the end of the third dosing interval). Remember that doses would be given at 0, 12, 24, and 36 hours.

Problem 1B. To achieve the desired concentrations rapidly, a loading dose can be given. Determine an appropriate loading dose for patient BW. Assume that the loading dose will be a 2-hour IV infusion.

To estimate a loading dose, we need to know the volume of distribution and the elimination rate constant. Because we do not know the patient-specific pharmacokinetic values, the population estimates can be used (V of 0.9 L/kg TBW [see **Equation 13-1**] and K of 0.06 hr^{-1} as previously determined [see **Equation 13-2**]). Then the equation as shown in Lesson 5 describing plasma concentration over time with an IV infusion is applied. Note that again we ignore the distribution phase and assume that a one-compartment model is adequate (**Figure 13-3**):

$$C_{\text{peak desired}} = \frac{X_0/t}{VK}(1 - e^{-Kt})e^{-Kt'}$$

(See **Equation 13-3**.)

where:

$C_{ss\,\text{peak}}$ = desired peak plasma concentration 2 hours after infusion

X_0 = dose (note: $X_0/t = K_0$)

t = duration of infusion (2 hours)

K = 0.06 hr^{-1}

V = 61.4 L

t' = time after end of infusion (2 hours)

Note: The term e$^{-Kt'}$ describes the decline in plasma concentration from the end of the infusion to some later time (2 hours in this example). Then, insertion of the known values gives the following:

$$30\,\text{mg/L} = \frac{(X_0/2\,\text{hr})(1 - e^{-0.06\,\text{hr}^{-1}(2\text{hr})})}{(61.4\,\text{L})(0.06\,\text{hr}^{-1})}e^{-0.06\,\text{hr}^{-1}(2\text{hr})}$$

$$= \frac{(X_0/2\,\text{hr})(0.113)}{(3.68\,\text{L/hr})}(0.887)$$

$$X_0 = \frac{(30\,\text{mg/L})(3.68\,\text{L/hr})(2\,\text{hr})}{(0.887)(0.113)}$$

Note: This 2 is from transposing the 2 in X$_0$/2 component indicating that the loading dose is infused over 2 hours

$$= 2203.6\,\text{mg LD (rounded to 2000 mg)}$$

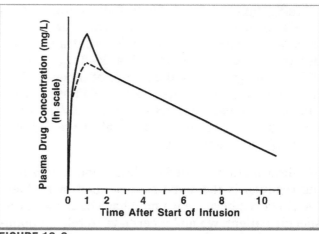

FIGURE 13-3.
Plasma concentrations over time for a loading dose. Dashed line represents simplification to one-compartment model.

Clinical Correlate

Note that although the calculated loading dose is 2203.6 mg, we would likely round to either 2 g or 2.5 g. Many institutions cap loading doses at 2.5 g (and initial maintenance regimens at 2 g every 12 hours) due to concern for alteration of kinetics in obesity (extremes of weight) and lack of specific information on if actual body weight is the best dosing weight to use for these patients. Therapeutic monitoring of vancomycin levels is important in obese patients for this reason and can be used to base dosing adjustments once they are known. Also, note how this calculated loading dose equation (above) compares to the easier method of using 20–25 mg/kg TBW.

Clinical Correlate

Close observation of Figure 13-3 confirms that we are not actually measuring a true peak concentration, as we did for aminoglycosides. We are, rather, measuring a 2-hour postpeak concentration that places this point on the straight-line portion of the terminal elimination phase.

Problem 1C. After administration of the loading dose and seven doses (1250 mg each) at 12-hour intervals, plasma vancomycin concentrations are determined to be 35 mg/L (2 hours after the end of the 2-hour infusion) and 23 mg/L at the end of the dosing interval. Calculate a new dose for BW (this time using actual patient-specific K and V) to attain the original target peak and trough concentrations (30 mg/L and 18 mg/L, respectively).

The information needed to determine a new dosing regimen is the same as described in Problem 1A. However, because we now have data about this specific patient, we no longer have to rely on population estimates. To begin, we should calculate the patient's vancomycin elimination rate constant, half-life, and volume of distribution from the plasma concentrations determined.

Calculation of K

First, K is easily calculated from the slope of the plasma drug concentration versus time curve during the elimination phase (**Figure 13-4**) (see Lesson 3) specifically **Equation 3-1** and Lesson 12:

$$K = -\frac{\ln C_2 - \ln C_1}{t_2 - t_1}$$

$$= -\frac{\ln\ 23\ \text{mg/L} - \ln\ 35\ \text{mg/L}}{10\ \text{hr} - 2\ \text{hr}}$$

$$= -\frac{3.14 - 3.56}{8\ \text{hr}}$$

$$= 0.053\ \text{hr}^{-1}$$

(See **Equation 3-1**.)

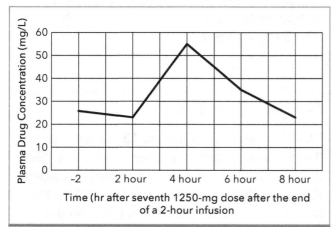

FIGURE 13-4.
Calculation of elimination rate constant given two plasma concentrations (35 mg/L at 2 hours after the infusion and 23 mg/L at 10 hours after the end of a 2-hour infusion).

Clinical Correlate

Be careful when selecting t_2 and t_1. In the above example, if dose one is begun at 8:00 AM and infused for 2 hours, then the patient would receive the entire dose by 10:00 AM. The peak plasma level would then be drawn 2 hours later, or 12:00 PM. Given that the trough concentration will be attained immediately before dose two (given at 8:00 PM), the total time elapsed between the plasma readings is 8 hours, or $(t_2 - t_1)$.

The half-life $(T\frac{1}{2})$ can then be calculated as follows:

$$T\frac{1}{2} = \frac{0.693}{K}$$

$$= \frac{0.693}{0.053\ \text{hr}^{-1}}$$

$$= 13.1\ \text{hr}$$

(See **Equation 3-3**.)

Calculation of V

Note that the elimination rate constant is lower, and the half-life is greater than originally estimated. Now the volume of distribution (V) can be estimated with the multiple-dose infusion equation for steady state:

$$C_{ss\,peak} = \frac{K_0(1 - e^{-Kt})}{VK(1 - e^{-K\tau})}e^{-Kt'}$$

(See **Equation 13-3**.)
where:

$C_{ss\,peak}$ = peak concentration 2 hours after infusion = 35 mg/L

K_0 = maintenance dose (1250 mg over 2 hours)

t = duration of infusion (2 hours)

t' = time between end of infusion and collection of blood sample (2 hours)

K = elimination rate constant (0.053 hr^{-1})

V = volume of distribution (to be determined)

τ = dosing interval (12 hours)

These values are then put into the equation:

$$C_{ss\,peak} = \frac{(1250\text{ mg/2 hr})(1-e^{-0.053\text{ hr}^{-1}(2\text{ hr})})}{V(0.53\text{ hr}^{-1})(1-e^{-0.053\text{ hr}^{-1}(12\text{ hr})})}e^{-0.053\text{ hr}^{-1}(2\text{ hr})}$$

$$35\text{ mg/L} = \frac{(1250\text{ mg/2 hr})(0.1006)}{V(0.053\text{ hr}^{-1})(0.471)}(0.8994)$$

Rearranging gives the following:

$$V = \frac{(1250\text{ mg/2 hr})(0.1006)(0.8994)}{(0.053\text{ hr}^{-1})(0.471)(35\text{ mg/L})}$$

$$= 64.8\text{ L or }0.95\text{ L/kg}$$

So the original estimate for the volume of distribution was slightly lower than the volume determined with the plasma concentrations.

Calculation of New τ

Before calculating a new maintenance dose, we can first check to see if we need to use a new dosing interval, as follows:

$$\tau_{desired} = \frac{1}{-K}[\ln C_{trough(desired)} - \ln C_{peak(desired)}] + t + t'$$

(See **Equation 13-4.**)
where:

t = duration of infusion (2 hours)

t' = time after end of infusion (2 hours)

τ = dosing interval, calculated as follows:

$$\tau = \frac{1}{-0.053\text{ hr}^{-1}}(\ln 18\text{ mg/L} - \ln 30\text{ mg/L}) + 2\text{ hr} + 2\text{ hr}$$

$$= \frac{1}{-0.053\text{ hr}^{-1}}(2.89 - 3.4) + 4\text{ hr}$$

$$= (-18.87)(-0.511)$$

$$= 13.64\text{ hr}$$

Therefore, our best new dosing interval is still approximately 12 hours.

Calculation of New K_0

$$C_{ss\,peak} = \frac{K_0(1-e^{-Kt})}{VK(1-e^{-K\tau})}e^{-Kt'}$$

$$30\text{ mg/L} = \frac{K_0(1-e^{-0.053\text{ hr}^{-1}(2\text{ hr})})}{(64.8\text{ L})(0.053\text{ hr}^{-1})(1-e^{-0.053\text{ hr}^{-1}(12\text{ hr})})}e^{-0.053\text{ hr}^{-1}(2\text{ hr})}$$

$$= \frac{K_0(0.101)}{(64.8\text{ L})(0.053\text{ hr}^{-1})(0.471)}(0.8994)$$

Rearranging gives the following:

$$K_0 = \frac{(30\text{ mg/L})(0.053\text{ hr}^{-1})(64.8\text{ L})(0.471)}{(0.101)(0.8994)}$$

$$= (538.7\text{ mg/hr})(2\text{-hr infusion})$$

$$= 534.2\text{ mg for 2 hours} = 1068.4\text{ mg},$$

which will round to 1000 mg.

$$\frac{1068.4}{30} = \frac{1000}{X}\text{ (where X is peak expected with 1000 mg dose)}$$

Resultant C_{peak} and C_{trough} concentrations for a 1000-mg every 12-hour dose would be ~28.1 mg/L and 18.4 mg/L, respectively.

$$C_{trough} = C_{peak}(e^{-Kt})$$

$$= 28.1\text{ mg/L }(e^{-(0.053)(8)})$$

$$= 18.4\text{ mg/L}$$

Clinical Correlate

One can easily see how this tedious, repetitive calculation of dose, dosing interval, and trough concentration can be made much simpler by using various computer software and mobile app dosing programs, allowing you to try many different combinations. It is still vitally important to understand the kinetic equations, assumptions and limitations, basis for software or shortcut methods, and what variables affect dosing strategies.

CASE 2

PS, a 75-year-old male, 170 lb, 5'10" tall, SCr 2.7 mg/dL, is admitted to the hospital for possible endocarditis. PS has a history of IV drug abuse and previous bacteremia associated with needle use for injecting drugs. He has a new heart murmur and has been spiking fevers for over a week. Two sets of blood cultures subsequently return with gram-positive cocci, resistant to methicillin but susceptible to vancomycin. The physician consults the pharmacy for vancomycin dosing and monitoring. A quick clinical assessment of this patient indicates that his renal function is extremely low, meaning time to steady state would be many days. Estimated pharmacokinetic parameters confirm this assumption: CrCl ~24.3 mL/min, estimated K of 0.024 hr^{-1}, V of 69.57 L, $T\frac{1}{2}$ of ~28.88 hours, and, therefore, a time to steady-state calculation of between 86.63 hours, using three half-lives, and 144.4 hours, using five half-lives.

Note: There are two opportunities to calculate patient-specific pharmacokinetic values: after the first dose or after steady state has been achieved. In this case, because the patient has such a long half-life, it is decided to calculate these parameters after the first dose, which allows for subsequent dose adjustments without waiting the many days necessary for steady state to be reached. The reason for calculating this patient's K and V is to predict how often a vancomycin dose will be needed, when the next dose should be given, and the size of the next dose.

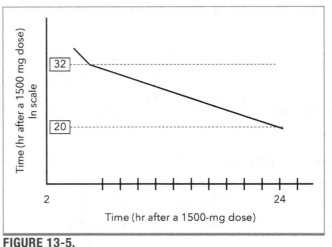

FIGURE 13-5.
Plasma concentrations after loading dose of vancomycin in a patient with renal impairment (32 mg/L at 2 hours and 20 mg/L at 24 hours after the end of the infusion).

$$K = -\text{slope of natural log of vancomycin}$$
$$\text{concentration versus time plot}$$

$$= -\frac{\ln C_2 - \ln C_1}{t_2 - t_1}$$

$$= -\frac{\ln 20 \text{ mg/L} - \ln 32 \text{ mg/L}}{24 \text{ mg} - 2 \text{ hr}}$$

$$= 0.0214 \text{ hr}^{-1}$$

(See **Equation 3-1**.)

Clinical Correlate

Remember that the second plasma level was taken 24 hours after the *end of the infusion*, not 24 hours after the first plasma level. Therefore, we must account for the 2 hours that elapsed between the end of the infusion and first plasma level.

Problem 2A. Two hours after the end of a 1500-mg loading dose administered over 2 hours, the vancomycin plasma concentration was 32 mg/L; it is 20 mg/L at 24 hours after the end of this infusion (**Figure 13-5**). Calculate the vancomycin K, half-life, and V in this patient.

First, we calculate the elimination rate constant (K) and half-life ($T\frac{1}{2}$):

The half-life in this case can be calculated as follows:

$$T\frac{1}{2} = \frac{0.693}{K}$$

$$= \frac{0.693}{0.022 \text{ hr}^{-1}}$$

$$= 31.5 \text{ hr}$$

(See **Equation 3-3**.)

Now the volume of distribution (V) can be estimated, using the simple relationship given below:

Loading dose = plasma concentration achieved
× volume of distribution

By rearranging, we get:

$$V = \frac{\text{loading dose}}{\text{plasma concentration achieved}}$$

$$= \frac{1500 \text{ mg}}{32 \text{ mg/L}}$$

$$= 46.88 \text{ L}$$

Note that the patient's calculated K of 0.022 hours and V of 46.88 L are both lower than our estimated values of 0.024 hours and 69.57 L, respectively.

Problem 2B. With the information just determined, calculate when the next vancomycin dose should be given and what it should be. Assume that the plasma vancomycin concentration should decline to 15 mg/L before another dose is given and that the plasma concentration desired 2 hours after the infusion is complete is 30 mg/L (i.e., desired C_{peak}).

First, we must know the time needed for the plasma concentration to decline to 15 mg/L. It can easily be calculated from the known plasma concentrations, the elimination rate constant, and the desired trough plasma concentration:

$$C_{trough} = C_{peak}e^{-Kt}$$

where:

C_{peak} = observed concentration of 32 mg/L

K = elimination rate constant (0.022 hr^{-1})

t = time between first observed concentration of 32 mg/L and the desired concentration of 15 mg/L (unknown)

Then:

15 mg/L = (32 mg/L)($e^{(-0.022 \text{ hr}^{-1})(t)}$)

To solve for t, we can first take the natural log of each side of the equation:

ln 15 mg/L = ln 32 mg/L (−0.022 hr^{-1})(t)

Rearranging gives the following:

$$t = \frac{\ln 15 \text{ mg/L} / \ln 32 \text{ mg/L}}{-0.022 \text{ hr}^{-1}}$$

$$= 35.5 \text{ hr}$$

Therefore, at approximately *35* hours after the plasma concentration of 32 mg/L is observed (or ~37 hours after the end of the infusion), the next vancomycin dose can be given.

Next, we determine dosing interval and maintenance dose as follows:

$$\tau = \frac{1}{-K}\left(\ln C_{trough(desired)} - \ln C_{peak(desired)}\right) + t + t'$$

$$= \frac{1}{-0.022}(\ln 15 \text{ mg/L} - \ln 30 \text{ mg/L}) + 2 \text{ hr} + 2 \text{ hr}$$

$$= \frac{1}{-0.022}(2.71 - 3.4) + 4$$

$$= \frac{1}{-0.022}(2.71 - 3.4) + 4$$

$$= (-45.5)(-0.69) + 4$$

$$= 35 \text{ hr, rounded up to } 36 \text{ hr}$$

Note: Additional 2 hr = extra time from end of infusion until level is drawn. Compare to **Equation 12-4.**

(See **Equation 13-4.**)

The maintenance dose can then be calculated as follows:

$$C_{ss \text{ peak}} = \frac{K_0(1-e^{-Kt})}{VK(1-e^{-K\tau})}e^{-Kt'}$$

(See **Equation 13-3.**)
where:

$C_{ss \text{ peak}}$ = concentration 2 hours after end of infusion

τ = 36 hours

t = duration of infusion (2 hours)

t' = time after end of infusion (2 hours)

V = 46.9 L

K = 0.022 hr^{-1}

Rearranging to solve for K_0:

$$K_0 = \frac{VK(C_{ss \text{ peak}})(1-e^{-K\tau})}{(1-e^{-Kt})(e^{-Kt'})}$$

$$= \frac{(46.9 \text{ L})(0.022 \text{ hr}^{-1})(30 \text{ mg/L})(1-e^{-0.022 \text{ hr}^{-1}(36 \text{ hr})})}{(1-e^{-0.022 \text{ hr}^{-1}(2 \text{ hr})})(e^{-0.022 \text{ hr}^{-1}(2 \text{ hr})})}$$

$$K_0 = \frac{16.92}{(0.043)(0.957)}$$

$$= 412 \text{ mg} \times 2 = 825 \text{ mg, rounded to } 1000 \text{ mg}$$

Finally, we must check to see what our trough concentration will be after rounding both dose and dosing interval. Remember that because we rounded the dose up to 1000 mg, we must calculate how the expected peak would change in proportion to the higher dose used.

$$\frac{825 \text{ mg}}{30 \text{ mg} / \text{L}} = \frac{1000 \text{ mg}}{X \text{ mg/L}}$$

where $X = 36$ mg/L

Now we can calculate what the trough from our 1000-mg dose would be at the end of the dosing interval.

$$C_{\text{trough}} = C_{\text{peak}} e^{-Kt''} \quad \text{(See Equation 13-5.)}$$

where:

$$t'' = \text{time between } C_{\text{trough}} \text{ and } C_{\text{peak}}$$

$$= \tau - t - t'$$

$$= 36 - 2 - 2 = 32 \text{ hr}$$

and:

$$C_{\text{trough}} = (36 \text{ mg/L}) e^{(-0.022 \text{ hr}^{-1})(32 \text{ hr})}$$

$$= 18 \text{ mg/L}$$

This is an appropriate trough level for treatment of suspected endocarditis (goal range 15–20 mg/L).

CASE 3

A 65-year-old woman, patient BA (weighing 75 kg, 5'7"), is being treated for a hospital-acquired MRSA bacteremia seeding from an infected sacral decubitus ulcer. MIC values for this organism are <1 mg/L. Her estimated CrCl is 36 mL/min. Her physician prescribed an initial 1250-mg vancomycin loading dose followed by a maintenance dose of 1000 mg (infused over 2 hours) every 24 hours. Per hospital protocol, you are required to check all vancomycin dosing and recommend changes as needed.

Problem 3A. Predict the steady-state C_{trough} from this dose, using population average values for K and V. Will this achieve a C_{trough} of >10 mg/L?

The equation for a one-compartment, intermittent-infusion drug can be used to solve for $C_{ss \text{ peak}}$ and $C_{ss \text{ trough}}$:

$$C_{ss \text{ peak}} = \frac{K_0(1 - e^{-Kt})}{VK(1 - e^{-K\tau})} e^{-Kt'}$$

(See **Equation 13-3.**)

where:

$C_{ss \text{ peak}}$ = peak plasma concentration at steady state

K_0 = drug infusion rate (also maintenance dose given over 2 hours)

V = volume of distribution (population estimate for vancomycin of 0.9 L/kg TBW)

K = elimination rate constant (population estimate for vancomycin)

t = infusion time (2 hours in this case)

τ = patient's current dosing interval

t' = time between end of infusion and collection of blood sample (2 hours)

First, we must calculate patient BA's K and V values for use in this equation. The estimated K would be as follows:

$$K = 0.00083 \text{ hr}^{-1} (\text{CrCl}) + 0.0044$$

(See **Equation 13-2.**)

$$= 0.00083 (36) + 0.0044$$

$$= 0.034 \text{ hr}^{-1}$$

The patient BA's estimated volume of distribution (V) is calculated from the population estimate of 0.9 L/kg TBW:

$$0.9 \text{ L/kg} \times 75 \text{ kg} = 67.5 \text{ L} \quad \text{(See Equation 13-1.)}$$

Now that we have these estimates of K and V, we can calculate the C_{peak} and C_{trough} values that would be obtained with this dose of 1000 mg every 24 hours. By application of the general equation for a one-compartment, first-order, intermittently infused drug, we get the following:

$$C_{ss\,peak} = \frac{K_0(1 - e^{-Kt})}{VK(1 - e^{-K\tau})}e^{-Kt'}$$

(See **Equation 13-3**.)

where:

$C_{ss\,peak}$ = concentration that would result from this dose at steady state

K_0 = drug infusion rate (maintenance dose per hour)

V = volume of distribution (population estimate for vancomycin)

K = elimination rate constant (population estimate for vancomycin)

t = duration of infusion

t' = time from end of infusion until concentration is determined (2 hours for peak)

τ = desired or most appropriate dosing interval

Therefore:

$$C_{ss\,peak} = \frac{(1000\text{ mg/2 hr})(1 - e^{-0.034\text{ hr}^{-1}(2\text{ hr})})}{(67.5\text{ L})(0.034\text{ hr}^{-1})(1 - e^{-0.034\text{ hr}^{-1}(24\text{ hr})})}e^{-0.034\text{ hr}^{-1}(2\text{ hr})}$$

$$= \frac{(1000\text{ mg/2 hr})(0.0657)}{(2.295\text{ L/hr})(0.558)}(0.934)$$

$$= (30.7 /)1.28$$

$$= 23.98\text{ mg/L}$$

The peak concentration, in this case, is primarily calculated to continue the math necessary to calculate her trough concentration and can be estimated with the following equation:

$$C_{ss\,trough} = C_{ss\,peak}e^{-Kt}$$

In this case, patient BA's C_{trough} will equal the C_{peak} (drawn 2 hours after the 2-hour infusion) multiplied by the fraction of this C_{peak} remaining after elimination has occurred for t' hours, which, in this case, is 20 hours (24-hour dosing interval minus 4 hours).

The patient's estimated $C_{ss\,trough}$ is calculated as follows:

$$C_{ss\,trough} = (23.9\text{ mg/L})e^{(-0.034\text{ hr}^{-1})(20\text{ hr})}$$

$$= (23.9)(0.51)$$

$$= 12.19\text{ mg/L}$$

Now that you know the eventual expected steady-state trough of 12.2 mg/L, which is below our target of 15 mg/L, a clinical decision can be made to either increase dose slightly or wait until patient's vancomycin level is at steady state and obtain a steady-state trough concentration.

Problem 3B. What vancomycin dose would you recommend for patient BA to attain a C_{peak} of 28 mg/L (drawn 2 hours after the end of a 2-hour infusion) and a C_{trough} of 15 mg/L?

Using the estimates of K (0.034 hr^{-1}) and V (67.5 L), we should first determine the best dosing interval (τ) for patient BA:

$$\tau = \frac{1}{-K}[\ln C_{trough(desired)} - \ln C_{peak(desired)}] + t + t'$$

(See **Equation 13-4**.)

where t is the time of infusion and t' is the time after the end of the infusion. Then:

$$\tau = \frac{1}{-0.034\text{ hr}^{-1}}(\ln 15\text{ mg/L} - \ln 28\text{ mg/L}) + 2\text{ hr} + 2\text{ hr}$$

$$= -29.4\text{ hr }(2.71 - 3.33) + 4\text{ hr}$$

$$= 18.23 + 4$$

$$= 22.23\text{ hours, and we will round to 24 hours}$$

$$C_{ss\,peak} = \frac{K_0(1 - e^{-Kt})}{VK(1 - e^{-K\tau})}e^{-Kt'}$$

(See **Equation 13-3**.)

where:

$C_{ss\,peak}$ = desired peak concentration at steady state

K_0 = drug infusion rate (also maintenance dose you are trying to calculate)

V = volume of distribution (population estimate for vancomycin)

K = elimination rate constant (population estimate for vancomycin)

t = duration of infusion

t' = time from end of infusion until concentration is determined (2 hours for peak)

τ = desired or most appropriate dosing interval

Then:

$$C_{ss\,peak} = \frac{K_0(1-e^{-Kt})}{VK(1-e^{-K\tau})}e^{-Kt'}$$

$$C_{ss\,peak} = \frac{(K_0/2)(1-e^{-(0.034\ hr^{-1})(2\ hr)})(e^{-(0.034\ hr^{-1})(2\ hr)})}{(67.5\ L)(0.034\ hr^{-1})(1-e^{-(0.034\ hr^{-1})(24\ hr)})}$$

$$28\ mg/L = \frac{(K_0/2)(0.066)}{(2.3)(0.56)}(0.93)$$

$$28\ mg/L = \frac{(K_0/2)(0.0611)}{1.288}$$

$$28/1.288 = (K_0/2)(0.611)$$

$$590.2\ mg = K_0/2$$

$K_0 = $ ⟨1180⟩ mg rounded up to 1250 mg because we rounded our interval up to 24 hours

Note: Answer of 596 mg/hr for two hour infusion = 1192 mg

Once again we will need to calculate the proportional change in expected peak for our rounded dose of 1250 mg (instead of the 1167.42 mg that was expected to give a peak of 28 mg/L).

$$\frac{1180\ mg}{28\ mg/L} = \frac{1250\ mg}{X\ mg/L}$$

$$X = 29.66\ mg/L$$

The expected trough concentration can now be calculated:

$$C_{ss\,trough} = C_{ss\,peak}e^{-Kt}$$

(See **Equation 13-5**.)

In this case, C_{trough} will equal the C_{peak} (drawn 2 hours after the 2-hour infusion is complete) multiplied by the fraction of this C_{peak} remaining after elimination has occurred for t hours, which, in this case, is 20 hours (24-hour dosing interval minus 2 hours minus 2 hours):

$$C_{ss\,trough} = (29.66\ mg/L)e^{(-0.034\ hr^{-1})(20\ hr)}$$

$$= 29.66(0.51)$$

$$= 15.1\ mg/L$$

Thus, a dose of 1250 mg every 24 hours will yield an estimated C_{peak} of 29.66 mg/L and an estimated C_{trough} of 15.1 mg/L, which should be adequate in BA's case.

Clinical Correlate

Don't let these equations intimidate you. Try to develop a step-by-step model to walk you through the calculations, such as below:

- Determine patient-specific K and V values. If these values are not known, use population estimates.
- Determine the dosing interval.
- Determine the drug infusion rate (K_0).
- Check the trough to make sure it is within your desired range.

Problem 3C. Despite your dosing recommendation, BA continued to receive her original dose of 1000 mg every 24 hours (infused over 2 hours) with resultant steady-state peak and trough levels of 22 and 9 mg/L, respectively (**Figure 13-6**). Adjust patient BA's dose, this time using her specific pharmacokinetic parameters, to give a C_{peak} of approximately 26 mg/L and a $C_{ss\,trough}$ of approximately 14 mg/L.

To adjust this patient's dose, we must first determine her real K and V values, then calculate a new dosing interval, and finally solve for a new maintenance dose.

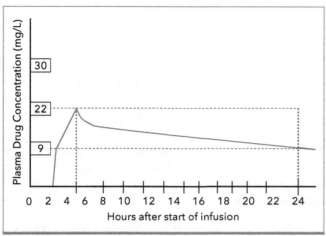

FIGURE 13-6.
Time between peak and trough.

To calculate K, we can use **Equation 3-1** and derived in Lesson 12:

$$K = -\frac{\ln C_{trough} - \ln C_{peak}}{\tau - t - t'}$$

$$= -\frac{\ln 9 \text{ mg/L} - \ln 22 \text{ mg/L}}{24 \text{ hr} - 2 \text{ hr} - 2 \text{ hr}}$$

$$= -\frac{2.197 - 3.09}{20 \text{ hr}}$$

$$= -\frac{0.893}{20 \text{ hr}}$$

$$= 0.0447 \text{ hr}^{-1}$$

(See **Equation 3-1**.)

To calculate V, we can use:

$$C_{ss \, peak} = \frac{K_0(1 - e^{-Kt})}{VK(1 - e^{-K\tau})}e^{-Kt'}$$

(See **Equation 13-3**.)

where:

$C_{ss \, peak}$ = measured steady state peak plasma concentration (22 mg/L) drawn 2 hours after end of a 2-hour infusion

K_0 = drug infusion rate (maintenance dose of 1000 mg, infused over 2 hours)

V = volume of distribution (unknown)

K = elimination rate constant calculated from C_{peak} and C_{trough} (0.0447 hr^{-1})

t = infusion time (2 hours)

t' = time from end of infusion until concentration is determined (2 hours for peak) (see Figure 13.6)

τ = dosing interval at time concentrations are obtained (24 hours)

By substituting the above values, we obtain:

$$22 \text{ mg/L} = \frac{(1000 \text{ mg/2 hr})(1 - e^{-0.0447 \text{ hr}^{-1}(2 \text{ hr})})}{V(0.0447 \text{ hr}^{-1})(1 - e^{-0.0447 \text{ hr}^{-1}(24 \text{ hr})})}e^{-0.0447 \text{ hr}^{-1}(2 \text{ hr})}$$

$$= \frac{(1000 \text{ mg/2 hr})(0.086)}{V(0.0447 \text{ hr}^{-1})(0.658)}(0.914)$$

$$(0.647 \text{ mg/L/hr})(V) = 39.08 \text{ mg/hr}$$

$$V = 60.74 \text{ L}$$

Note the differences between the previously estimated K and V of 0.034 hr^{-1} and 67.5 L and the calculated values of 0.0447 hr^{-1} and 60.74 L. The K value is larger, while the V is smaller than originally calculated.

Now, to calculate the best dosing interval, infused over 2 hours in this case, to get a C_{peak} of 28 mg/L and a $C_{ss \, trough}$ of approximately 15 mg/L, we would use the following:

$$\tau = \frac{1}{-K}[\ln C_{trough(desired)} - \ln C_{peak(desired)}] + t + t'$$

$$= \frac{1}{-0.0447 \text{ hr}^{-1}}[\ln 15 \text{ mg/L} - \ln 28 \text{ mg/L}] + 2 \text{ hr} + 2 \text{ hr}$$

$$= \frac{1}{-0.0447 \text{ hr}^{-1}}[2.71 - 3.33] + 4 \text{ hr}$$

$$= 17.9 \text{ hr}$$

we will use 18 hours in this case (though in practice it would be preferred to do every 12 or every 24 hours if possible)

(See **Equation 13-4**.)

The new maintenance dose now can be calculated:

$$C_{ss \, peak} = \frac{K_0(1 - e^{-Kt})}{VK(1 - e^{-K\tau})}e^{-Kt'}$$

(See **Equation 13-3**.)

where:

$C_{ss\,peak}$ = desired peak concentration at steady state (28 mg/L)

K_0 = drug infusion rate (also maintenance dose you are trying to calculate, in milligrams per hour)

V = volume of distribution (60.74 L)

K = elimination rate constant calculated from C_{peak} and C_{trough} (0.0447 hr^{-1})

t = infusion time (2 hours)

t' = time from end of infusion until concentration is determined (2 hours for peak)

τ = desired or most appropriate dosing interval (18 hours)

Then:

$$C_{ss\,peak} = \frac{K_0/2(1 - e^{-0.0447\,hr^{-1}(2\,hr)})}{(60.74\,L)(0.0447\,hr^{-1})(1 - e^{-0.0447\,hr^{-1}(18\,hr)})}e^{-0.0447\,hr^{-1}(2\,hr)}$$

$$28\,mg/L = \frac{(K_0/2)(0.0855)}{(1.5)}(0.914)$$

$$28 = \frac{K_0/2(0.0781)}{1.5}$$

$$42.04 = K_0/2\,(0.0781)$$

$$K_0/2 = 538.3\,mg \times 2 = 1076.57\,mg,$$
round to 1000 mg q 18 hr

We would round this dose to 1000 mg, which would slightly lower the actual peak value from 28 to approximately 26 mg/L. This calculation is shown below:

$$(1076.57\,mg/28\,mg/L) = 1000\,mg/X\,mg/L$$

where X = 26 mg/L

Problem 3D. Calculate the $C_{ss\,trough}$ for patient BA if she receives the new dose of 1000 mg every 18 hours. We can use the following equation, where t'' is now the number of hours between the peak and trough $(t'' = \tau - t - t')$. Therefore, $t'' = 14$ hours.

$$C_{ss\,trough} = C_{ss\,peak}e^{-t''}$$

(See **Equation 13-5.**)

$$= (26\,mg/L)\,e^{(-0.0447\,hr^{-1})(14\,hr)}$$

$$= 13.9\,mg/L$$

This new dose of 1000 mg every 18 hours based on patient-specific PK parameters will then give a C_{peak} of approximately 26 mg/L and a C_{trough} of approximately 13.9 mg/L.

Problem 3E. Suppose BA had been given 1 g every 12 hours (given as a 1-hour infusion) initially instead of 1g every 24 hours and the resulting steady state peak and trough were 35 and 23.8, respectively. Assume the previously calculated patient specific K and V for BA are the same (K = 0.0447, V = 60.47 L). Because the dose of 1 g every 12 hours resulted in a trough that was too high (23.8 mg/L), we will need to calculate how long the dose should be held before resuming the new dose of 1 g every 18 hours. The formula for calculating the number of hours to hold the dose is as follows:

$$C_{ss\,trough} = C_{trough(actual)}e^{-Kt} \quad \text{(See **Equation 3-2.**)}$$

where t is the amount of time to hold the dose. This formula is an application of the general formula (see Lesson 3) that the concentration at any time equals a previous concentration multiplied by the fraction remaining:

$$C = C_0e^{-Kt}$$

where:

C = drug concentration at time t (in this example, we will want to restart vancomycin when the level drops to around 15 mg/L (i.e., our goal trough level/ desired concentration at the end of the dosing interval for this patient)

C_0 = drug concentration at some earlier time or time zero (in this case the concentration at the end of the last dosing interval from the prescribed 1 g every 12 hours dose)

e^{-Kt} = fraction of original or previous concentration remaining

In patient BA's case:

$$15 \text{ mg/L} = (23.8 \text{ mg/L})e^{(-0.0447 \text{ hr}^{-1})(t)}$$

$$0.63 \text{ mg/L} = e^{(0.0447 \text{ hr}-1)(t)}$$

Next, take the natural logarithm of both sides:

$$\ln 0.63 = \ln \left(e^{-0.0447\text{hr}-1)(t)}\right)$$

$$-0.0462 = -0.0447(t)$$

$$t = 10.34 \text{ hr (could round to 11 hours)}$$

We should hold this patient's dose for an additional 11 hours after the next C_{trough} and then begin her new dose. The same equation can be used to determine the amount of time to hold the dose from the last C_{peak} of 35 mg/L. Again, the general equation is as follows:

$$C = C_0 e^{-Kt} \quad \text{(See Equation 3-2.)}$$

where:

C = drug concentration at time t (representing here the desired C_{trough} of 15 mg/L)

C_0 = drug concentration at some earlier time (representing here C_{peak} of 35 mg/L)

e^{-Kt} = fraction of previous concentration remaining

In patient BA's case:

$$15 \text{ mg/L} = (35 \text{ mg/L})e^{(-0.0447 \text{ hr}^{-1})(t)}$$

$$0.43 \text{ mg/L} = e^{(-0.0447 \text{ hr}^{-1})(t)}$$

Next, take the natural logarithm of both sides:

$$\ln 0.42 = \ln \left(e^{(-0.0447 \text{ hr}^{-1})(t)}\right)$$

$$-0.85 = -0.0447(t)$$

$$18.96 \text{ hr rounded to 19 hr} = T$$

We should hold this patient's dose for an additional 19 hours after the C_{peak} and then begin her new dose. Note that you can calculate time to hold using either C_{peak} or C_{trough}; both methods give the correct answer,

but you *must* examine where you are in the dosing versus serum concentration sequence.

A more intuitive method for estimating the time to hold patient BA's dose is by examination of the vancomycin half-life. We know that the drug concentration decreases by half over each half-life. We can estimate how many drug half-lives to wait for her concentration to approach our desired amount of 15 mg/L as follows. For patient BA (C_{trough} of 23.8 mg/L and $T\frac{1}{2}$ of 15.5 hours [0.693/]0.0447), the concentration will drop by one half from 23.8 to 11.9 (around 12) mg/L in one half-life of 15.5 hours. Because a concentration of 12 mg/L would be an acceptable time to restart, we need to hold only the *next scheduled dose* for an additional 15.5 hours before beginning the new dose of 1000 mg every 18 hours (although ideally therapy would be restarted around a concentration of 15 mg/L so therapy could technically restart closer to the 11 hours we calculated above using the equation $C_{\text{trough(desired)}} = C_{\text{trough(actual)}}e^{-Kt}$).

CASE 4

A 65-year-old man, patient RK, has a history of chronic lymphedema and recurrent skin and soft tissue infections. He is currently hospitalized with MRSA cellulitis. He has been treated with 1250 mg of vancomycin every 18 hours for the last 10 days. His most recent C_{peak} was 24 mg/L (drawn 2 hours after a 2-hour vancomycin infusion), and his most recent C_{trough} was 13 mg/L.

Problem 4. Patient RK's physician wants to discharge him and allow a local home infusion company to administer his vancomycin on a once-a-day basis for the remaining four days of therapy. You are asked to determine if it is possible to obtain a C_{trough} of >10 mg/L with a once-a-day dose. What is your response?

Before answering this question, we must be sure we know what the question is asking. Basically, this question is asking whether, based on the patient's pharmacokinetic parameters, a dose can be given to obtain a satisfactory C_{peak} and C_{trough} given a dosing interval of 24 hours.

First, we must determine patient RK's pharmacokinetic parameters based on his C_{peak} of 24 mg/L and C_{trough} of 13 mg/L. To calculate K, we can use the following:

$$-K = \frac{\ln C_{trough(measured)} - \ln C_{peak(measured)}}{\tau - t - t'}$$

(See **Equation 3-1**.)

where t' represents 2 hours, the number of hours after the infusion that the C_{peak} was drawn. Then:

$$K = -\frac{\ln 13 \text{ mg/L} - \ln 24 \text{ mg/L}}{18-2-2 \text{ hr}}$$

$$= -\frac{2.565 - 3.18}{14 \text{ hr}}$$

$$= 0.044$$

To calculate V, we can use the following:

$$C_{ss\,peak} = \frac{K_0(1-e^{-Kt})}{VK(1-e^{-K\tau})}e^{-Kt'}$$

(See **Equation 13-3**.)

where:

$C_{ss\,peak}$ = measured peak plasma concentration (24 mg/L)

K_0 = drug infusion rate (also maintenance dose of 1250 mg)

V = volume of distribution (unknown)

K = elimination rate constant calculated from C_{peak} and C_{trough} (0.044 hr^{-1})

t = duration of infusion (2 hours)

t' = time from end of infusion until concentration is determined (2 hours for peak)

τ = dosing interval at time concentrations are obtained (18 hours)

By substituting the above values, we obtain as follows:

$$24 \text{ mg/L} = \frac{(1250 \text{ mg/2})(1-e^{-0.044 \text{ hr}^{-1}(2 \text{ hr})})}{V(0.044 \text{ hr}^{-1})(1-e^{-0.044 \text{ hr}^{-1}(18 \text{ hr})})}e^{-0.044 \text{ hr}^{-1}(2 \text{ hr})}$$

$$= \frac{(1250 \text{ mg/2})(0.084)}{V(0.044)(0.547)}(0.916)$$

$$V = 83.44 \text{ L}$$

Next, we use our general equation to solve for K_0 (maintenance dose) with our predetermined 24-hour dosing interval:

$$C_{ss\,peak} = \frac{K_0(1-e^{-Kt})}{VK(1-e^{-K\tau})}e^{-Kt'}$$

where:

$C_{ss\,peak}$ = desired peak concentration at steady state (33 mg/L)

K_0 = drug infusion rate (also maintenance dose you are trying to calculate, in milligrams per hour infused for 2 hours)

V = calculated volume of distribution (83.44 L)

K = elimination rate constant calculated from C_{peak} and C_{trough} (0.044 hr^{-1})

t = duration of infusion time (2 hours)

t' = time from end of infusion until concentration is determined (2 hours for peak)

τ = dosing interval desired (24 hours)

By substituting the above values, we obtain as follows:

$$33 \text{ mg/L} = \frac{(K_0/2)(1-e^{-0.044 \text{ hr}^{-1}(2 \text{ hr})})}{(83.44 \text{ L})(0.044 \text{ hr}^{-1})(1-e^{-0.044 \text{ hr}^{-1}(24 \text{ hr})})}e^{-0.044 \text{ hr}^{-1}(2 \text{ hr})}$$

$$33 \text{ mg/L} = \frac{(K_0/2)(0.0842)}{(3.67)(0.652)}(0.915)$$

$$K_0/2 = 1026 \text{ mg}$$

$$K_0 = 2052 \text{ mg, round to 2000 mg, infused over 2 hours}$$

Finally, we must check to see that our C_{trough} concentration with this dose is acceptable.

$$C_{ss\,trough} = C_{ss\,peak}e^{-Kt''}$$

(See **Equation 13-5**.)

In this case, patient RK's C_{trough} will be equal to his C_{peak} of 33 mg/L (actually 32.2 because we rounded down to 2000 mg from the 2052 mg calculated in our equation) multiplied by the fraction of the C_{peak} remaining after elimination has occurred for t'' hours, which, in this case, is 20 hours (24-hour dosing interval minus t [2 hours] minus t' [2 hours]).

Therefore:

$$C_{ss\ trough} = (32.2\ mg/L)e^{(-0.044\ hr^{-1})(20\ hr)}$$

$$= 13.36\ mg/L$$

We can conclude that 2000 mg every 24 hours will yield a trough concentration >10 mg/L. In fact, it will be 13.4 mg/L. This is sufficient for treatment of a skin and soft tissue infection to complete the remaining days of therapy. If we needed to reach a goal trough of 15–20 mg/L (for infections when this is recommended) once daily dosing would likely not be feasible for this patient.

Trough-Only Vancomycin Pharmacokinetics

Because the trough vancomycin concentration has been shown to be most associated with drug efficacy and decreased development of microorganism resistance and yet also associated with nephrotoxicity, many practitioners simply use a ratio and proportion method of dosing adjustment based solely on the trough level. For instance, if trough = 8 on a dose of 750 mg every 12 hours, they simply double both values and give 1500 mg every 12 hours to yield a trough of approximately twice the previous value (from 8 to 16 mg/L). This method is accurate due to vancomycin having first-order or linear pharmacokinetics elimination. The first level must have been drawn at or after steady state. Unfortunately, single-trough-level-only dosing methods do not allow for calculation of individual patient-specific values for vancomycin clearance (CL_{vanco}), V, K, or estimated C_{peakss}, and therefore, makes a concomitant change in dosing interval somewhat of a guessing game. Consequently, several methods have been devised that attempt to estimate one vancomycin population estimate such as K or Vd and solve for the other estimate to obtain a "better" C_{peakss}. Although there are many iterations of this method, these single-trough methods estimate either K or Vd and then solve for

the other. For instance, some practitioners use the Matzke equation (as shown in **Equation 13-3**) to estimate K and solve for V or vice-versa.

Another popular and intuitive method is the Ambrose-Winter method, which uses the simple equation below[4]:

$$C\,peak_{ss} = (dose/V) + C\,trough_{ss}$$

This equation allows you to estimate a peak concentration based on the simple relationship that Concentration = amount of drug (or dose)/Volume and then using this value of C_{peakss} (but now written as [dose/V] + $C_{troughss}$) where (dose/V) + $C_{troughss}$ is simply a re-expression of C_{peakss} as also shown above.

Although these methods are not as accurate as having both a "real" peak and trough serum concentration, they are more accurate than using estimates for both K and Vd and may be adequate in most clinical situations.

References

1. Rybak MJ, Lomaestro BM, Rotscahfer JC, et al. Therapeutic monitoring of vancomycin in adult patients: A consensus review of the American Society of Health-System Pharmacists, the Infectious Diseases Society of America, and the Society of Infectious Diseases Pharmacists. *Am J Health-Syst Pharm.* 2009;66(1):82–98.

2. Hong J, Krop LC, Johns T, Pai MP. Individualized vancomycin dosing in obese patients: a two-sample measurement approach improves target attainment. *Pharmacotherapy.* 2015;35(5):455–63.

3. Pai MP, Bearden DT. Antimicrobial dosing considerations in obese patients. *Pharmacotherapy.* 2017;27(8):1081-91.

4. Ambrose PJ, Winter ME. Vancomycin. In: Winter ME, ed. *Basic Clinical Pharmacokinetics.* 5th ed. Philadelphia, PA: Lippincott Williams & Wilkins; 2010:459-87.

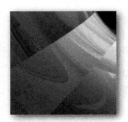

Discussion Points

D-1. In Case 1, Problem 1A, suppose BW is actually 6' 2" tall, weighs 106 kg, and has an estimated creatinine clearance of 61 mL/min. How would your maintenance dose differ to achieve plasma concentrations of 22 mg/L for the peak (2 hours after a 2-hour infusion) and approximately 12 mg/L for the trough?

D-2. Steady-state serum concentrations resulting from the maintenance dose you calculated in D-1 were reported by the laboratory as: peak, 17.8 mg/L and trough, 10.2 mg/L. Calculate a new maintenance dose to give our desired peak and trough concentrations of 22 mg/L and approximately 12 mg/L, respectively.

D-3. Assume that BA in Case 3 actually received a vancomycin 1250-mg loading dose followed by a maintenance dose of 1000 mg (over 2 hours) every 12 hours. Predict the steady state peak and trough levels that would result from this maintenance dose, using population average values for K and V.

D-4. Assume that the first dose for a patient (a 41-year-old female, 5' 6", 148 lb, with positive blood cultures for MRSA; SCr, 1.2 mg/dL; white blood cell count, 18,300/mm^3, 10% bands; receiving 1000 mg of vancomycin IV every 12 hours) is scheduled for 8:00 AM on 12/1. Describe in detail the process of how you determine when serum levels (and what type of levels) should be obtained. Then write an order as it would appear in the Physician's Order section of the patient's medical record for how serum levels should be obtained. This order should be grammatically correct, include only approved abbreviations, and provide sufficient detail that nursing services can easily follow your instructions without having to contact you for further clarification.

D-5. Based on your experience in the provision of direct patient care, design a pharmacy-managed vancomycin dosing protocol that could be used in your practice setting. This protocol should be written from the standpoint that the pharmacist is providing complete dosing and monitoring of vancomycin in a patient case (instead of simply providing recommendations to a physician to manage). All steps required to effectively dose and monitor (including equations used) a patient for whom vancomycin is prescribed should be included. Describe in detail how you would monitor this drug using serum concentrations. Write the order for this drug as it would appear in the Physician's Order section of the patient's medical record.

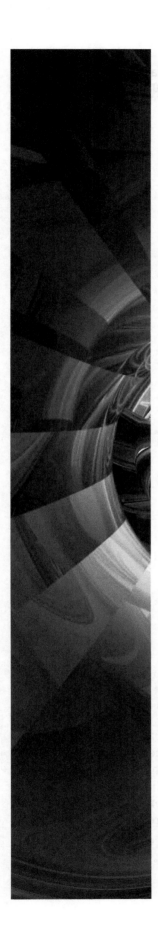

Theophylline

Methylxanthines, including theophylline and aminophylline, have been used in the management of asthma and chronic obstructive pulmonary disease (COPD) for more than five decades. With time, the use of these agents has declined as a result of the advent of alternative therapy, including beta-2 agonists, anticholinergics, corticosteroids, mast cell stabilizers, leukotriene modifiers, and immunomodulators. Although methylxanthines produce little therapeutic benefits for the patient with asthma, these agents may reduce dyspnea, increase exercise tolerance, and improve respiratory drive in patients with COPD.[1,2] At the same time, theophylline is an excellent agent for illustrating pharmacokinetic concepts associated with the continuous intravenous (IV) infusion model. Cases in this lesson focus on patient-specific dosing of aminophylline and theophylline.

Theophylline typically follows first-order pharmacokinetics in most patients with serum concentrations within the therapeutic range of 5–15 mg/L. It may undergo nonlinear, or Michaelis–Menten, pharmacokinetics (see Lesson 10) when serum concentrations are within this range; however, this is more likely to occur at concentrations exceeding 15 mg/L.[3]

Theophylline is eliminated from circulation through hepatic oxidative metabolism (cytochrome P450) and has a low intrinsic clearance (see Lesson 9). Therefore, total hepatic clearance of theophylline is determined by the intrinsic clearance of the liver and is not dependent on liver blood flow. Disease states, drugs, and other factors that may influence theophylline clearance are found in **Table 14-1**.

Theophylline is usually administered intravenously or orally. When theophylline derivatives are used, the theophylline dose equivalent should be calculated. For example, aminophylline is 80% theophylline. Therefore, to obtain the theophylline dose equivalent, the aminophylline dose should be multiplied by 0.8.

Many different oral formulations of theophylline are available. Some of these are rapidly absorbed after administration. Others are designed to slowly release drug in the gastrointestinal tract for up to 24 hours. The type of oral product used directly affects pharmacokinetic calculations.

TABLE 14-1. Factors and Drugs That Alter Theophylline Clearance

Factors	Total Body Clearance (L/kg/hr)	Clearance Adjustment (× 0.04 L/kg/hr)
Hepatic disease	0.02	0.5
Acute pulmonary edema	0.02	0.5
Severe chronic obstructive pulmonary disease	0.03	0.8
Heart failure	0.016	0.5
Cor pulmonale	0.028	0.7
Cigarette smoking	0.063	1.6
Former cigarette smoking (quit >2 years)	0.051	1.2
Marijuana smoking	0.072	1.7
Marijuana and cigarettes	0.09	2.2
Elderly cigarette smokers	0.045	1.1

Drugs	Clearance Adjustment (× 0.04 L/kg/hr)
Cimetidine (after 2 or more days)	0.5–0.7
Oral contraceptives	0.7
Interferon	0.15
Ciprofloxacin	0.7–0.75
Diltiazem	0.8–0.9
Norfloxacin	0.85
Phenytoin	1.35–1.5
Phenobarbital	1.35–1.5
Erythromycin	0.75–0.8
Propranolol	0.5–0.7
Verapamil	0.8–0.9
Rifampin	1.35–1.5
Phenytoin + smoking	1.9

CASE 1

MA is a 62-year-old, 65-kg man with a 30-year history of mild COPD that has been satisfactorily controlled with beta-2 agonist, ipratropium, and inhaled steroid therapy. However, over the past 2 months, MA has experienced increased difficulty in breathing. His physician wishes to admit him to the hospital and initiate IV aminophylline.

Problem 1A. Calculate an appropriate loading dose of aminophylline for MA that will result in a theophylline concentration of 14 mcg/mL.

To calculate a loading dose of aminophylline requires that we know the desired theophylline plasma concentration, the patient's theophylline volume of distribution, the aminophylline salt equivalent for theophylline, and the fraction of drug administered that reaches the systemic circulation.

In this case, the desired plasma theophylline concentration is 14 mcg/mL, the aminophylline salt equivalent (*S*) is 0.8, and the fraction of drug administered reaching the systemic circulation (*F*) is 1.

The one remaining factor that is necessary to make this loading dose calculation is the patient's theophylline volume of distribution (*V*). This is calculated from the patient's weight and the expected volume (in liters per kilogram) from published literature:

14-1
$$V(L) = \text{weight (kg)} \times 0.5 \text{ L/kg}$$

$$= 65 \text{ kg } (0.5 \text{ L/kg})$$

$$= 32.5 \text{ L}$$

Clinical Correlate

For theophylline, the patient's actual body weight should be used to calculate the volume of distribution unless the patient's actual weight is more than 50% above his or her ideal body weight. In patients more than 50% above ideal body weight, volume of distribution should be calculated using ideal body weight.

Based on the information we now have, we can calculate an aminophylline loading dose for MA. The basic loading dose equation can be derived from the plasma concentration equation we learned in Lesson 1:

$$\text{Concentration} = \frac{\text{amount of drug in body}}{\text{volume in which drug is distributed}}$$

$$C = \frac{X}{V}$$

(See **Equation 1-1**.)

We can rewrite this equation as below:

$$D = C \times V$$

Taking into consideration the *S* and *F* values for aminophylline, we can rewrite the above variation of **Equation 1-1** as follows:

14-2
$$D = \frac{Cpd\,V}{SF}$$

where:

D = the loading dose (milligrams)

Cpd = the desired concentration (milligrams per liter [L] or micrograms per milliliter [mL])

V = the volume of distribution (liters)

S = salt form

F = bioavailability, which is equal to 1 for drugs given intravenously

Substituting known values for these parameters:

$$D = \frac{14 \text{ mg/L} \times (32.5 \text{ L})}{0.8 \times 1}$$

$$= 568.75 \text{ mg}$$

$$= 570 \text{ mg}$$

This 570-mg aminophylline loading dose will produce a serum concentration slightly >14 mcg/mL. ***Note:*** Remember, aminophylline is a salt form of theophylline and contains approximately 80% theophylline equivalents. Aminophylline infusions are often rounded to the nearest 25 mg due to available products, so the dose would likely be changed to 575 mg.

Problem 1B. The loading dose is to be administered over a 30-minute interval. An aminophylline maintenance infusion is to be started immediately on completion of the loading dose. Suggest an aminophylline infusion rate for MA that will achieve a plasma theophylline concentration of 12 mcg/mL.

STEP A

The first step in solving this problem is to estimate MA's theophylline clearance. This can be accomplished by using the following equation:

14-3
$$Cl = (0.04 \text{ L/kg/hr}) \times \text{weight (kg)}$$

where:

Cl = clearance (L/hr; clearance is based on the patient's actual body weight)

0.04 L/kg/hr = population estimate found in the literature

Therefore:

$$Cl = (0.04 \text{ L/kg/hr}) \times \text{weight (kg)}$$

$$= (0.04 \text{ L/kg/hr}) \times 65 \text{ kg}$$

$$= 2.6 \text{ L/hr}$$

STEP B

To solve for a maintenance dose (milligrams per hour), we can rearrange and slightly modify **Equation 4-3** to **Equation 14-4** as follows:

$$\overline{C} = \frac{\text{dose}}{\text{Cl}_t \times \tau}$$

(See **Equation 4-3.**)

14-4 $$D = \frac{\overline{C}p_{ss} \, \text{Cl}\tau}{SF}$$

where:

D = the maintenance dose (milligrams per hour)

$\overline{C}_{pss}$ = average steady-state concentration desired (micrograms per milliliter)

Cl = clearance (liters per hour)

S = salt form

F = bioavailability

τ = dosing interval, which is 1 hour for a continuous IV infusion

After inserting the Cl value calculated in Step A, the S and F values, a dosing interval of 1 hour, and our desired serum concentration for $\overline{C}p_{ss}$, $\overline{C}pss$ we can solve for the maintenance dose:

$$D = \frac{12 \text{ mcg/mL} \times 2.6 \text{ L/hr} \times 1 \text{ hr}}{0.8}$$

$$= 39.0 \text{ mg/hr}$$

$$= 39 \text{ mg/hr}$$

Figure 14-1 demonstrates the relationship between serum levels achieved with the loading and maintenance doses of theophylline or aminophylline.

Problem 1C. How long will it take for MA's theophylline therapy to reach steady state?

• Steady state is reached once a given dose of a drug is administered for 5 half-lives of the drug.

• Half-life is determined by the equation $T\frac{1}{2} = 0.693/K$.

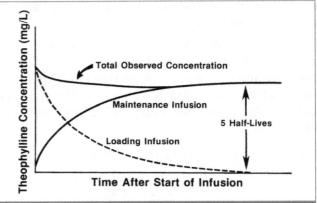

FIGURE 14-1.
Plasma concentrations with a loading dose and continuous infusion of theophylline or aminophylline.

• This requires that we know the value for K in this patient.

Using the equation $\text{Cl} = K \times V$, we can use our estimated values for Cl and V to estimate K.

$$\text{Cl} = K \times V$$

$$2.6 \text{ L/hr} = K \times (0.5 \text{ L/kg} \times 65 \text{ kg})$$

$$= K \times 32.5 \text{ L}$$

$$K = 0.08 \text{ hr}^{-1}$$

Now, substituting K into our half-life equation, we can solve for half-life.

$$T\frac{1}{2} = 0.693/K$$

$$= 0.693/0.08$$

$$= 8.7 \text{ hours}$$

Steady state will be reached in 3–5 half-lives. Therefore, steady state would be reached between 3×8.7 hours = 26.1 hours to 5×8.7 hours = 43.5 hours.

Problem 1D. MA's steady-state theophylline serum concentration is 11.6 mcg/mL. Is there any reason to change his dose at this time?

As long as MA is improving clinically and not experiencing theophylline adverse effects, it would be appropriate to leave his dose as is.

CASE 2

CJ is a 58-year-old, 72-kg, woman who is admitted to the hospital for treatment of severe chronic bronchitis. She has a history of cigarette smoking since age 14 and is currently receiving verapamil for high blood pressure.

Problem 2A. Estimate CJ's volume of distribution and clearance for theophylline.

To estimate CJ's volume of distribution (see **Equation 14-1**):

$$V(L) = \text{weight}(kg) \times 0.5 \text{ L/kg}$$

$$= 72 \text{ kg}(0.5 \text{ L/kg})$$

$$= 36 \text{ L}$$

To estimate CJ's clearance (see **Equation 14-3**):

$$Cl = (0.04 \text{ L/kg/hr}) \times \text{weight}(kg) \times (\text{adjustment factors})$$

$$= (0.04 \text{ L/kg/hr}) \times 72 \text{ kg} \times (0.8) \times (1.6) \times (0.8)$$

$$= 2.95 \text{ L/hr}$$

The clearance adjustment factors of 0.8, 1.6, and 0.8 are found in **Table 14-1** for severe bronchitis (severe COPD), cigarette smoking and verapamil, respectively. While useful, these adjustment factors are approximations and do not replace the need for therapeutic drug monitoring. It is unclear whether the use of more than two adjustments improves accuracy.

Problem 2B. Calculate an aminophylline loading dose for CJ that will achieve an initial plasma concentration of 12 mcg/mL. The dose will be given as an infusion over 30 minutes.

To calculate the loading dose:

$$D = \frac{Cpd\,V}{SF}$$

(See **Equation 14-2**.)

$$D = \frac{12 \text{ mcg/mL} \times 36 \text{ L}}{0.8}$$

$$= 540 \text{ mg}$$

Problem 2C. Calculate an infusion rate of aminophylline that will maintain CJ's serum concentration at 12 mcg/mL.

To determine the infusion rate:

$$D = \frac{\bar{C}\,p_{ss}\,Cl\tau}{SF}$$

(See **Equation 14-4**.)

$$D = \frac{12 \text{ mcg/mL} \times 2.95 \text{ L/hr} \times 1 \text{ hr}}{0.8}$$

$$= 44.25 \text{ mg / hr}$$

$$= 44 \text{ mg / hr}$$

Problem 2D. A steady-state theophylline serum concentration is reported by the laboratory as 18.2 mcg/mL. Calculate a new aminophylline maintenance dose to achieve a steady-state theophylline serum concentration of 12 mcg/mL.

STEP A

The first step in calculating a new aminophylline maintenance dose for CJ is to solve for her actual theophylline clearance. When calculating her initial maintenance dose, we estimated clearance using a population value. Now that we have a measured steady-state serum concentration, we can calculate an actual value.

To determine CJ's actual theophylline clearance, we can rearrange **Equation 14-4** in Problem 1B and calculate this parameter as follows:

$$D = \frac{\bar{C}\,p_{ss}\,Cl\tau}{SF}$$

Rearrange to solve for Cl:

$$Cl = \frac{DSF}{\bar{C}\,p_{ss}\tau}$$

(See **Equation 14-4**.)
where:

　　Cl = clearance (liters per hour)

　　D = maintenance dose (milligrams per hour)

　　S = salt form

F = bioavailability

$\bar{C}p_{ss}$ = average steady-state concentration (micrograms per milliliter)

$$Cl = \frac{44 \text{ mg/hr} \times 0.8 \times 1}{18.2 \text{ mcg/mL}}$$

$$= 1.93 \text{ L/hr}$$

Notice that we estimated CJ's theophylline Cl as 2.95 L/hr, but her actual value is 1.93 L/hr.

STEP B

Now that we have CJ's actual theophylline clearance, we can calculate a new maintenance dose that will give us the desired theophylline serum concentration of 12 mcg/mL:

$$D = \frac{\bar{C} \, p_{ss} \, Cl\tau}{SF}$$

(See **Equation 14-4**.)

$$D = \frac{12 \text{ mcg/mL} \times 1.93 \text{ L/hr} \times 1 \text{ hr}}{0.8 \times 1}$$

$$= 28.95 \text{ mg / hr}$$

$$= 29 \text{ mg / hr}$$

STEP C

Before we can begin this new maintenance dose of aminophylline in CJ, it is necessary to determine how long we must hold her current dose until her serum theophylline concentration declines to an acceptable value. We will choose a level of 12 mcg/mL. To determine how long it will be necessary to wait before starting this new maintenance dose, we need to determine CJ's theophylline elimination rate. We will make the calculation using her actual clearance value. Using the following formula:

$$K = \frac{Cl}{V}$$

(See **Equation 3-4**.)

where:

K = elimination rate constant (hr^{-1})

Cl = clearance (liters per hour)

V = volume of distribution (liters)

$$K = 1.93 \text{ L/hr/36 L}$$

$$= 0.054 \text{ hr}^{-1}$$

Next we can determine the time we need to wait by using the following equation:

$$C = C_0 e^{-Kt} \quad \text{(See Equation 3-2.)}$$

where:

t = time to wait (hours)

C = desired concentration (micrograms per milliliter)

C_0 = current concentration (micrograms per milliliter)

K = elimination rate constant (hr^{-1})

Therefore:

$$12 = 18.2e^{-0.054t}$$

$$12/18.2 = e^{-0.054t}$$

$$0.659 = e^{-0.054t}$$

$$\ln 0.659 = \ln e^{-0.054t}$$

$$-0.417 = -0.054t$$

$$t = 7.7 \text{ hours}$$

CJ would receive the new infusion of 25 mg/hr starting 8 hours after discontinuing the previous infusion of 44 mg/hr.

Clinical Correlate

The most significant side effects from theophylline occur at serum concentrations higher than 20 mcg/mL. These include nausea, vomiting, headache, diarrhea, irritability, and insomnia. At concentrations higher than 35 mcg/mL, major adverse effects include hyperglycemia, hypotension, cardiac arrhythmias, seizures, brain damage, and death. Side effects may differ depending upon whether it is an acute overdose or chronic accumulation of theophylline.[4]

CASE 3

SR is a 47-kg patient admitted to the emergency department with difficulty breathing. He has been prescribed theophylline for resistant asthma on an outpatient basis but admits his compliance to his medication regimen is poor. A STAT theophylline level is reported as 3.9 mcg/mL.

Problem 3A. Calculate an appropriate theophylline loading dose to give SR a serum level of 14 mcg/mL.

STEP A

Estimate SR's theophylline volume of distribution.

$$V = \text{weight}(kg) \times 0.5 \text{ L/kg}$$

$$= 47 \text{ kg} \times 0.5 \text{ L/kg}$$

$$= 23.5 \text{ L}$$

STEP B

Using SR's estimated V, calculate an appropriate theophylline loading dose. In this situation, we will slightly modify the loading dose **Equation 14-2** to the following:

$$D = \frac{(\text{Cpd} - \text{Cpi})V}{SF}$$

(See **Equation 14-2.**)

where:

D = the loading dose

Cpd = the desired concentration (milligrams per liter)

Cpi = the initial concentration (milligrams per liter)

V = the volume of distribution (liters)

S = salt form

F = bioavailability, which is equal to 1 for drugs administered intravenously

$$D = \frac{(14 \text{ mcg/mL} - 3.9 \text{ mcg/mL}) \times 23.5 \text{ L}}{1 \times 1}$$

$$= 237.4 \text{ mg}$$

$$= 240 \text{ mg}$$

This 240-mg theophylline loading dose will result in a serum concentration slightly >14 mg/L. Notice in this situation we are using a value of 1 for S (theophylline is not in a salt form).

Problem 3B. Calculate a theophylline maintenance dose that will maintain SR's serum concentration at 12 mcg/mL.

STEP A

As we saw in Case 1, the first step in solving this problem is to estimate SR's theophylline clearance. This can be accomplished by using the following equation:

14-3 $\qquad \text{Cl} = (0.04 \text{ L/kg/hr}) \times \text{weight}(kg)$

where:

Cl = clearance (L/hr; clearance is based on the patient's actual body weight)

0.04 L/kg/hr = population estimate found in the literature

Therefore:

$$\text{Cl} = (0.04 \text{ L/kg/hr}) \times \text{weight (kg)}$$

$$= (0.04 \text{ L/kg/hr}) \times 47 \text{ kg}$$

$$= 1.88 \text{ L/hr}$$

STEP B

To solve for a maintenance dose (milligrams per hour), we can rearrange and slightly modify **Equation 4-3** to **Equation 14-4** as follows:

$$\overline{C} = \frac{\text{dose}}{\text{Cl}_t \times \tau}$$

(See **Equation 4-3.**)

14-4 $\qquad D = \frac{\overline{C}p_{ss} \, \text{Cl}\tau}{SF}$

where:

D = the maintenance dose (milligrams per hour)

$\overline{C}p_{ss}$ = average steady-state concentration desired (micrograms per milliliter)

Cl = clearance (liters per hour)

S = salt form

F = bioavailability

τ = dosing interval, which is 1 hour for a continuous IV infusion

After inserting the Cl value calculated in Step A, S and F values, a dosing interval of 1 hour, and our desired serum concentration for $\bar{C}p_{ss}$, we can solve for the maintenance dose:

$$D = \frac{12 \text{ mcg/mL} \times 1.88 \text{ L/hr} \times 1 \text{ hr}}{1 \times 1}$$

$$= 22.56 \text{ mg / hr}$$

$$= 23 \text{ mg / hr}$$

Notice that both S and F for theophylline are 1.

Problem 3C. SR has been stabilized on his 23 mg/hr of theophylline regimen, and his steady-state serum theophylline level is now 13.2 mcg/mL. Calculate a dose of sustained-release theophylline for SR to maintain a theophylline serum concentration of 12 mcg/mL.

Many theophylline sustained-release formulations follow the same pharmacokinetic profile as continuous IV infusions. Therefore, we can easily make a conversion from a continuous infusion to an oral sustained-release formulation as follows:

STEP A

Calculate SR's theophylline clearance.

$$Cl = \frac{DSF}{\bar{C}p_{ss}\tau}$$

(See **Equation 14-4.**)

$$Cl = \frac{23 \text{ mg/hr} \times 1 \times 1}{13.2 \text{ mcg/mL} \times 1}$$

$$= 1.74 \text{ L/hr}$$

STEP B

Calculate the dose to be given orally every 12 hours.

$$D = \frac{\bar{C}p_{ss} \, Cl\tau}{SF}$$

(See **Equation 14-3.**)

where:

D = the maintenance dose (milligrams)

$\bar{C}p_{ss}$ = the desired average steady-state concentration (micrograms per milliliter)

Cl = clearance (liters per hour)

τ = dosing interval (hours)

S = salt form

F = bioavailability

$$D = \frac{12 \text{ mcg/mL} \times 1.74 \text{ L/hr} \times 12 \text{ hr}}{1 \times 1}$$

$$= 250.56 \text{ mg}$$

$$= 250 \text{ mg}$$

SR should receive a total daily dose of 500 mg of sustained-release theophylline orally split into two doses given every 12 hours. The dose could be given as 300 mg in the morning and 200 mg in the evening. Note that F for many oral sustained-release theophylline preparations is 1.

References

1. Sorkness CA, Kelly HW. Asthma. In: DiPiro JT, Talbert RL, Yee GC, et al., eds. *Pharmacotherapy: A Pathophysiologic Approach*. 10th ed. www.accesspharmacy.com. Accessed December 5, 2017.

2. Bourdet SV, Williams DN. Chronic obstructive pulmonary disease. In DiPiro JT, Talbert RL, Yee GC, et al., eds. *Pharmacotherapy: A Pathophysiologic Approach*. 10th ed. www.accesspharmacy.com. Accessed December 5, 2017.

3. Wagner JG. Theophylline: pooled Michaelis–Menten behavior of theophylline and its parameters (V_{max} and K_m) among asthmatic children and adults. *Ther Drug Monit*. 1987;9(1):11–20.

4. Hazardous Substances Data Bank [online database]. Theophylline. Bethesda, MD: U.S. National Library of Medicine. http://toxnet.nlm.nih.gov/cgi-bin/sis/htmlgen?HSDB. Accessed July 26, 2018.

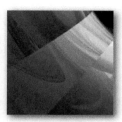

Discussion Points

D-1. Assume MA in Case 1 is a 64-year-old man with significant liver disease due to alcoholism and has uncontrolled severe COPD. How would these factors affect the maintenance dose you calculated for him?

D-2. In Case 2, assume CJ does not smoke tobacco but is started on Levofloxacin for her bronchitis. How would these changes affect her aminophylline maintenance dose?

D-3. If SR in Case 3 had a serum theophylline level of 15.9 mcg/mL as a result of his theophylline continuous infusion maintenance dose, what dose of oral sustained-release theophylline administered every 8 hours would he need to achieve a steady-state average plasma concentration of 12 mcg/mL?

D-4. Based on your experience in the provision of direct patient care, design a pharmacy-managed theophylline/aminophylline dosing protocol that could be used in your practice setting. This protocol should be written from the standpoint that the pharmacist is providing complete dosing and monitoring of theophylline/aminophylline in a patient case (instead of simply providing recommendations to a physician to manage). All steps (including equations used) required to effectively dose and monitor a patient for which theophylline/aminophylline is prescribed should be included. Describe in detail how you would monitor this drug using serum concentrations. Write the order for this drug as it would appear in the Physician's Order section of the patient's medical record.

D-5. Assume that a 49-year-old female, 5' 8" and 203 lb, with a serum creatinine of 1.34 mg/dL and white blood cell count of 18,300/mm^3 is receiving aminophylline as a continuous infusion in the dose of 38 mg/hr. This dose was initiated at 8:00 AM on 12/1. Describe in detail how you would determine when a serum level (and what type of level) should be obtained. Then write an order as it would appear in the Physician's Order section of the patient's medical record for how the serum level should be obtained. This order should be grammatically correct, include only approved abbreviations, and provide sufficient detail so that nursing services can easily follow your instructions without having to contact you for further clarification.

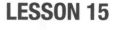

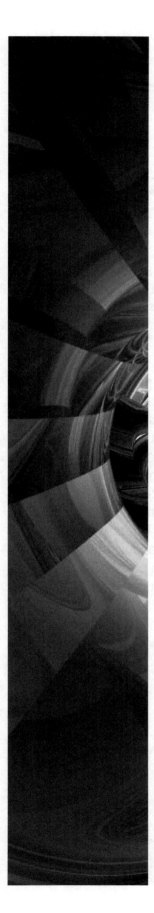

Phenytoin and Digoxin

Phenytoin

Phenytoin is an anticonvulsant medication used for many types of seizure disorders. Phenytoin is usually administered either orally or intravenously and exhibits nonlinear, or Michaelis–Menten, kinetics (see Lesson 10). Unlike drugs undergoing first-order elimination (**Figure 15-1**), the plot of the natural logarithm of concentration versus time is nonlinear with phenytoin (**Figure 15-2**). Phenytoin is 90% protein bound; only the unbound fraction is active. (Note that patients with low serum albumin concentrations will have a higher unbound, or active, fraction of phenytoin. This should be factored in when dosing these patients.)

Phenytoin is metabolized by hepatic enzymes that can be saturated with the drug at concentrations within the therapeutic range. Consequently, as the phenytoin dose increases, a disproportionately greater increase in plasma concentration is achieved. This enzyme saturation process can be characterized with an enzyme-substrate model first developed by the biochemists Michaelis and Menten in 1913. In this metabolic process, drug clearance is constantly changing (in a nonlinear fashion) as dose changes. Drug clearance decreases as drug concentration increases (**Figures 15-3** and **15-4**).

To describe the relationship between concentration and dose, a differential equation can be written as shown below:

$$\frac{dX}{dt} = \frac{V_{max} \times C_{ss}}{K_m + C_{ss}}$$

(See **Equation 10-1**.)

where:

   dX = change in amount of drug

   dt = change in time

   V_{max} = maximum amount of drug that can be metabolized per unit time, usually expressed as milligrams per day

   K_m = Michaelis–Menten constant, representing the concentration of phenytoin at which the rate of this enzyme-saturable hepatic metabolism is one-half of maximum

   C_{ss} = average steady-state phenytoin concentration

Next, this differential equation can be re-expressed algebraically by assuming that we are at steady state and dX/dt is held constant. Then dX/dt, the change in the amount of drug (X) over time (t), can be expressed as

231

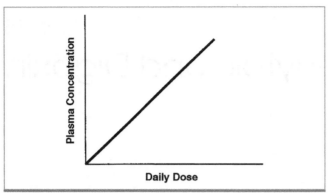

FIGURE 15-1.
First-order elimination model.

X_0/τ (dose over dosing interval), as shown in the following equation:

$$(X_0/\tau)(S) = \frac{V_{max} \times C_{ss}}{K_m + C_{ss}}$$

(See **Equation 10-1.**)

where:

X_0/τ = amount of phenytoin free acid divided by dosing interval (which can also be expressed as X_d, meaning daily dose of phenytoin free acid)

S = the salt factor or the fraction of phenytoin free acid in the salt form used; S equals 0.92 for phenytoin sodium injection, fosphenytoin when dose is expressed as phenytoin equivalents and capsules, 1 for phenytoin suspension and chewable tablets (i.e., the free acid form of phenytoin), and 0.66 for fosphenytoin injection if expressed as fosphenytoin (not phenytoin equivalents).

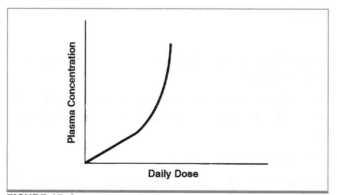

FIGURE 15-2.
Michaelis–Menten elimination model.

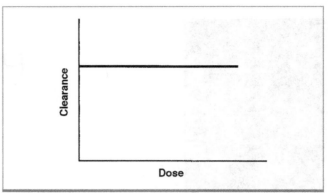

FIGURE 15-3.
First-order elimination model.

The oral bioavailability of phenytoin is considered to be 100%, so an *F* factor is not needed in these calculations.

Clinical Correlate

Although fosphenytoin is a prodrug containing only 66% phenytoin free acid, it is correctly prescribed and labeled in units of PE (phenytoin sodium equivalents). The commercial fosphenytoin product is packaged to be very similar to phenytoin sodium injection; it contains 150-mg fosphenytoin per 2-mL ampule, providing 100 mg PE (100-mg phenytoin sodium equivalents). Fosphenytoin is readily transformed to phenytoin free acid by various phosphatases throughout the body. When performing dose calculations, care must be taken to represent doses in the correct salt form (66% for fosphenytoin or 92% for phenytoin equivalents).

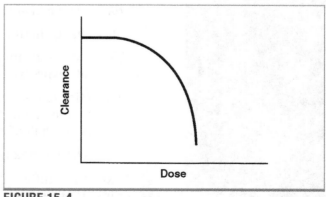

FIGURE 15-4.
Michaelis–Menten elimination model.

This Michaelis–Menten equation (MME) can then be rearranged to solve for C_{ss} as follows:

$$(X_0/\tau)(S) = \frac{V_{max} \times C_{ss}}{K_m + C_{ss}}$$

(See **Equation 10-1**.)

First, cross-multiply by the denominator:

$$\left[(X_0/\tau)(S) \times K_m\right] + \left[(X_0/\tau)(S) \times C_{ss}\right] = V_{max} \times C_{ss}$$

Then transpose $[(X_0/\tau)(S) \times C_{ss}]$ to the right side of the equation:

$$\left[(X_0/\tau)(S) \times K_m\right] = \left[V_{max} \times C_{ss}\right] - \left[(X_0/\tau)(S) \times C_{ss}\right]$$

Factor out C_{ss}:

$$\left[(X_0/\tau)(S) \times K_m\right] = C_{ss}\left[V_{max} - X_0/\tau \times (S)\right]$$

Transpose $[V_{max} - (X_0/\tau)(S)]$ to the left side of the equation:

$$C_{ss} = \frac{(X_0/\tau)(S) \times K_m}{V_{max} - (X_0/\tau)(S)}$$

The two representations of the MME below can now be used for phenytoin dosing, as illustrated in the following cases:

$$(X_0/\tau)(S) = \frac{V_{max} \times C_{ss}}{K_m + C_{ss}}$$

(See **Equation 10-1**.)

 $$C_{ss} = \frac{(X_0/\tau)(S) \times K_m}{V_{max} - (X_0/\tau)(S)}$$

Phenytoin Pharmacokinetic Parameters

In contrast to first-order drugs that use pharmacokinetic parameters for K and V, phenytoin dose calculations use population estimates for K_m and V_{max}. A K_m population estimate of 4 mg/L and a V_{max} estimate of 7 mg/kg/day are commonly used. Note, however, that K_m can range from 1 to 15 mg/L while V_{max} can range from 3 to >10 mg/kg/day in selected patients. Phenytoin's volume of distribution is usually estimated as 0.65 L/kg total body weight. Last, phenytoin trough serum drug concentrations

(meaning in this case, at least 8–12 hours after last oral dose) are usually used in dosing adjustment calculations to avoid unpredictable rates and extent of drug absorption from various dosage forms.

CASE 1

RW, a 50-year-old black man, is admitted to the hospital with status epilepticus that was successfully treated with intravenous (IV) lorazepam. His physician has written an order for the pharmacy to calculate and order an IV phenytoin loading dose, recommend an initial oral maintenance dose, and order timing of plasma concentrations. Other pertinent clinical data include weight, 85 kg; height, 6'0"; serum creatinine, 1.6 mg/dL; and serum albumin, 4.6 g/dL.

Problem 1A. What IV loading dose and oral maintenance dose would you recommend to achieve and maintain a phenytoin concentration of approximately 20 mg/L?

Calculation of the loading dose is not affected by the nonlinear pharmacokinetics of multiple-dose phenytoin regimens. The loading dose calculation is based on the patient's weight, estimated volume of distribution, serum albumin concentration, renal function assessment, and the salt form (i.e., salt factor) of phenytoin used. The generally accepted population parameter for phenytoin's volume of distribution is 0.65 L/kg of body weight.

The loading dose (X_0) formula is as follows:

$$X_0 = \frac{V \times C_{desired}}{S}$$

(See **Equation 1-1**.)

where:

> V = volume of distribution estimate of 0.65 L/kg [V = 0.65 L/kg (85 kg) = 55.25 L for RW]
>
> $C_{desired}$ = concentration desired 1 hour after the end of the infusion (20 mg/L for RW)
>
> S = salt factor (0.92 for injection). Note that this dose falls within the empiric loading dose range of 15–20 mg/kg.

Therefore:

$$X_0 = \frac{(55.25\ L)(20\ mg/L)}{0.92}$$

$$= 1200\ mg\ of\ phenytoin\ sodium$$
$$or\ fosphenytoin\ PE\ injection$$

We could then order a dose of 1200 mg of phenytoin mixed in 100 mL of normal saline given intravenously via controlled infusion. The administration rate for phenytoin sodium injection should not exceed 50 mg/min to avoid potential cardiovascular toxicity associated with the propylene glycol diluent of the phenytoin injection. The accuracy of this loading dose estimate can be checked by obtaining a phenytoin plasma drug concentration approximately 1 hour after the end of the loading dose infusion. Alternatively, we could give this 1200 mg of phenytoin sodium as the fosphenytoin salt (Cerebyx) also at a dose of 1200 mg PE of fosphenytoin at a rate of 150 PE mg/min. Both doses will deliver the same amount (1104 mg) of phenytoin free acid.

Clinical Correlate

Phenytoin sodium injection uses a propylene glycol base as its vehicle and will precipitate in most IV fluids. It is most compatible in normal saline but can even precipitate in this fluid and clog an existing inline IV filter. Propylene glycol is a cardiotoxic agent and can cause various complications, such as bradycardia and hypotension. An alternative is to use the newer fosphenytoin injection, which is compatible with many IV fluids and can also be administered safely at a faster rate (up to 150 mg/min).

Maintenance Dose Calculations

Several methods to calculate maintenance dose are described, with each method requiring more serum drug concentrations and yielding more accurate dosing estimates. Phenytoin dosage adjustments using these methods are more commonly done in the outpatient setting because they require steady-state concentrations that may take more than 2 weeks to be attained.

There are two methods to calculate an initial daily maintenance dose (X_d): an empiric method and a method based on estimating the patient's V_{max} and K_m.

Clinical Correlate

The Phenytoin Cheat Sheet at the end of the Maintenance Dose Calculations section is a concise review of the equations and sequencing for the three dose calculation methods.

Method 1A *(Empiric)*

Multiply RW's weight of 85 kg by 5 mg/kg/day to get an estimated dose of 425 mg of phenytoin free acid or 462 mg of phenytoin sodium, which would be rounded to 460 mg. This dose of 460 mg/day may be divided into 230 mg twice daily, if necessary, to decrease the likelihood of enzyme saturation and reduce concentration-dependent side effects. This assumes that the patient has an average K_m and V_{max}.

Method 1B *(Population Parameters)*

Substitute population estimates for V_{max} and K_m into the MME and solve for the dose as follows:

$$X_d \times S = \frac{V_{max} \times C_{ss}}{K_m + C_{ss}}$$

(See **Equation 10-1**.)

Therefore:

$$X_d(0.92) = \frac{595\ mg/day \times 15\ mg/L}{4\ mg/L + 15\ mg/L}$$

$$= \frac{8925\ mg^2\ L/day}{19\ mg/L}$$

$$= 470\ mg/day\ of\ phenytoin\ free\ acid$$

$$X_d = \frac{470\ mg/day}{0.92}$$

$$= 510\ mg/day\ of\ sodium\ salt\ rounded\ to\ 500\ mg$$

500 mg phenytoin sodium provides 460 mg phenytoin free acid

where:

V_{max} = population estimate of maximum rate of drug metabolism (7 mg/kg/day × 85 kg = 595 mg/day)

K_m = population estimate of Michaelis–Menten constant (4 mg/L)

C_{ss} = desired average steady-state plasma concentration of 15 mg/L

S = salt factor (0.92 for phenytoin sodium capsules)

Note how the units in the equation cancel out, yielding mg/day as the final units.

This calculation of 470 mg of phenytoin free acid (510 mg sodium salt) by use of population estimates is larger than our empiric estimate of 425 mg/day (460 mg sodium salt), showing that the empiric method of 5 mg/kg/day results in a lower value for RW's initial phenytoin maintenance dose. In RW's case, although the population estimate dose would equal a daily dose of five 100-mg phenytoin sodium capsules, a patient would usually be started on 460 mg/day (230 mg twice daily) and titrated up to 500 mg if needed based on plasma phenytoin drug concentrations and clinical response. Next we will evaluate when a serum drug concentration would reflect a steady-state value. A daily dose of phenytoin 423 mg free acid (460 mg sodium salt) will be utilized for our next calculations.

Problem 1B. When would you recommend that steady-state plasma concentrations be drawn?

It is difficult to calculate when multiple dosing with phenytoin will reach steady state because the time to steady state is concentration dependent. With drugs that undergo first-order elimination, steady state can be reached in three to five drug half-lives because this model assumes that clearance and volume of distribution are constant. However, because of its capacity-limited metabolism, phenytoin clearance decreases with increasing concentration. Therefore, the calculation of time to reach steady state is quite complicated and cannot be based on half-life. In fact, phenytoin does not have a true half-life; its half-life is dependent on drug concentration.

The major factor in determining how long it will take to attain steady state is the difference between V_{max} and the daily dose. The closer V_{max} is to the dose, the longer it will take to achieve steady state. This relationship between V_{max} and concentration can be derived mathematically by examining the equations used to calculate dose for first- and zero-order models. We will start by rearranging two definitions in the first-order model:

$$C_{ss} = \frac{X_0}{V} \quad \text{rearranges to} \quad X_0 = C_{ss} \times V$$

(See **Equation 1-1**.)

and

$$Cl_t = VK \quad \text{rearranges to} \quad V = \frac{Cl_t}{K}$$

so, by substituting for V:

$$X_0 = \frac{C_{ss} \times Cl_t}{K} \quad \text{or} \quad X_0 \times K = C_{ss} \times Cl_t$$

$C_{ss} \times Cl_t$ from our first-order equation can be substituted for X_0/τ in the zero-order equation derived in the introduction:

$$X_0/\tau = \frac{V_{max} \times C_{ss}}{K_m + C_{ss}}$$

(See **Equation 10-1**.)

Substituting $C_{ss} \times Cl_t$ for X_0/τ yields:

$$Cl_t \times C_{ss} = \frac{V_{max} \times C_{ss}}{K_m + C_{ss}}$$

Solving for Cl_t:

$$(C_{ss} \times Cl_t \times K_m) + (Cl_t \times C_{ss}^2) = V_{max} \times C_{ss}$$

$$\frac{C_{ss} \times Cl_t \times K_m}{C_{ss}} + \frac{Cl_t \times C_{ss}^2}{C_{ss}} = V_{max}$$

$$(Cl_t \times K_m) + (Cl_t \times C_{ss}) = V_{max}$$

$$Cl_t(K_m + C_{ss}) = V_{max}$$

This equation can now be rearranged to represent clearance in terms of V_{max} and C_{ss} as shown:

$$Cl_t = \frac{V_{max}}{K_m + C_{ss}}$$

where:

    Cl_t = clearance of phenytoin

    V_{max} = maximum rate of drug metabolism, usually expressed as milligrams per day

    K_m = Michaelis–Menten constant, representing the concentration of phenytoin at which the rate of this enzyme-saturable hepatic metabolism is half of maximum

    C_{ss} = average steady-state phenytoin concentration

Examination of this equation shows that when C_{ss} is very small compared to K_m, Cl_t will approximate V_{max}/K_m, a relatively constant value. Therefore, at low concentrations, the metabolism of phenytoin follows a first-order process. However, as C_{ss} increases to exceed K_m, as is usually seen with therapeutic concentrations of phenytoin, Cl_t will decrease and metabolism will convert to zero order.

We can calculate an estimate of the time it takes to get to 90% of steady state using the following equation:

$$t_{90\%} = \frac{K_m \times V}{(V_{max} - X_d)^2}[(2.3 \times V_{max}) - (0.9 \times X_d)]$$

(See **Equation 10-4.**)

where:

    $t_{90\%}$ = estimated number of days to get to 90% of steady state

    X_d = daily dose of phenytoin (in mg/day)

    V = volume of distribution

    V_{max} = maximum rate of drug metabolism (in milligrams per day)

    K_m = Michaelis–Menten constant

This equation is derived from a complex integration of the differential equation describing the difference between the rate of drug coming in (i.e., the daily dose) and the rate of drug going out of the body. This equation gives us an estimate of when to draw steady-state plasma concentrations and assumes that the beginning phenytoin concentration is zero. In patients such as RW, who have previously received a loading dose, $t_{90\%}$ may be different, usually shorter, unless the loading dose yielded an initial concentration greater than that desired, in which case $t_{90\%}$ would be even longer.

Clinical Correlate

The $t_{90\%}$ equation is a very rough estimate of time to 90% of steady state and should be used only as a general guide. The clinician should check nonsteady-state phenytoin concentrations before this time to avoid serious subtherapeutic or supratherapeutic concentrations.

In patient RW's case, $t_{90\%}$ is calculated as follows:

$$t_{90\%} = \frac{K_m \times V}{(V_{max} - X_d)^2}[(2.3 \times V_{max}) - (0.9 \times X_d)]$$

(See **Equation 10-4.**)

where:

    K_m = 4 mg/L

    V_{max} = 7 mg/kg/day × 85 kg = 595 mg/day

    X_d = 423 mg/day of phenytoin (free acid = 460mg sodium salt)

    V = 0.65 L/kg × 85 kg = 55.25 L

Therefore:

$$t_{90\%} = \frac{4 \text{ mg/L} \times 55.25 \text{ L}}{(595 \text{ mg/day} - 423 \text{ mg/day})^2}$$
$$\times [(2.3 \times 595 \text{ mg/day}) - (0.9 \times 423 \text{ mg/day})]$$
$$= \frac{221}{29584}[(1368.5) - (0.9 \times 423)]$$
$$= 0.007(988)$$
$$= 7.4 \text{ days}$$

Note how the units cancel out in this equation, leaving the answer expressed in days, not hours. This equation estimates that it will take RW approximately 7 days for his phenytoin concentration to reach steady state with a desired C_{ss} concentration of 15 mg/L.

Close inspection of this calculation illustrates the impact that the denominator—the difference of V_{max} and daily dose—has on the time it takes to reach steady state. For example, if we assume that

RW's daily dose was 550 mg/day, we can resolve the $t_{90\%}$ equation with the new dose.

$$t_{90\%} = \frac{4 \text{ mg/L} \times 55.25 \text{ L}}{(595 \text{ mg/day} - 550 \text{ mg/day})^2}$$
$$\times [(2.3 \times 595 \text{ mg/day}) - (0.9 \times 550 \text{ mg/day})]$$

$$= \frac{4(55.25)}{(595 - 550)^2}[2.3(595) - 0.9(550)]$$

$$= \frac{221}{2025}(1368.5 - 495)$$

$$= 0.109(873.5)$$

$$= 95.2 \text{ days}$$

This means that, theoretically, it would now take approximately 95 days for patient RW to reach steady state on a dose of 550 mg/day. Of course, RW would actually show signs of toxicity long before he reached steady state, but this illustrates the effect the difference of dose (and V_{max}, similarly) has on the calculation of time to steady state. In fact, if the daily dose exceeds V_{max}, steady state is never achieved.

CASE 2

For this case, we use the data presented in Case 1 and continue treating patient RW. A phenytoin plasma concentration (free acid) of 6 mg/L is drawn 18 days after the beginning of therapy. Although RW's seizure frequency has decreased, he is still having occasional seizures, and his physician has decided to adjust his dosing regimen to attain a plasma concentration of 15 mg/L.

Method 2 (One Steady-State Level)

Problem 2A. Calculate an appropriate dosing regimen to attain our desired concentration of 15 mg/L.

Now that we have one steady-state concentration, we can calculate a new maintenance dose for RW. This is done using the basic MME with two unknowns, V_{max} and K_m. We can use a population

estimate for one of the unknowns (usually K_m), solve for the other unknown, and then recalculate the new dose once again using the MME. This method is preferred over using population estimates for both unknowns. For RW, this calculation is as follows:

$$X_d \times S = \frac{V_{max} \times C_{ss}}{K_m + C_{ss}}$$

(See **Equation 10-1**.)

First, rearrange the MME to isolate V_{max}:

$$V_{max} = \frac{(X_d \times S)(K_m + C_{ss})}{C_{ss}}$$

$$V_{max} = \frac{(423 \text{ mg/day} \times 1)(4 \text{ mg/L} + 6 \text{ mg/L})}{(6 \text{ mg/L})}$$

$$= \frac{(423 \text{ mg/day})(10 \text{ mg/L})}{(6 \text{ mg/L})}$$

$$= \frac{(4230 \text{ mg}^2/\text{day} \times L)}{(6 \text{ mg/L})}$$

$$= 705 \text{ mg/day as free acid, rounded to 706 mg/day}$$

(See **Equation 10-1**.)
where:

V_{max} = calculated estimate of patient's V_{max}

K_m = population estimate of 4 mg/L

$X_d \times S$ = patient's daily dose of phenytoin (423 mg/day of free acid)

C_{ss} = reported steady-state concentration (6 mg/L)

So RW's new estimated V_{max} is 705 mg/day, which is larger than the population estimate of 595 mg/day, meaning that he has a greater phenytoin clearance than first estimated.

We now take the new V_{max} and the MME for our new dose and use it in the MME to solve for X_d as follows:

$$X_d \times S = \frac{V_{max} \times C_{ss}}{K_m + C_{ss}}$$

(See **Equation 10-1**.)

$$X_d \times S = \frac{705 \text{ mg/day} \times 15 \text{ mg/L}}{4 \text{ mg/L} + 15 \text{ mg/L}}$$

$$= \frac{10575 \text{ mg}^2/\text{day} \times \text{L}}{19 \text{ mg/L}}$$

$$= 556.5 \text{ mg/day}$$

$$X_d \, (0.92) = 556 \frac{\text{mg}}{\text{day}} \text{ of phenytoin free acid}$$

$$X_d = 604 \frac{\text{mg}}{\text{day}} \text{ of phenytoin sodium,}$$
rounded to 600 mg/day

where:

$X_d \times S$ = new dose of phenytoin sodium ($S = 0.92$)

C_{ss} = desired steady-state concentration of 15 mg/L

K_m = population estimate of 4 mg/L

V_{max} = calculated estimate (705 mg/day)

Therefore, RW's new dose would be 600 mg/day as phenytoin sodium capsules in divided doses, which is equivalent to 552 mg of phenytoin free acid. Because this is a large increase in dose, it may saturate the patient's hepatic enzymes, causing the plasma concentration to increase disproportionately. The practitioner may decide to give a lower dose initially based on the risk benefit of adverse events versus the need for improved seizure control. Again, note how units cancel out in this equation, yielding mg/day.

Clinical Correlate

Phenytoin doses are usually increased by 25–100 mg/day. Because the clinical accuracy using this pharmacokinetic modeling is not as accurate and predictive as those for the aminoglycosides and theophylline, good clinical judgment is required when recommending a dose.

Problem 2B. When should a plasma phenytoin concentration be drawn?

We can recalculate when RW's phenytoin concentration will reach steady state on this new dose. Remember, time to 90% of steady state ($t_{90\%}$) is dependent on plasma drug concentration. RW's new estimate of $t_{90\%}$ is calculated as follows:

$$t_{90\%} = \frac{K_m \times V}{(V_{max} - X_d)^2}[(2.3 \times V_{max}) - (0.9 \times X_d)]$$

(See **Equation 10-4.**)
Therefore:

$$t_{90\%} = \frac{4 \text{ mg/L} \times 55.25 \text{ L}}{(705 \text{ mg/day} - 552 \text{ mg/day})^2}$$
$$\times [(2.3 \times 705 \text{ mg/day}) - (0.9 \times 552 \text{ mg/day})]$$

$$t_{90\%} = \frac{221 \text{ mg}}{(153 \text{ mg/day})^2}[(1621.5 \text{ mg/day}) - (496.8 \text{ mg/day})]$$

$$= 0.0094(1124.7)$$

$$= 10.6 \text{ days for new } t_{90\%} \text{ to be reached}$$

where:

K_m = population estimate (4 mg/L)

V_{max} = calculated estimate based on one steady-state concentration (780 mg/day)

X_d = daily dose of 552 mg/day phenytoin-free acid or 600 mg/day phenytoin sodium.

V = population estimate of volume of distribution (55.25 L)

Note that our new $t_{90\%}$ is slightly smaller than the previous estimate because the difference between V_{max} and dose is now greater.

Method 3 *(Two Steady-State Levels)*

Problem 2C. Three weeks later, RW's plasma phenytoin concentration is 20 mg/L on his regimen of phenytoin sodium 300 mg twice daily (600 mg daily sodium salt providing 552 mg daily of free acid). He is now seizure free, and his physician wants to adjust his dose to get his plasma concentration back to 15 mg/L. Note that RW states that he has been taking his phenytoin exactly as prescribed. What dose would you now recommend to achieve a plasma phenytoin concentration of 15 mg/L?

Now that we have measured two different steady-state concentrations at two different doses, we can make an even more accurate dosing change. As shown in Lesson 14, clearance can be expressed as X_d/C_{ss}, resulting in the plot in **Figure 15-5.**

We can now plot both steady-state doses (X_1 of 423 mg/day and X_2 of 552 mg/day) on the y-axis and both steady-state X_d/C_{ss} values ($X_1/C_1 = 423/6$ L/day and $X_2/C_2 = 552/20$ L/day) on the x-axis, thus linearizing these relationships. This allows us to express the relationship in the algebraic form for a straight line, $Y = mX + b$, where m, the slope of the line, equals the negative value of the patient's K_m (i.e., $m = -K_m$) and the y-intercept is the patient's V_{max}. For RW, this graph is drawn as in **Figure 15-6.**

The slope of the line, which represents $-K_m$, can now be calculated as follows:

$$-K_m = \frac{X_1 - X_2}{\dfrac{X_1}{C_1} - \dfrac{X_2}{C_2}}$$

$$= \frac{423 \text{ mg/day} - 552 \text{ mg/day}}{\dfrac{423 \text{ mg/day}}{6 \text{ mg/L}} - \dfrac{552 \text{ mg/day}}{20 \text{ mg/L}}}$$

$$-K_m = \frac{-129}{(70.5) - (27.6)}$$

$$K_m = 3 \text{ mg/L}$$

(See **Equation 10-2.**)

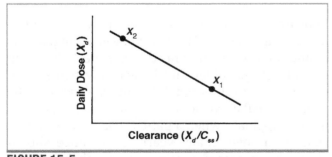

FIGURE 15-5.
Relationship of daily dose to clearance.

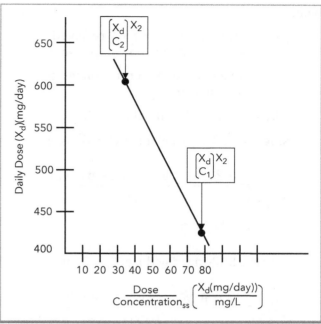

FIGURE 15-6.
Relationship of daily dose to the dose divided by steady-state concentration achieved.

Clinical Correlate

It is best to use the free acid amount of phenytoin, not the sodium salt, when calculating K_m in the above equation and in all subsequent calculations. The calculated free acid dose can then be converted to the appropriate dose form accounting for its salt form.

Next, we substitute this new value for K_m into the MME and solve for an even more accurate V_{max} than calculated previously, as follows:

$$V_{max} = \frac{(X_d \times S)(K_m + C_{ss})}{C_{ss}}$$

(See **Equation 10-1.**)

where:

$X_d \times S$ = either of the doses RW received (423 or 552 mg/day of free acid)

C_{ss} = steady-state concentration at the dose selected

K_m = calculated value of 2 mg/L

Using the 423-mg/day dose, C_{ss} = 6 mg/L.

$$V_{max} = \frac{(423 \text{ mg/day})(3 \text{ mg/L} + 6 \text{ mg/L})}{6 \text{ mg/L}}$$

$$= 634.5 \text{ mg/day}$$

Using the 552-mg/day dose, C_{ss} = 20 mg/L.

$$V_{max} = \frac{(552 \text{ mg/day})(3 \text{ mg/L} + 20 \text{ mg/L})}{20 \text{ mg/L}}$$

$$= 634.8 \text{ mg/day}$$

which we will round to 635 mg/day. Note that either set of doses and concentrations will give the same V_{max}.

Finally, we substitute our new V_{max} of 634 mg/day (rounded down to reduce risk of overestimation of dose) and our calculated K_m of 3 mg/mL into the MME and solve for X_d as follows:

$$X_d \times S = \frac{V_{max} \times C_{ss}}{K_m + C_{ss}}$$

(See **Equation 10-1**.)

$$X_d(0.92) = \frac{(634 \text{ mg/day})(15 \text{ mg/L})}{3 \text{ mg/L} + 15 \text{ mg/L}}$$

$$X_d(0.92) = 528 \text{ mg/day of phenytoin free acid}$$

$$X_d = 573.9 \text{ mg/day of phenytoin sodium}$$

where

V_{max} = 634 mg/day of phenytoin free acid

K_m = 3 mg/L

C_{ss} = desired average steady-state plasma concentration of 15 mg/L

S = salt factor (0.92 for phenytoin sodium capsules)

Once again the challenge of administering our calculated dose requires dose rounding. Therefore, we could give RW 560 mg (five 100-mg phenytoin capsules plus two 30-mg phenytoin capsules) daily in divided doses. This would require the use of two dose strengths (phenytoin sodium 100-mg and 30-mg capsules) and would give slightly less than the calculated amount of 575 mg/day of sodium salt.

Clinical Correlate

It is important to dose phenytoin correctly so side effects do not occur. Dose-related side effects at serum concentrations >20 mg/L include nystagmus, whereas concentrations >30 mcg/mL may result in nystagmus and ataxia. Concentrations >40 mg/L may produce ataxia, lethargy, seizures, and diminished cognitive function. Adverse effects that may occur at therapeutic concentrations include gingival hyperplasia, folate deficiency, peripheral neuropathy, hypertrichosis, and thickening of facial features.

Long-Term Phenytoin Monitoring

Repeated use of Method 3 (above) allows for continued dosing adjustments over many years in patients maintained on phenytoin; this is especially useful as children get older and bigger. Any two sets of drug concentrations and different dose pairs can be used to calculate an adjusted dose, which makes for interesting math when a patient has dozens of concentrations over many years. Compliance should always be assessed before trusting these dosage adjustment calculations.

Clinical Correlate

When interpreting phenytoin concentrations, there are several considerations. It is important to determine if the reported level is a free or total phenytoin level. Free phenytoin levels do not require any adjustment. Total levels must be corrected when hypoalbuminemia, acid base disturbances, or renal dysfunction exist—as all of these conditions may affect protein binding.[6] While equations exist to "correct" phenytoin levels in these populations, it is preferable to monitor free phenytoin levels instead.

Phenytoin Cheat Sheet

The Phenytoin Cheat Sheet contains the equations and sequencing for the three dosing methods detailed in the Maintenance Dose Calculations Section above. Equations are presented for calculating doses when you have no phenytoin serum drug concentration, one phenytoin serum drug concentration, and, finally, two phenytoin serum drug concentrations obtained on two different doses.

PHENYTOIN DOSING CHEAT SHEET

DOSING METHOD 1A:

Use 5 mg/kg/day

DOSING METHOD 1B:

Use population estimates for the Michaelis–Menten values for K_m of 4 mg/L and V_{max} of 7 mg/kg/day and solve the general MME formula as shown below:

Equation 1 MME:

$$X_d \times S = \frac{V_{max}(C_{ss\ (desired)})}{(K_m + C_{ss\ (desired)})}$$

K_m estimate = 4 mg/L

V_{max} estimate = 7 mg/kg/day

S = salt form factor (either 1, 0.92, or 0.66)

DOSING METHOD 2: ONE STEADY-STATE LEVEL

Use this method as in Equation 2 below after you have one steady-state phenytoin serum drug concentration to **solve for** V_{max} while still using the population parameter for K_m of 4 mg/L.

After solving for this better value for V_{max}, use it plus the old K_m value in the MME to re-solve for dose, as shown below.

To solve for V_{max}:

Equation 2:

This is simply a **rearrangement of MME (Equation 1):**

$$V_{max} = \frac{(X_d \times S)(K_m + C_{ss(lab)})}{C_{ss(lab)}}$$

To solve for dose:

Use Equation 1 again.

Equation 1 (MME) again:

$$X_d \times S = \frac{\textit{\textbf{better}}V_{max}(C_{ss(desired)})}{(\textbf{population parameter for}\ K_m + C_{ss(desired)})}$$

K_m estimate = 4 mg/L

V_{max} estimate = as solved for mg/kg/day

S = salt form factor (either 1, 0.92, or 0.66)

DOSING METHOD 3: TWO STEADY-STATE LEVELS ON TWO DIFFERENT DOSES

Use after you have **two steady-state** phenytoin concentrations from two different phenytoin doses. You can now work Equation 3 to solve for **an even better value for** K_m (shown below).

Use this better K_m value to once again re-solve for a better V_{max} value than used in Method 2. Once you get new V_{max} (i.e., real K_m and V_{max}), re-solve Equation 1 (MME) again for dose.

Equation 3:

Use this to solve for real K_m:

X_d = dose

C = concentration

To solve for real V_{max}:

Use Equation 2 again.

To solve for dose:

Use Equation 1 (MME) again.

To solve for real V_{max}:

Use Equation 2 once again.

$$\textit{\textbf{real}}V_{max} = \frac{X_d \times S(\textit{\textbf{real}}K_m + C_{ss(lab)})}{C_{ss(lab)}}$$

To solve for dose:

Use Equation 1 again.

Equation 1 (MME) yet again:

$$\textit{\textbf{best}}X_d \times S = \frac{\textit{\textbf{real}}V_{max}(C_{ss(desired)})}{\textit{\textbf{real}}K_m(C_{ss(desired)})}$$

real K_m (mg/L)

real V_{max} (mg/kg/day)

S = salt form factor (either 1, 0.92, or 0.66)

Digoxin

Digoxin is an inotropic medication that may be useful in the treatment of patients with heart failure (HF) to decrease hospitalizations and a limited role as therapy for supraventricular tachycardia. Desired serum concentrations in these patients range from 0.5 to 0.9 ng/mL.[1] This conservative target has been associated with a decline in the overall incidence of digoxin toxicity. Notice that the units of plasma concentrations for digoxin are different (nanograms per milliliter) from those of other commonly monitored drugs (usually milligrams per liter).

Digoxin may also be used in the management of arrhythmias such as atrial fibrillation (AF) and atrial flutter. It is effective in controlling heart rate at rest in patients with AF and may be used in patients with concomitant HF, left ventricular dysfunction, and a sedentary lifestyle. Digoxin is an acceptable treatment for slowing a rapid ventricular response and improving left ventricular function in patients with acute myocardial infarction and AF associated with severe left ventricular dysfunction and HF. In combination with a beta-blocker or nondihydropyridine calcium channel antagonist, digoxin may be used to control heart rate during exercise in patients with AF, as well as in the pregnant patient with AF. Digoxin may also be used to terminate paroxysmal supraventricular tachycardia (PSVT).[2,3]

In patients with normal left ventricular function, digoxin is less effective for ventricular rate control than calcium channel blockers or beta-blockers. However, it may be used in combination with these agents in patients with less than satisfactory ventricular rate control from monotherapy.[3]

Doses of digoxin are usually administered orally or intravenously. Loading doses are no longer recommended in HF patients.[1] Although digoxin loading doses have been used extensively in patients with AF, atrial flutter, and PSVT, other drugs are more effective and/or have a more rapid onset of action. Therefore, digoxin loading doses are rarely needed unless alternative therapy is contraindicated or not effective in a given patient.[2] The current recommended loading dose of digoxin for ventricular rate control is 0.25 mg IV every 2 hours up to a total of 1.5 mg. For PSVT, the loading dose is 8–12 mcg/kg given as follows: one half of the dose is given over 5 minutes; 25% is given in 4–8 hours; and the final 25% given 4–8 hours later.[3]

Electrocardiogram monitoring is performed during loading dose administration to assess for toxicity.[4] The recommended maintenance dose of digoxin for ventricular rate control is 0.125–0.375 mg per day. With declining renal function, these doses may be further reduced or administered as alternate day therapy.[3]

Steady-state volume of distribution (V_{ss}) of digoxin is large and extremely variable. Differences in renal function account for some of the interpatient variation.

15-2
$$V_{ss} = 4{-}9 \text{ L/kg ideal body weight (IBW)}$$
$$\text{(average adult, 7 L/kg IBW)}^4$$

When calculating an oral digoxin dose, the bioavailability (F) of the dosage form used must be considered. For patients with normal oral absorption, digoxin tablets are 50% to 90% (average, 70%) absorbed ($F = 0.7$), and digoxin elixir is 75% to 85% absorbed (average, $F = 0.8$).

Systemic clearance (Cl_t) of digoxin can be calculated as follows[5]:

15-3
$$Cl_t = (1.303 \times CrCl) + Cl_m$$

where:

Cl$_m$ = metabolic clearance

= 40 mL/min for patients with no or mild HF

= 20 mL/min for patients with moderate to severe HF

Several methods have been proposed for calculating doses of digoxin that have been described in detail elsewhere. Recent investigators have developed a nomogram for determining digoxin doses that achieve lower serum concentrations.[6]

CASE 3

BH is a 72-year-old, 5'3", 145-lb female who has a diagnosis of HF for which she currently receives a beta-blocker, an angiotensin-converting enzyme inhibitor (ACEI), and a diuretic. She has been hospitalized three times in the past year for her HF; at this time, her physician wishes to initiate digoxin therapy. Her current serum creatinine is 1 mg/dL.

Problem 3A. Calculate a maintenance dose of digoxin tablets to be given to BH to achieve a satisfactory steady-state serum digoxin level.

Clinical Correlate

Patients with HF usually do not require a loading dose of digoxin before initiating maintenance dose therapy.[1]

The relationship between the steady-state plasma concentration, maintenance dose, and total systemic clearance is shown below:

15-4
$$C_{ss} = \frac{X_d \times 10^6 \times F}{Cl_t \times \tau}$$

(See **Equation 4-3**.)

The above equation can be rearranged and written as follows:

$$X_d = \frac{C_{ss} \times Cl_t \times \tau}{10^6 \times F}$$

where:

X_d = maintenance dose of digoxin, in milligrams per day

C_{ss} = steady-state plasma concentration, in nanograms per milliliter

Cl_t = total body clearance

τ = dosing interval, in minutes (1440 minutes = 1 day)

10^6 = conversion from nanograms to milligrams (i.e., 10^6 ng = 1 mg)

F = 0.7 for tablets

We have previously established that the desired steady-state serum digoxin concentration in the patient with HF ranges from 0.5 to 0.9 ng/mL. We will choose a level of 0.8 ng/mL for BH.

To determine systemic clearance, we must first estimate BH's creatinine clearance. We use the Cockcroft–Gault equation:

$$CrCl_{(female)} = (0.85)\frac{(140 - age)(BW)}{72 \times SCr}$$

(See **Equation 9-1**.)

where:

CrCl = creatinine clearance, in milliliters per minute

BW = body weight, in kilograms

SCr = serum creatinine, in milligrams per deciliter

Therefore:

$$CrCl_{(female)} = \frac{(0.85)(140 - 72)(58 \text{ kg})}{72 \times 1.00}$$

$$= 46.6 \text{ mL/min}$$

Total body clearance of digoxin would be as follows:

$Cl_t = (1.303 \times CrCl) + Cl_m$ (See **Equation 15-3**.)

$= (1.303 \times 46.6 \text{ mL/min}) + 20 \text{ mL/min}$

$= 80.7 \text{ mL/min}$

The daily maintenance dose required to achieve a steady-state concentration of 0.8 ng/mL would be as follows:

$$X_d = \frac{C_{ss} \times Cl_t \times \tau}{10^6 \times F}$$

$$X_d = \frac{0.8 \text{ ng/mL} \times (80.7 \text{ mL/min}) \times 1440 \text{ min}}{10^6 \text{ ng/mg} \times 0.7}$$

$$= 0.133 \text{ mg}$$

(See **Equation 15-4**.)

Therefore, BH should receive 0.125 mg of digoxin daily to achieve a steady-state digoxin concentration of slightly <0.8 ng/mL.

Problem 3B. Two months later, BH has a steady-state serum digoxin level drawn. The laboratory reports this value as 0.5 ng/mL. Although this value is within the therapeutic range for HF, BH's physician desires to increase the dose to achieve a slightly higher serum concentration. Calculate a new maintenance dose for BH that will achieve a serum concentration of 0.8 ng/mL.

The first step to solving this problem is to calculate BH's actual serum digoxin clearance. We can do this as follows:

$$Cl_t = \frac{X_d \times 10^6 \times F}{C_{ss} \times \tau}$$

where:

Cl_t = total body clearance

X_d = maintenance dose of digoxin, in milligrams per day

C_{ss} = steady-state plasma concentration, in nanograms per milliliter

τ = 1440 minutes (1 day)

10^6 = conversion from nanograms to milligrams (i.e., 10^6 ng = 1 mg)

F = bioavailability (0.7 for digoxin tablets)

Plugging in our values for patient BH:

$$Cl_t = \frac{0.125 \text{ mg} \times 10^6 \text{ ng/mg} \times 0.7}{0.5 \text{ ng/mL} \times 1440 \text{ min}}$$

$$= 121.5 \text{ mL/min}$$

From this we see that BH's total body clearance of digoxin is slightly higher than the value we calculated using population estimates.

Now, we can use this clearance value to calculate a new maintenance dose to achieve our desired serum concentration of 0.8 ng/mL.

$$X_d = \frac{C_{ss} \times Cl_t \times \tau}{10^6 \times F}$$

$$X_d = \frac{0.8 \text{ ng/mL} \times (121.5 \text{ mL/min}) \times 1440 \text{ min}}{10^6 \text{ ng/mg} \times 0.7}$$

$$= 0.199 \text{ mg}$$

This dose can be achieved by alternating 0.25 mg with 0.125 mg every other day. This would be the equivalent of administering 0.1875 mg per day.

Problem 3C. BH begins her new digoxin regimen. Three months later she reports to her physician's office complaining of nausea and vomiting. A serum digoxin level (10 hours after her last dose) and serum creatinine are drawn. Her digoxin concentration is 1.6 ng/mL, and her serum creatinine has risen to 1.92 mg/dL. Her physician tells her to hold her digoxin for the next two days and come back to the office to have her serum digoxin concentration repeated. Her serum level (48 hours after the last serum level was drawn) is now 1.1 ng/mL. Calculate a new digoxin dose that will achieve a steady-state serum concentration of 0.8 ng/mL.

BH appears to now be experiencing declining renal function (rise in serum creatinine). To determine a new dose, we must first calculate her actual Cl_t. As before, we can do this by rearranging the following equation:

$$C_{ss} = \frac{X_d \times 10^6 \times F}{Cl_t \times \tau}$$

(See **Equation 15-4**.)

to:

$$Cl_t = \frac{X_d \times 10^6 \times F}{C_{ss} \times \tau}$$

where:

Cl_t = total body clearance

X_d = maintenance dose of digoxin, in milligrams per day

C_{ss} = steady-state plasma concentration, in nanograms per milliliter

τ = 1440 minutes (1 day)

10^6 = conversion from nanograms to milligrams (i.e., 10^6 ng = 1 mg)

F = bioavailability (0.7 for digoxin tablets)

Plugging in our values for patient BH:

$$Cl_t = \frac{0.1875 \text{ mg} \times 10^6 \text{ ng/mg} \times 0.7}{1.6 \text{ ng/mL} \times 1440 \text{ min}}$$

$$= 57 \text{ mL/min}$$

In making this determination, it is important that we use the average daily dose BH is receiving as well as the serum value resulting from this dose (and not the serum value reported 2 days later with doses held). It is of interest to note a significant decline in digoxin total body clearance with declining renal function.

Then we use patient BH's actual Cl_t to calculate the appropriate dose to achieve our desired C_{ss} of 0.8 ng/mL.

$$X_d = \frac{C_{ss} \times Cl_t \times \tau}{10^6 \times F}$$

$$X_d = \frac{0.8 \text{ ng/mL} \times (57 \text{ mL/min}) \times 1440 \text{ min}}{10^6 \text{ ng/mg} \times 0.7}$$

$$= 0.094 \text{ mg/day}$$

This dose can be achieved by alternating 0.125 mg with 0.0625 mg (one half of a 0.125-mg tablet) every other day.

Problem 3D. How much longer do we need to wait until we can begin BH's new digoxin maintenance dose?

Because BH's latest serum digoxin concentration is elevated (1.1 ng/mL), we cannot begin her new maintenance dose until this value decreases to approximately 0.8 ng/mL. To calculate the amount of time that must elapse until this occurs, we can use the following equation:

$$C_{\text{level 2(steady state)}} = C_{\text{level 1(steady state)}}e^{-Kt}$$

where:

$C_{\text{level 2(steady state)}}$ = the serum concentration we desire before the new maintenance dose is started (0.8 ng/mL)

$C_{\text{level 1(steady state)}}$ = the serum concentration the patient currently has (1.1 ng/mL)

K = the elimination rate constant

t = the time we must wait until $C_{\text{level 2(steady state)}}$ is reached

We can calculate K as follows:

$$K = \frac{\ln 1.1 - \ln 1.6}{48 \text{ hr}}$$

$$= 0.008 \text{ hr}^{-1}$$

Now, we can solve for time t:

$$C_{\text{level 2(steady state)}} = C_{\text{level 1(steady state)}}e^{-Kt}$$

$$0.8 \text{ ng/mL} = 1.1 \text{ ng/mL } e - 0.008t$$

$$0.727 = e - 0.008t$$

$$\ln 0.727 = \ln e - 0.008t$$

$$-0.319 = -0.008t$$

$$39.9 \text{ hr} = t$$

So we need to wait another 40 hours before we begin BH's new digoxin maintenance dose.

CASE 4

JW is a 56-year-old, 6' 4" tall, 200-lb patient with HF. He is currently receiving a beta-blocker and an ACEI. His physician wishes to add digoxin to this regimen. His current serum creatinine is 1.1 mg/dL.

Problem 4A. Calculate a maintenance dose of digoxin tablets that will achieve a steady-state serum concentration of 0.7 ng/mL for JW.

The first step in solving this problem is to determine JW's total body clearance for digoxin. To determine this, we must first estimate his creatinine clearance.

$$CrCl_{\text{male}} = \frac{(140 - \text{age})(BW)}{72 \times SCr}$$

(See **Equation 9-1**.)

where:

CrCl = creatinine clearance, in milliliters per minute

BW = body weight, in kilograms; see lesson 12 for review of weight to use.

SCr = serum creatinine, in milligrams per deciliter

Therefore:

$$CrCl_{\text{male}} = \frac{(140 - 56)(86.8 \text{ kg})}{72 \times 1.1}$$

$$= 92 \text{ mL/min}$$

Total body clearance of digoxin would be as follows:

$$Cl_t = (1.303 \times CrCl) + Cl_m \quad \text{(See **Equation 15-3**.)}$$

$$= (1.303 \times 92 \text{ mL/min}) + 40 \text{ mL/min}$$

$$= 160 \text{ mL/min}$$

The daily maintenance dose required to achieve a steady-state concentration of 0.7 ng/mL would be:

$$X_d = \frac{C_{ss} \times Cl_t \times \tau}{10^6 \times F}$$

$$X_d = \frac{0.7 \text{ ng/mL} \times (160 \text{ mL/min}) \times 1440 \text{ min}}{10^6 \text{ ng/mg} \times 0.7}$$

$$= 0.23 \text{ mg}$$

(See **Equation 15-4**.)

Therefore, JW should receive 0.25 mg of digoxin daily.

Problem 4B. Suppose JW had to initially receive his daily digoxin maintenance dose by IV administration. Calculate this dose.

$$X_d = \frac{C_{ss} \times Cl_t \times \tau}{10^6 \times F}$$

$$X_d = \frac{0.7 \text{ ng/mL} \times (160 \text{ mL/min}) \times 1440 \text{ min}}{10^6 \text{ ng/mg} \times 1}$$

$$= 0.16 \text{ mg}$$

Note: $F = 1$ for IV administered drugs. Because digoxin injection is available in a 0.25-mg/mL concentration, the potential for errors when the dose is drawn from the vial are a concern. So the patient's dose would be 0.16 mg/0.64 mL.

Clinical Correlate

IV administration of digoxin should be given by slow IV push. This method of administration prevents the propylene glycol contained in this formulation from causing cardiovascular collapse.

Problem 4C. JW is currently receiving digoxin 0.25 mg orally daily. He has a steady-state serum digoxin level reported as 1.2 ng/mL. If all doses are held, predict how long it will take for his serum concentration to fall to 0.7 ng/mL.

In Problem 3C, we encountered a similar situation in which we solved for the time to wait before an elevated serum concentration declined to an acceptable value with doses held. In that situation, we had two steady-state serum concentrations to solve for

a K value. In the current problem, we will address how we can estimate a K value and, therefore, time to wait, with only one steady-state serum concentration available.

The first step to solving this problem is to calculate JW's actual serum digoxin clearance. We can do this as follows:

$$Cl_t = \frac{X_d \times 10^6 \times F}{C_{ss} \times \tau}$$

where:

Cl_t = total body clearance

X_d = maintenance dose of digoxin, in milligrams per day

C_{ss} = steady-state plasma concentration, in nanograms per milliliter

τ = 1440 minutes (1 day)

10^6 = conversion from nanograms to milligrams (i.e., 10^6 ng = 1 mg)

F = bioavailability (0.7 for digoxin tablets)

Plugging in our values for patient JW:

$$Cl_t = \frac{0.25 \text{ mg} \times 10^6 \text{ ng/mg} \times 0.7}{1.2 \text{ ng/mL} \times 1440 \text{ min}}$$

$$= 101 \text{ mL/min}$$

Step 2 to solving this problem is to use the equation below to calculate time to wait:

$$C_{\text{level 2(steady state)}} = C_{\text{level 1(steady state)}} e^{-Kt}$$

where:

$C_{\text{level 2(steady state)}}$ = the serum concentration we desire before the new maintenance dose is started (0.7 ng/mL)

$C_{\text{level 1(steady state)}}$ = the serum concentration the patient currently has (1.2 ng/mL)

K = the elimination rate constant

t = the time we must wait until $C_{\text{level 2(steady state)}}$ is reached

To use this equation requires that we know the value for K. We can estimate this from the following equation:

$$K = \frac{Cl}{V}$$

We can estimate V as 7 L/kg IBW. (See **Equation 15-2**.)

$$V = 7 \ \text{L/kg} \times 91 \ \text{kg}$$

$$= 637 \ \text{L}$$

Now, we can estimate K.

K is in units of hr^{-1}

V is in units of liters

Cl therefore must be converted to units of liters per hour (L/hr):

$$101 \ \text{mL/min} \times 60 \ \text{min/hr} = 6060 \ \text{mL/hr}$$

$$6060 \ \text{mL/hr divided by } 1000 \ \text{mL/L} = 6.06 \ \text{L/hr}$$

$$K = \frac{Cl}{V}$$

$$= \frac{6.06 \ \text{L/hr}}{637 \ \text{L}}$$

$$= 0.0095 \ \text{hr}^{-1}$$

Using the equation:

$$C_{\text{level 2(steady state)}} = C_{\text{level 1(steady state)}} e^{-Kt}$$

$$0.7 \ \text{ng/mL} = 1.2 \ \text{ng/mL} \ e^{-0.0095t}$$

$$0.583 = e^{-0.0095t}$$

$$\ln 0.583 = \ln e^{-0.0095t}$$

$$-0.54 = -0.0095t$$

$$56.8 \ \text{hr} = t$$

So we must wait an additional 57 hours for JW's serum digoxin level to drop to 0.7 ng/mL. Before initiating a new maintenance dose, it would be prudent to repeat a serum digoxin level to ensure his elimination rate has not changed during this waiting period and that his serum concentration is an acceptable value.

References

1. Yancy CW, Jessup M, Bozkurt B, et al. 2013 ACCF/AHA guideline for the management of heart failure: a report of the American College of Cardiology Foundation/American Heart Association Task Force on Practice Guidelines. *J Am Coll Cardiology.* 2013;62(16):e147–239. http://content.onlinejacc.org. Accessed December 21, 2017.

2. January CT, Wann S, Alpert JS, et al. 2014 AHA/ACC/HRS guideline for management of patients with atrial fibrillation: a report of the American College of Cardiology/American Heart Association Task Force on Practice Guidelines and Heart Rhythm Society. *Circulation.* 2014;130(23):2071–104. http://circ.ahajournals.org/content/130/23/e199. Accessed December 21, 2017.

3. Parker RB, Nappi JM, Cavallar LH. Chapter 14: the arrhythmias. In: DiPiro JT, Talbert RL, Yee GC, et al., eds. *Pharmacotherapy: A Pathophysiologic Approach.* 10th ed. New York, NY: McGraw-Hill. http://accesspharmacy.mhmedical.com/content.aspx?bookid=1861&sectionid=146028752. Accessed January 28, 2018.

4. Koup JR, Jusko WJ, Elwood CM, et al. Digoxin pharmacokinetics: role of renal failure in dosage regimen design. *Clin Pharmacol Ther.* 1975;18(1):9–21.

5. Bauman JJ, DiDomenico RJ, Viana M, et al. A method of determining the dose of digoxin for heart failure in the modern era. *Arch Intern Med.* 2006;166(22):2539–45.

6. Soriano VV, Tesoro EP, Kane SP. Characterization of free phenytoin concentrations in end-stage renal disease using the Winter-Tozer equation. *Ann Pharmacother.* 2017;51(8):669–74.

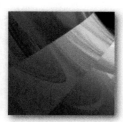

Discussion Points

Phenytoin

D-1. Suppose RW in Case 1, Problem 1A was 60 years old, weighed 85 kg, and had a serum albumin level of 2.6 mg/L. What would be his oral maintenance dose of phenytoin based on these changes?

D-2. Based on your calculations in Discussion Point 1, calculate a new maintenance dose for RW that would result in a steady-state plasma concentration of 15 mg/L.

D-3. The laboratory reports a serum phenytoin concentration of 20 mg/L from the dose you calculated in Discussion Point 2. Calculate a new dose that will result in a serum concentration of 15 mg/L (i.e., use Method 2).

D-4. Based on your experience in the provision of direct patient care, design a pharmacy-managed phenytoin dosing protocol that could be used in your practice setting. This protocol should be written from the standpoint that the pharmacist is providing complete dosing and monitoring of phenytoin in a patient case (instead of simply providing recommendations to a physician to manage). All steps required (including equations used) to effectively dose and monitor a patient for whom phenytoin is prescribed should be included. Describe in detail how you would monitor this drug using serum concentrations. Write the order for this drug as it would appear in the Physician's Order section of the patient's medical record.

D-5. A 41-year-old female, 5' 2" and 160 lb, presents to the emergency department with uncontrolled seizures (serum creatinine, 1.4 mg/dL; serum albumin, 3.6 g/dL; white blood cell count 18,300/mm^3, receiving phenytoin 300 mg daily at home). Assuming that phenytoin 200 mg every 12 hours orally is initiated at 8:00 AM on 12/1, describe in detail the process for how you determine when serum levels (and what type of levels) should be obtained. Then write an order as it would appear in the Physician's Order section of the patient's medical record for how serum levels should be obtained. This order should be grammatically correct, include only approved abbreviations, and provide sufficient detail that nursing services can easily follow your instructions without having to contact you for further clarification.

Digoxin

D-6. Suppose BH's serum digoxin concentration in Problem 3B had been 1.2 ng/mL. What maintenance dose would be required to achieve a serum concentration of 0.8 ng/mL?

D-7. Explain how to administer an appropriate digoxin loading dose to a patient with atrial fibrillation.

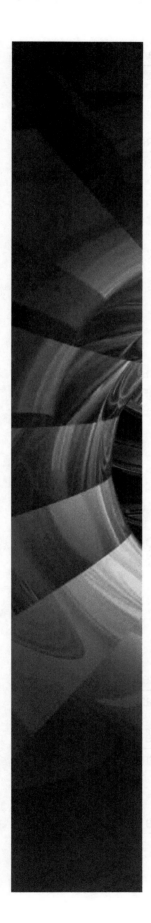

Basic and Drug-Specific Pharmacokinetic Equations

Basic Pharmacokinetic Equations

Equation Showing the Relationship of Drug Concentration (mg/L), Drug Dose (mg), and Volume of Distribution (L)

1-1
$$\text{concentration} = \frac{\text{amount of drug in body}}{\text{volume in which drug is distributed}}$$

$$C = \frac{X}{V}$$

(See p. 10.)

Equation for Calculating Total Body Clearance

2-1
$$Cl_t = Cl_r + Cl_m + Cl_b + Cl_{other}$$

(See p. 23.)

Equation for Calculating Organ Clearance of a Drug

2-2
$$Cl_{organ} = Q \times \frac{C_{in} - C_{out}}{C_{in}} \text{ or } Cl_{organ} = QE$$

(See p. 24.)

Elimination Rate Constant (K) for First-Order, One-Compartment Model

3-1
$$\text{slope} = -K = \frac{\ln C_1 - \ln C_0}{t_1 - t_0}$$

(See p. 34.)
or:

$$-K = \frac{\ln \dfrac{C_1}{C_0}}{t_1 - t_0}$$

Concentration at Any Given Time, Based on a Previous Concentration (C_0) and K for First-Order, One-Compartment Model

3-2
$$C = C_0 e^{-Kt}$$

(See p. 34.)

where:

C = plasma drug concentration at time = t

C_0 = plasma drug concentration at time = 0

K = elimination rate constant

t = time after dose

e^{-Kt} = percent or fraction remaining after time (t)

Note: Used often to calculate Cp_{min} from Cp_{max}.

Calculation of $T\frac{1}{2}$ from K, or K from $T\frac{1}{2}$ for First-Order, One-Compartment Model

3-3
$$T\frac{1}{2} = \frac{0.693}{K}$$

(See p. 36.)

or:

$$K = \frac{0.693}{T\frac{1}{2}}$$

Mathematical Relationship Between Systemic Clearance (Cl_t) to Both V and K for First-Order, One-Compartment Model

3-4
$$Cl_t/V = K$$

(See p. 37.)

or:

$$Cl_t = V \times K \text{ or } V = Cl_t/K$$

Calculation of Area Under the Plasma Drug Concentration Curve (AUC) and Its Relationship to Both Drug Clearance ($K \times V$) and Dose Administered

3-5
$$AUC = \frac{dose\ administered}{drug\ clearance}$$

(See pp. 37–38.)

or:

$$drug\ clearance = \frac{dose\ administered}{AUC}$$

or:

$$AUC = \frac{initial\ concentration\ (C_0)}{elimination\ rate\ constant\ (K)}$$

Accumulation Factor When Not at Steady State for a One-Compartment, First-Order Model

4-1
$$accumulation\ factor = \frac{(1 - e^{-nK\tau})}{(1 - e^{-K\tau})}$$

(See p. 52.)

Accumulation Factor When at Steady State for a One-Compartment, First-Order Model

4-2
$$\frac{1}{(1 - e^{-K\tau})}$$

(See p. 56.)

Calculation of Average Drug Concentration from AUC and Dosing Interval or from Dose/Cl

$$\bar{C} = \frac{AUC}{\tau}$$

and because:

$$AUC = \frac{dose}{drug\ clearance}$$

$$\bar{C} = \frac{dose}{drug\ clearance \times \tau}$$

or:

4-3
$$\bar{C} = \frac{dose}{Cl_t \times \tau}$$

(See p. 57.)

Cockcroft–Gault Equations for Calculating Creatinine Clearance (CrCl) in Men and Women

9-1
$$CrCl_{male} = \frac{(140 - age)IBW}{72 \times SCr}$$

(See p. 138.)

or:

$$CrCl_{female} = \frac{(0.85)(140 - age)IBW}{72 \times SCr}$$

Note: IBW = ideal body weight.

Equations for Estimating IBW in Men and Women

9-2 IBW_{males} = 50 kg + 2.3 kg for each inch over 5 feet in height

(See p. 139.)

$IBW_{females}$ = 45.5 kg + 2.3 kg for each inch over 5 feet in height

Adjusted Body Weight (AdjBW) Equation for Patients Whose Total Body Weight (TBW) Is More Than 20% over Their IBW for CGEQ

9-3 $AdjBW = IBW + 0.4(TBW - IBW)$

(See p. 139.)

Michaelis–Menten Equation (MME)

10-1
$$\text{Daily dose} = \frac{V_{max}C}{K_m + C}$$

(See p. 148.)

or:

$$\text{Daily dose }(K_m + C) = V_{max}C$$

$$\text{Daily dose }(K_m) + \text{daily dose }(C) = V_{max}C$$

$$\text{Daily dose }(C) = V_{max}C - \text{daily dose }(K_m)$$

Note: Relates V_{max}, K_m, plasma drug concentration, and daily dose (at steady state) for zero-order (i.e., nonlinear) model.

Calculation of K_m, the Michaelis Constant (mg/L), Representing the Drug Concentration at Which the Rate of Elimination Is Half the Maximum Rate (V_{max}) for Zero-Order (i.e., nonlinear) Model

10-2 $$\text{Slope} = -K_m = \frac{dose_{initial} - dose_{increased}}{dose/C_{initial} - dose/C_{increased}}$$

(See p. 148.)

Calculating Steady-State Concentration from Estimates of K_m, V_{max}, and Dose (Rearrangement of the MME) for Zero-Order (i.e., nonlinear) Model

10-3
$$C = \frac{K_m(\text{daily dose})}{V_{max} - \text{daily dose}}$$

(See p. 149.)

Aminoglycoside Dosing Equations

Calculation of Population Estimates for K Based on CrCl

12-1 $K = 0.00293\ (CrCl) + 0.014$

(See p. 181.)

Calculation of Population Estimates for Volume of Distribution (V) Based on Body Weight or AdjBW$_{AG}$

12-2 $V = 0.24$ L/kg (IBW)

(See p. 181.)

or:

$V = 0.24$ L/kg (AdjBW$_{AG}$)

where:

12-3 $AdjBW_{AG} = IBW + 0.4(TBW - IBW)$

(See p. 181.)

Note: Use if patient is >30% above ideal body weight

Calculation of Best Dosing Interval (τ) Based on Desired Peak and Trough Concentrations

$$\boxed{12\text{-}4} \quad \tau = \frac{1}{-K}\left(\ln C_{trough(desired)} - \ln C_{peak(desired)}\right) + t$$

(See pp. 183 and 191.)

where t is the duration of the infusion in hours.

Note: Should be rounded off to a practical dosing interval such as every 8 hours, every 12 hours, etc.

Calculation of Initial Maintenance Dose (K_0) Based on Estimates of K, V, Desired C_{peak}, and τ

$$\boxed{5\text{-}1} \quad C_{ss\,peak} = \frac{K_0(1 - e^{-Kt})}{VK(1 - e^{-K\tau})}$$

(See p. 74.)

where:

$C_{ss\,peak}$ = desired peak drug concentration at steady state (milligrams per liter)

K_0 = drug infusion rate (also maintenance dose you are trying to calculate, in milligrams per hour)

V = volume of distribution (population estimate for aminoglycosides, in liters)

K = elimination rate constant (population estimate for aminoglycosides, in reciprocal hours)

t = duration of infusion (hours)

τ = desired or most appropriate dosing interval (hours)

Calculation of Expected Concentration from Known Concentration (C_0), Dose (K_0), and Dosing Interval Used

$$\boxed{3\text{-}2} \quad C = C_0 e^{-Kt}$$

(See p. 34.)

or:

$$C_{ss\,trough} = C_{ss\,peak}e^{-Kt'}$$

(See p. 34 and **Equation 3-2**.)

where $t' = \tau -$ time of infusion (t), or the change in time from the first concentration to the second.

Calculation of Loading Dose Based on Initial Calculated Maintenance Dose and Accumulation Factor

$$\boxed{12\text{-}5} \quad \text{loading dose} = \frac{K_0}{(1 - e^{-K\tau})}$$

(See p. 189.)

where:

K_0 = estimated maintenance dose

$1/(1 - e^{-K\tau})$ = accumulation factor at steady state

τ = dosing interval at which estimated maintenance dose is given

Calculation of Patient-Specific (i.e., actual) K Based on Two Drug Concentrations and Dosing Interval

$$\boxed{3\text{-}1} \quad K = \frac{\ln C_{trough} - \ln C_{peak}}{\tau - t}$$

(See p. 34.)

or:

$$-K = \frac{\ln C_{peak} - \ln C_{trough}}{\tau - t}$$

Remembering a rule of logarithms: $\ln a - \ln b = \ln (a/b)$, we can simplify this equation for hand-held calculators:

$$K = -\frac{\ln\left(\dfrac{C_{trough}}{C_{peak}}\right)}{\tau - t}$$

or:

$$-K = \frac{\ln\left(\dfrac{C_{peak}}{C_{trough}}\right)}{\tau - t}$$

Either equation may be used to calculate K.

Calculation of Patient-Specific (i.e., actual) V Based on Actual K, and Dose (K_0), τ

5-1
$$C_{ss\,peak} = \frac{K_0(1 - e^{-Kt})}{VK(1 - e^{-K\tau})}$$

(See p. 74.)

where:

$C_{ss\,peak}$ = C_{peak} measured at steady state

K_0 = maintenance dose infused at time C_{peak} and C_{trough} were measured

V = patient's actual volume of distribution that you are trying to determine based on C_{peak} and C_{trough} values

K = elimination rate constant calculated from patient's C_{peak} and C_{trough} values

t = duration of infusion (hours)

τ = patient's dosing interval at time C_{peak} and C_{trough} were measured

Calculation of Actual (i.e., new) Dosing Interval Based on Patient-Specific Value for K

12-4
$$\tau = \frac{1}{-K}(\ln C_{trough(desired)} - \ln C_{peak(desired)}) + t$$

(See pp. 186 and 194.)

where t is the duration of infusion in hours and K is the actual elimination rate calculated from patient's peak and trough values.

Calculation of Patient-Specific or Adjusted Maintenance Dose (K_0) Based on Actual Values for K and V

5-1
$$C_{ss\,peak} = \frac{K_0(1 - e^{-Kt})}{VK(1 - e^{-K\tau})}$$

(See p. 74.)

where:

$C_{ss\,peak}$ = desired steady-state C_{peak}

K_0 = drug infusion rate (also adjusted maintenance dose you are trying to calculate, in milligrams per hour)

V = actual volume of distribution determined from patient's measured C_{peak} and C_{trough} values, in liters

K = actual elimination rate constant calculated from patient's measured C_{peak} and C_{trough} values, in reciprocal hours

t = infusion time, in hours

τ = adjusted dosing interval rounded to a practical number

Calculation of New Expected $C_{ss\,trough}$ That Would Result Based on a Known or Estimated $C_{ss\,peak}$ and Interval Used

$$C_{ss\,trough} = C_{ss\,peak}e^{-Kt'}$$

(See p. 34 and **Equation 3-2**.)

where K is actual patient-specific K (for example, after calculating a new maintenance dose and C_{peak} has been estimated).

Calculation of Time to Hold Dose When Actual C_{trough} from Laboratory Is Too High

$$C_{ss\,trough\,(desired)} = C_{ss\,trough}e^{-Kt'}$$

where t' is the amount of time to hold the dose after the end of the dosing interval.

Next, take the natural log of both sides:

number = number (t') and then simply solve for t', which is now not an exponent.

Average Dose for Gentamicin or Tobramycin When Given as an Extended-Interval (i.e., once daily) Dose Based on Actual Body Weight

X_0 = 5.1 mg/kg actual body weight or adjusted body weight if IBW exceeds actual weight by ≥30%

Vancomycin Dosing Equations

Calculation of Population Estimate for *K* Based on CrCl

13-2 $K = 0.00083 \text{ hr}^{-1} [\text{CrCl (in mL/min)}] + 0.0044$

(See p. 204.)

Calculation of Population Estimate for Volume of Distribution (*V*) Based on TBW

13-1 $V = 0.9 \text{ L/kg TBW}$

(See p. 204.)

Note that, unlike the aminoglycosides, it is recommended that TBW be used to calculate the volume of distribution.

Calculation of Best Dosing Interval (τ) Based on Desired Peak and Trough Concentrations

13-4 $\tau = \dfrac{1}{-K}\left[\ln C_{\text{trough(desired)}} - \ln C_{\text{peak(desired)}}\right] + t + t'$

(See p. 205 and **Equation 12-4**.)

where:

   t = duration of infusion (usually 1 or 2 hours for vancomycin)

   t' = time between end of infusion and collection of blood sample (usually 2 hours)

Calculation of Initial Maintenance Dose (*K₀*) Based on Estimates of *K*, *V*, Desired *C*peak, τ, and *t*

13-3 $C_{ss\,\text{peak}} = \dfrac{K_0(1 - e^{-Kt})}{VK(1 - e^{-K\tau})} e^{-Kt'}$

(See p. 205 and **Equation 5-1**.)

where:

$C_{ss\,\text{peak}}$ = desired peak concentration (usually 2 hours after end of infusion)

K_0 = drug infusion rate (dose/infusion time)

   t = duration of infusion (usually 1 or 2 hours for vancomycin)

   K = estimated elimination rate constant

   V = estimated volume of distribution

   t' = time between end of infusion and collection of blood sample (usually 2 hours) (inclusion of t' is different from the calculation for aminoglycosides because sampling time for vancomycin is often at least 4 hours after the beginning of the infusion)

   τ = desired dosing interval, as determined above

Calculation of *C*trough Concentration Expected from Dose (*K₀*) and Dosing Interval Used (τ)

13-5 $C_{\text{trough}} = C_{ss\,\text{peak}} e^{-Kt''}$

(See p. 206 and **Equation 3-2**.)

where t'' is the difference in time between the two plasma concentrations.

Calculation of Patient-Specific (i.e., actual) *K* Based on Two Drug Concentrations and Dosing Interval

$$K = -\dfrac{\ln C_{\text{trough}} - \ln C_{\text{peak}}}{\tau - t - t'}$$

(See **Equation 3-1**.)

Calculation of Patient-Specific (i.e., actual) *V* Based on Actual *K* from Two Drug Concentrations, Dose (*K₀*), and τ

13-3 $C_{ss\,\text{peak}} = \dfrac{K_0(1 - e^{-Kt})}{VK(1 - e^{-K\tau})} e^{-Kt'}$

(See p. 205.)

where $C_{ss\,\text{peak}}$ = measured steady-state peak plasma concentration drawn 2 hours after end of infusion.

Calculation of Actual (i.e., new) Dosing Interval Based on Patient-Specific Value for K

13-4 $\tau = \dfrac{1}{-K}[\ln C_{\text{trough(desired)}} - \ln C_{\text{peak(desired)}}] + t + t'$

(See p. 205.)

Calculation of Patient-Specific Maintenance Dose (K_0) Based on Actual Values for K and V

13-3 $C_{ss\,\text{peak}} = \dfrac{K_0(1 - e^{-Kt})}{VK(1 - e^{-K\tau})} e^{-Kt'}$

(See p. 205.)

where:

$C_{ss\,\text{peak}}$ = desired peak concentration at steady state

$\quad K_0$ = drug infusion rate (also maintenance dose you are trying to calculate, in milligrams per hour)

$\quad V$ = volume of distribution

$\quad K$ = elimination rate constant calculated from C_{peak} and C_{trough}

$\quad t$ = infusion time (usually 1 or 2 hours)

$\quad t'$ = time from end of infusion until concentration is determined (usually 2 hours for peak)

$\quad \tau$ = desired or most appropriate dosing interval

Calculation of New Expected $C_{ss\,\text{trough}}$ That Would Result Based on a Known or Estimated $C_{ss\,\text{peak}}$ and Interval Used

13-5 $C_{ss\,\text{trough}} = C_{ss\,\text{peak}} e^{-Kt''}$

(See p. 206.)

where t'' is now the number of hours between the peak and trough ($t'' = \tau - t - t'$).

Calculation of Time to Hold Dose When Actual C_{trough} from Laboratory Is Too High

$$C_{\text{trough(desired)}} = C_{\text{trough(actual)}} e^{-Kt}$$

(See p. 34 and **Equation 3-2**.)

where t is the amount of time to hold the dose.

Next, take the natural log of both sides: number = number (t') and then simply solve for t' which is now not an exponent.

Theophylline Dosing Equations

Equation for Calculating the Volume of Distribution for Theophylline and Aminophylline

14-1 $V(\text{L}) = \text{weight (kg)} \times 0.5\ \text{L/kg}$

(See p. 223.)

Equation for Calculating a Loading Dose of Theophylline or Aminophylline

14-2 $D = \dfrac{(\text{Cpd})(V)}{SF}$

(See p. 223.)

Equation for Calculating Clearance for Theophylline or Aminophylline

14-3 $Cl = (0.04\ \text{L/kg/hr}) \times \text{weight (kg)}$

(See p. 223.)

Equation for Calculating a Theophylline or Aminophylline Maintenance Dose

14-4 $D = \dfrac{(\overline{C}p_{ss})(Cl\tau)}{SF}$

(See p. 224.)

Phenytoin Dosing Equations

Calculation of Population Estimate for Volume of Distribution (*V*)

$$V = 0.65 \text{ L/kg}$$

Michaelis–Menten Constant, Representing the Concentration of Phenytoin at Which the Rate of Enzyme-Saturable Hepatic Metabolism Is One-Half of Maximum (½*V*max)

$$K_m = 4 \text{ mg/L}$$

Maximum Amount of Drug That Can Be Metabolized per Unit Time

$$V_{max} = 7 \text{ mg/kg/day}$$

Note: Usually expressed as mg/day.

Calculation of Phenytoin Loading Dose

`1-1`
$$X_0 = \frac{V \times C_{desired}}{S}$$

(See p. 10.)

where:

V = volume of distribution estimate of 0.65 L/kg

$C_{desired}$ = concentration desired 1 hour after the end of the infusion

S = salt factor

Two Representations of Michaelis–Menten Equation Used to Calculate Daily Dose [*X*₀/τ (*S*)] or Expected Serum Concentration *C*ss

`10-1`
$$(X_0/\tau)(S) = \frac{V_{max} \times C_{ss}}{K_m + C_{ss}}$$

(See p. 148.)

`15-1`
$$C_{ss} = \frac{(X_0/\tau)(S)(K_m)}{V_{max} - X_0/\tau(S)}$$

(See p. 233.)

Calculation of Time (in Days) for Phenytoin Dosing Regimen to Reach Approximately 90% of Its Steady-State Concentration

`10-4`
$$t_{90\%} = \frac{K_m \times V}{(V_{max} - X_d)^2}[(2.3 \times V_{max}) - (0.9 \times X_d)]$$

(See p. 150.)

where:

X_d = daily dose of phenytoin (in milligrams per day)

V = volume of distribution

V_{max} = maximum rate of drug metabolism (in milligrams per day)

K_m = Michaelis–Menten constant

Phenytoin Dosing Methods

Method 1A (Empiric)

Use 5 mg/kg/day.

Method 1B (Population Parameters)

Use population estimates for the Michaelis–Menten values for K_m of 4 mg/L and V_{max} of 7 mg/kg/day and solve the general MME formula as shown below:

$$X_d = (X_0/\tau)(S) = \frac{V_{max} \times C_{ss\,desired}}{K_m + C_{ss\,desired}}$$

Method 2 (One Steady-State Level)

Use this method after you have one steady-state phenytoin serum drug concentration to solve for V_{max} while still using the population parameter for K_m.

First, to solve for V_{max}:

$$\boxed{10\text{-}1} \quad V_{max} = \frac{(X_d \times S)(K_m + C_{ss-lab})}{C_{ss-lab}}$$

(See p. 148.)

where:

V_{max} = calculated estimate of patient's V_{max}

K_m = population estimate of 4 mg/L

$X_d \times S$ = patient's daily dose of phenytoin free acid

C_{ss} = reported steady-state concentration

Second, after solving for this "better" value for V_{max}, use it plus the old K_m value in the MME to re-solve for dose, as shown below:

$$\boxed{10\text{-}1} \quad X_d \times S = \frac{V_{max} \times C_{ss}}{K_m + C_{ss}}$$

(See p. 148.)

where:

$X_d \times S$ = new dose of phenytoin (either free acid or salt)

C_{ss} = desired steady-state concentration (usually 15 mg/L)

K_m = population estimate of 4 mg/L

V_{max} = calculated estimate from above

Method 3 (Two Steady-State Levels)

Use after you have two steady-state phenytoin concentrations from two different phenytoin doses. You can now work another equation to solve for a better value for K_m (shown below). Then use this better K_m value to once again resolve for an even better V_{max} value than used in Method 2. Once you get new (i.e., real) K_m and V_{max}, resolve the MME equation for dose.

First, solve for "real" K_m. The slope of the line, which represents $-K_m$, can now be calculated as follows:

$$\boxed{10\text{-}2} \quad -K_m = \frac{X_1 - X_2}{\dfrac{X_1}{C_1} - \dfrac{X_2}{C_2}}$$

(See p. 148.)

where:

X = dose (where X is milligrams of free acid)

C = concentration

Next, we substitute this new value for K_m into the MME and solve for a V_{max} as follows:

$$\boxed{10\text{-}1} \quad V_{max} = \frac{(X_d \times S)(K_m + C_{ss})}{C_{ss}}$$

(See p. 148.)

where:

$X_d \times S$ = either of the doses the patient received, expressed as free acid

C_{ss} = steady-state concentration at the dose selected

K_m = calculated value

Finally, we substitute our new V_{max} value (mg/day) and our calculated K_m value (mg/mL) into the MME and solve for X_d as follows:

$$\boxed{10\text{-}1} \quad X_d \times S = \frac{V_{max} \times C_{ss}}{K_m + C_{ss}}$$

(See p. 148.)

Digoxin Dosing Equations

Volume of Distribution of Digoxin in Patients with Normal Renal Function

15-2 V_{ss} = 4 to 9 L/kg IBW (average, 7 L/kg IBW)

(See p. 243.)

Equation for Estimating Total Systemic Clearance for Digoxin

15-3 $Cl_t = (1.303 \times CrCl) + Cl_m$

(See p. 243.)

where:

 Cl_t is expressed as mL/min

 Cl_m = 40 mL/min in patients with no or mild heart failure

 = 20 mL/min in patients with moderate-to-severe heart failure

Equation Showing Relationship between Steady-State Plasma Concentration, Maintenance Dose, and Total Systemic Clearance

15-4 $$C_{ss} = \frac{X_d \times 10^6 \times F}{Cl_t \times \tau}$$

(See p. 244.)

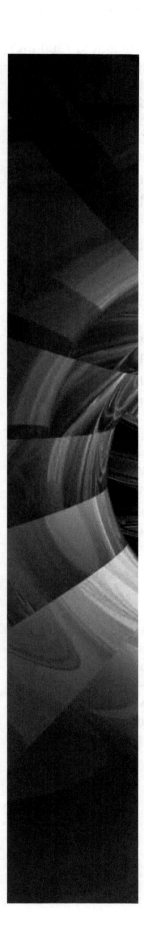

Supplemental Problems*

QUESTIONS

SP1.   Quinidine (a drug used for cardioversion in patients with atrial fibril-
       lation) was administered at a dose of 648 mg orally. After one dose of
       quinidine, the patient's sinus rhythm was restored. The following plasma
       drug concentration and time data were collected:

Time after Dose (hr)	Plasma Drug Concentration (mg/L)
5	46.1
7	44.3
14	40.7
24	34.2
38	28.6
54	24.3

Determine the approximate time after the dose when the plasma drug
concentration falls to 20 mg/L.

A. 32

B. 40

C. 60

D. 65

SP2.   Using the same data for quinidine dosing above, estimate the volume of
       distribution.

A. 16.4 L

B. 13.2 L

C. 10.9 L

D. 20.6 L

*These problems supplement material presented in Lessons 1–11.

SP3. Just after an IV dose of antibiotic X, the plasma drug concentration was 6.9 mg/L. Seven hours later, the concentration was 3.3 mg/L. Predict the plasma drug concentration at 12 hours after the dose.

A. 3.3 mg/L

B. 2.1 mg/L

C. 1.95 mg/L

D. 1.1 mg/L

SP4. The following plasma drug concentration and time data were obtained after an IV bolus dose of procainamide (420 mg):

Time after Dose (hr)	Plasma Drug Concentration (mg/L)
0	3.92
0.5	3.41
1	3.27
2	2.34
3	1.88
5	1.26
7	0.71
10	0.36

Calculate clearance by the area method.

A. 25.75 L/hr

B. 19.4 L/hr

C. 33.6 L/hr

D. 11.8 L/hr

SP5. What will be the minimum concentration after the tenth IV dose of drug X if C_{max} equals 175 mg/L after the first dose, K equals 0.5 hr^{-1}, and τ equals 8 hours? (Assume an IV bolus dose model.)

A. 2.56 mg/L

B. 4.85 mg/L

C. 3.26 mg/L

D. 7.56 mg/L

SP6. An IV bolus dose of antibiotic Q (500 mg) was administered to a patient on an every-8-hour schedule. Predict the plasma drug concentrations at 4 and 8 hours after dosing. Assume: (1) a one-compartment model, (2) $T\frac{1}{2} = 5.35$ hours, (3) $Cl_t = 12.9$ L/hr, and (4) the attainment of steady state.

A. 4.68 and 2.78 mg/L, respectively

B. 7.87 and 4.67 mg/L, respectively

C. 5.53 and 2.52 mg/L, respectively

D. 2.78 and 2.32 mg/L, respectively

SP7. For the same patient, predict the plasma concentrations at 4 and 8 hours after the second dose.

A. 6.93 and 3.34 mg/L, respectively

B. 3.32 and 2.19 mg/L, respectively

C. 7.87 and 4.12 mg/L, respectively

D. 4.12 and 2.45 mg/L, respectively

SP8. An 80-kg patient receives 1000 mg of drug Y intravenously by bolus injection every 6 hours. Assume that $V = 0.5$ L/kg, and $T\frac{1}{2} = 6.4$ hours. Predict the steady-state peak and trough concentrations.

A. 28.6 and 14.7 mg/L, respectively

B. 52.4 and 27.4 mg/L, respectively

C. 24.3 and 12.9 mg/L, respectively

D. 19.8 and 9.6 mg/L, respectively

SP9. Calculate the theophylline clearance (Cl_t) for a 52-kg patient receiving a continuous IV infusion of aminophylline at 60 mg/hr. The patient's steady-state plasma theophylline concentration with this dose rate is 20.2 mg/L. Assume that the patient's $V = 0.45$ L/kg. Remember, aminophylline = 80% theophylline.

A. 2.38 L/hr

B. 3.75 L/hr

C. 3.71 L/hr

D. 2.37 L/hr

SP10. The following plasma concentration and time data were collected after a single 500-mg IV dose of amikacin:

Time after Dose (hr)	Amikacin Concentration (mg/L)
2	25.4
4	19.3
8	13.7
16	7.8
24	4
36	1.6
48	0.75

Calculate K, V_{area}, and Cl_t for this patient.

A. 0.18 hr^{-1}, 16.5 L, and 1.49 L/hr, respectively

B. 0.01 hr^{-1}, 1.65 L, and 0.1493e L/hr, respectively

C. 0.09 hr^{-1}, 16.5 L, and 1.49 L/hr, respectively

D. 0.09 hr^{-1}, 165 L, and 16.5 L/hr, respectively

SP11. Seven healthy female subjects were each given 1500 mg of an experimental drug (BB-K8) by IV bolus administration. The drug follows first-order kinetics. The following mean plasma concentration and time data were obtained:

Time after Dose (hr)	Mean Plasma Drug Concentration (mg/L)
0	116
0.08	108.3
0.17	92.8
0.25	83.3
0.5	59.2
0.75	38.2
1	30.6
1.5	22.9
2	19.7
3	13.2
4	9.3
5	7.3
6	5.1
7	4.1
8	2.8

Plot the plasma concentration versus time profile on semilog paper. From your graph, determine A, B, α, β, V_{area}, and Cl_t (in milliliters per minute).

A. -3.60 hr^{-1}, 0.41 hr^{-1}, 39.1 L, and 11 L/hr, respectively

B. -2.60 hr^{-1}, 0.31 hr^{-1}, 29.1 L, and 9 L/hr, respectively

C. -1.60 hr^{-1}, 0.21 hr^{-1}, 19.1 L, and 7 L/hr, respectively

D. -4.60 hr^{-1}, 0.35 hr^{-1}, 49.1 L, and 12 L/hr, respectively

SP12. Calculate V_{area} given the data in Supplemental Problem 1. Compare it with the V calculated (using the back-extrapolation method) in Supplemental Problem 2.

A. 24.6 L

B. 12.9 L

C. 8.3 L

D. 33.7 L

SP13. An outpatient had been taking 500 mg of phenytoin per day for 1 month and had a plasma concentration of 7 mg/L when sampled 6 hours after the dose. Because of continued seizures, the dose was increased to 600 mg/day. Four weeks later, the patient was seen in a clinic, and the plasma drug concentration 6 hours after the dose was 10 mg/L (assume steady state). The physicians asked that the dose be increased to provide a plasma concentration of 13 mg/L 6 hours after the dose. What dose would you recommend?

A. 652 mg phenytoin free acid/day

B. 700 mg phenytoin free acid/day

C. 752 mg phenytoin free acid/day

D. 900 mg phenytoin free acid/day

ANSWERS

SP1. A, B, C. *Incorrect answers*

D. **CORRECT ANSWER**

$$K = -\frac{(\ln 44.3 - \ln 28.6)}{(38 - 7 \text{ hr})} = 0.014 \text{ hr}^{-1}$$

$$C_2 = C_1 e^{-Kt}$$

$$20 \text{ mg/dL} = (46.1 \text{ mg/L})e^{-0.014 \text{ hr}^{-1}(t)}$$

$$t = 60 \text{ hours}$$

Since the serum drug concentration was drawn 5 hours after the dose, and the question asks how long after dose administration,

$$t = 60 + 5 = 65 \text{ hours}$$

Your answer may vary slightly due to differences in how your graph was drawn. This is why using known points to calculate K is more accurate.

SP2. A, C, D. *Incorrect answers*

B. **CORRECT ANSWER**

$$C_0 = 49 \text{ mg/L}$$

$$V = \frac{\text{dose}}{C_0} = \frac{648 \text{ mg}}{49 \text{ mg/L}} = 13.2 \text{ L}$$

SP3. A, B, D. *Incorrect answers*

C. **CORRECT ANSWER.** First, calculate the elimination rate constant (K):

First, calculate the elimination rate constant (K):

$$K = -\frac{(\ln 6.9 - \ln 3.3)}{(0 - 7 \text{ hr})} = 0.105 \text{ hr}^{-1}$$

Then use these equations:

$$C = C_0 e^{-Kt}$$

$$C_{\text{at 12 hr}} = (6.9 \text{ mg/L})e^{-0.105 \text{ hr}^{-1}(12 \text{ hr})}$$

$$= 1.95 \text{ mg/L}$$

SP4. A. **CORRECT ANSWER.** To calculate clearance by the area method, we need to know the area under the plasma concentration curve (AUC) and the dose (X_0). Therefore, it is first necessary to calculate AUC using the trapezoidal method as shown below. Note that one way to indicate an AUC from one time point to another is as $AUC_{0 \to 0.5}$, which means AUC from 0 to 0.5 hour.

$$AUC_{0 \to 0.5} = \frac{(3.92 \text{ mg/L} + 3.41 \text{ mg/L})}{2} \times (0.5 - 0 \text{ hr})$$

$$= 1.83 \text{ (mg/L)} \times \text{hr}$$

$$AUC_{0.5 \to 1} = \frac{(3.41 + 3.27)}{2} \times (1 - 0.5) = 1.67 \text{ (mg/L)} \times \text{hr}$$

$$AUC_{1 \to 2} = \frac{(3.27 + 2.34)}{2} \times (2 - 1) = 2.81 \text{ (mg/L)} \times \text{hr}$$

$$AUC_{2 \to 3} = \frac{(2.34 + 1.88)}{2} \times (3 - 2) = 2.11 \text{ (mg/L)} \times \text{hr}$$

$$AUC_{3 \to 5} = \frac{(1.88 + 1.26)}{2} \times (5 - 3) = 3.14 \text{ (mg/L)} \times \text{hr}$$

$$AUC_{5 \to 7} = \frac{(1.26 + 0.71)}{2} \times (7 - 5) = 1.76 \text{ (mg/L)} \times \text{hr}$$

$$AUC_{7 \to 10} = \frac{(0.71 + 0.36)}{2} \times (10 - 7) = 1.61 \text{ (mg/L)} \times \text{hr}$$

$$AUC_{10 \to \infty} = \frac{C_{10 \text{ hr}}}{K} = \frac{0.36 \text{ mg/L}}{0.26 \text{ hr}^{-1}} = 1.38 \text{ (mg/L)} \times \text{hr}$$

$$AUC = 1.83 + 1.67 + 2.81 + 2.11 + 3.14 + 1.76 + 1.61 + 1.38$$

$$= 16.31 \text{ (mg/L)} \times \text{hr}$$

$$Cl_t = \frac{X_0}{AUC} = \frac{420 \text{ mg}}{16.31 \text{ (mg/L)} \times \text{hr}} = 25.75 \text{ L/hr}$$

B, C, D. *Incorrect answers*

SP5. A, B, D. *Incorrect answers*

C. CORRECT ANSWER. To determine C_{min} after the tenth dose, first calculate C_{max} after the tenth dose using the multiple-dose equation:

$$C_{max(n\text{th dose})} = C_{max(n\text{th dose})}\frac{(1-e^{-nK\tau})}{(1-e^{-K\tau})}$$

$$C_{max\,10} = C_{max\,1}\frac{(1-e^{-10K\tau})}{(1-e^{-K\tau})}$$

$$= (175 \text{ mg/L})\frac{(1-e^{(-10)(0.5\text{ hr}^{-1})(8\text{ hr})})}{(1-e^{(-0.5\text{ hr}^{-1})(8\text{ hr})})}$$

$$= 178 \text{ mg/L}$$

Then:

$$C_{min\,10} = C_{max\,10}e^{-K\tau} = (178 \text{ mg/L})e^{(-0.5\text{ hr}^{-1})(8\text{ hr})}$$

$$= 3.26 \text{ mg/L}$$

SP6. A. CORRECT ANSWER. To predict plasma concentrations 4 and 8 hours after a dose at steady state, we should first estimate the C_{max} (at 0 hour after the dose) using the steady-state IV equation:

$$C_{max} = \frac{X_0}{V(1-e^{-K\tau})}$$

So we first need to estimate V and K. V can be estimated from:

$$Cl_t = VK$$

Note that:

$$K = \frac{0.693}{T_{1/2}} = 0.129 \text{ hr}^{-1}$$

Then:

$$V = \frac{Cl_t}{K} = \frac{12.9 \text{ L/hr}}{\left(\dfrac{0.693}{5.35 \text{ hr}}\right)}$$

$$V = 100 \text{ L}$$

Then:

$$C_{max} = \frac{500 \text{ mg}}{(100 \text{ L})(1-e^{-0.129\text{ hr}^{-1}(8\text{ hr})})}$$

$$= 7.77 \text{ mg/L}$$

From C_{max}, the concentration at any time after a dose can be calculated by:

$$C_t = C_{max}e^{-Kt}$$

So:

$$C_{4\text{ hr}} = (7.77 \text{ mg/L})(e^{-0.129\text{ hr}^{-1}(4\text{ hr})})$$

$$= 4.64 \text{ mg/L}$$

and:

$$C_{8\text{ hr}} = (7.77 \text{ mg/L})(e^{-0.129\text{ hr}^{-1}(8\text{ hr})})$$

$$= 2.77 \text{ mg/L}$$

B, C, D. *Incorrect answers*

SP7. A, B, C. *Incorrect answers*

D. CORRECT ANSWER. The equations used to solve Supplemental Problem 5 can be used here, with the number of doses (n) equal to 2 rather than 13:

$$C_{max(2\text{nd dose})} = \frac{X_0(1-e^{-nK\tau})}{V(1-e^{-K\tau})}$$

$$= \frac{(500 \text{ mg})(1-e^{(-2)(-0.13\text{ hr}^{-1})(8\text{ hr})})}{(97.69 \text{ L})(1-e^{(-0.13\text{ hr}^{-1})(8\text{ hr})})}$$

$$= 6.93 \text{ mg/L}$$

Then:

$$C_t = C_{max}e^{-Kt}$$

$$C_{4\,hr} = (6.93 \text{ mg/L})(e^{(-0.13 \text{ hr}^{-1})(4 \text{ hr})})$$

$$= 4.64 \text{ mg/L}$$

$$C_{8\,hr} = (6.93 \text{ mg/L})(e^{(-0.13 \text{ hr}^{-1})(8 \text{ hr})})$$

$$= 2.45 \text{ mg/L}$$

SP8.   A, C, D. *Incorrect answers*

B.   CORRECT ANSWER. First, determine K and total V:

$$V = 0.5 \text{ L/kg} \times 80 \text{ kg} = 40 \text{ L}$$

$$K = \frac{0.693}{T \frac{1}{2}} = \frac{0.693}{6.4 \text{ hr}} = 0.108 \text{ hr}^{-1}$$

Then use the steady-state multiple-dose equation (for IV bolus doses):

$$C_{peak} = \frac{X_0}{V}\left(\frac{1}{1-e^{-K\tau}}\right)$$

$$= \frac{1000 \text{ mg}}{(40 \text{ L})(1-e^{-0.108 \text{ hr}^{-1}(6 \text{ hr})})}$$

$$= 52.4 \text{ mg/L}$$

$$C_{trough} = C_{peak}e^{-K\tau}$$

$$= (52.4 \text{ mg/L})e^{-0.108 \text{ hr}^{-1}(6 \text{ hr})}$$

$$= 27.4 \text{ mg/L}$$

SP9.   A.   CORRECT ANSWER. To calculate clearance, use the relationship:

$$Cl_t = \frac{K_0}{C_{ss}} = \frac{60 \text{ mg/hr} (0.80)}{20.2 \text{ mg/L}} = 2.38 \text{ L/hr}$$

B, C, D. *Incorrect answers*

SP10.   A, B, D. *Incorrect answers*

C.   CORRECT ANSWER. First, the data should be plotted on semilog graph paper to determine if they are linear or nonlinear. When the points are determined to make a straight line, any two may be chosen to calculate K. (It is best, however, to choose two that are not close to each other, such as 2 and 4 hours.) So:

$$K = -\left(\frac{\Delta Y}{\Delta X}\right) = -\left(\frac{\ln 1.6 - \ln 25.4}{36 \text{ hr} - 2 \text{ hr}}\right) = 0.08 \text{ hr}^{-1}$$

Then:

$$T \frac{1}{2} = \frac{0.693}{K} = 8.7 \text{ hr}$$

To calculate V_{area} and Cl_t, we should first estimate the AUC. With a one compartment, first-order model after IV administration, the calculation of AUC is simplified. In this case:

$$AUC = \frac{C_0}{K}$$

where C_0 is determined by $C_t = C_0e^{-Kt}$. For $t = 2$ hours:

$$25.4 \text{ mg/L} = C_0e^{-0.08 \text{ hr}^{-1}(2 \text{ hr})}$$

Then:

$$C_0 = 29.88 \text{ mg/L}$$

and:

$$AUC = \frac{29.88 \text{ mg/L}}{0.08 \text{ hr}^{-1}}$$

$$= 374 \text{ mg/L} \times \text{hr}$$

Then:

$$V_{area} = \frac{X_0}{AUC \times K}$$

$$= \frac{500 \text{ mg}}{(374 \text{ mg/L} \times hr)(0.08 \text{ hr}^{-1})}$$

$$= 16.71 \text{ L}$$

$$Cl_t = \frac{X_0}{AUC}$$

$$= \frac{500 \text{ mg}}{(374 \text{ mg/L} \times hr)} = 1.34 \text{ L/hr}$$

Note that the use of AUC for calculation of clearance generally produces a more accurate estimate than the use of $Cl_t = K \times V$.

SP11. A, C, D. *Incorrect answers*

B. CORRECT ANSWER. A, B, α, and β will be calculated using residuals. First, back-extrapolate the terminal (straight-line) portion of the plot and estimate the back-extrapolated points. Determine the residual points by subtracting the back-extrapolated concentrations from the actual concentrations.

Actual Points		Back Extrapolated Points		Residual Points
108.3	–	32	=	76.3 mg/L
92.8	–	31	=	61.8 mg/L
83.3	–	30	=	53.3 mg/L
59.2	–	28	=	31.2 mg/L
38.2	–	26	=	12.2 mg/L
30.6	–	24	=	6.6 mg/L
22.9	–	21	=	1.9 mg/L

Then *plot the* residual points on the same graph. From the back-extrapolated line, the intercept = B (equals 33 mg/L) and the terminal slope gives β:

$$\beta = \frac{\ln 2.8 - \ln 13.2}{8 \text{ hr} - 3 \text{ hr}} = -0.31$$

$$= -0.31 \text{ hr}^{-1}$$

Then from the residual line, the intercept = A (equals 84 mg/L) and the slope gives α:

$$\alpha = \frac{\ln 1.9 - \ln 76.3}{1.5 \text{ hr} - 0.08 \text{ hr}} = -2.60$$

$$= -2.60 \text{ hr}^{-1}$$

To calculate V_{area} and Cl_t, the AUC must first be determined. The AUC can be estimated using the trapezoidal rule or by adding the area of each exponential equation:

$$AUC = \frac{A}{\alpha} + \frac{B}{\beta} = 32.3 + 106.5$$

$$= 138.8 \text{ (mg/L)} \times hr$$

Then:

$$V_{area} = \frac{dose}{AUC \times \beta}$$

$$= \frac{1500 \text{ mg}}{[138.8 \text{ (mg/L)} \times hr](0.31 \text{ hr}^{-1})} = 34.9 \text{ L}$$

$$Cl_t = \frac{dose}{AUC}$$

$$= \frac{1500 \text{ mg}}{138.8 \text{ mg/L}} = 10.8 \text{ L/hr}$$

SP12. A, B, C. *Incorrect answers*

D. CORRECT ANSWER.

$$V_{area} = \frac{dose}{AUC \times K}$$

$$K = 0.014 \text{ hr}^{-1}$$

To calculate the AUC, the C_0 must first be estimated from the plot ($C_0 = 49$ mg/L):

$$\text{AUC}_{0\to5} = \frac{(49.0 + 46.1)(5 - 0)}{2} = 237.7 \text{ (mg/L)} \times \text{hr}$$

$$\text{AUC}_{5\to7} = \frac{(46.1 + 44.3)(7 - 5)}{2} = 90.4 \text{ (mg/L)} \times \text{hr}$$

$$\text{AUC}_{7\to14} = \frac{(44.3 + 40.7)(14 - 7)}{2} = 297.5 \text{ (mg/L)} \times \text{hr}$$

$$\text{AUC}_{14\to24} = \frac{(40.7 + 34.2)(24 - 14)}{2} = 374.5 \text{ (mg/L)} \times \text{hr}$$

$$\text{AUC}_{24\to38} = \frac{(34.2 + 28.6)(38 - 24)}{2} = 439.6 \text{ (mg/L)} \times \text{hr}$$

$$\text{AUC}_{38\to54} = \frac{(28.6 + 24.3)(54 - 38)}{2} = 423.2 \text{ (mg/L)} \times \text{hr}$$

$$\text{AUC}_{54\to\infty} = \frac{C_{54}}{K} = \frac{24.3 \text{ mg/L}}{0.014 \text{ hr}^{-1}} = 1735.7 \text{ (mg/L)} \times \text{hr}$$

Then:

$$\text{AUC} = 237.7 + 90.4 + 297.5 + 374.5$$
$$+ 439.6 + 423.2 + 1735.7$$

$$= 3598.6 \text{ (mg/L)} \times \text{hr}$$

$$V_{\text{area}} = \frac{X_0}{\text{AUC} \times K}$$

$$= \frac{648 \text{ mg}}{[3598.6 \text{ (mg/L)} \times \text{hr}](0.014 \text{ hr}^{-1})}$$

$$= 12.86 \text{ L}$$

So, in this case, the two estimates for V are similar.

SP13. A, C, D. *Incorrect answers*

B. CORRECT ANSWER. Phenytoin follows Michaelis–Menten (saturable) pharmaco- kinetics. To determine V_m and K_m, the daily dose must be plotted (y-axis) versus the daily dose divided by the resulting steady-state concentrations (x-axis). From a plot of the dose (y-axis) versus dose/concentration (x-axis), the following are observed:

$V_m = 1200$ mg daily (which is equal to the y-intercept)

$K_m = 8.8$ mg/L (which equals –slope)

Then:

$$\text{dose} = \frac{V_m C_{ss}}{K_m + C_{ss}}$$

where:

$C_{ss} = 13$ mg/L, the desired concentration:

$$= \frac{(1200 \text{ mg})(13 \text{ mg/L})}{8.8 \text{ mg/L} + 13 \text{ mg/L}} = 715 \text{ mg/day}$$

Therefore, the likely daily dose would be 700 mg/day.

Alternatively, you can use **Equation 10-2 on page 148** to calculate $-K_m$ from these two doses and two levels. Both methods should give the same answer.

Glossary

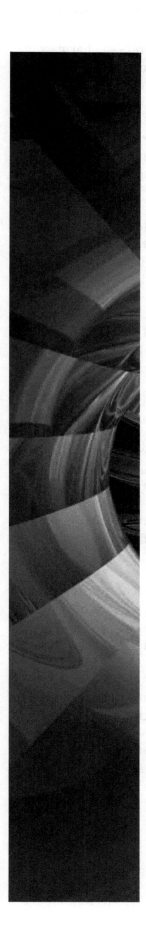

Area under the first moment curve (AUMC)—the area under the first moment curve (drug concentration × time) versus time (moment) curve, an important model-independent pharmacokinetic parameter.

Area under the plasma concentration versus time curve (AUC)—the area formed under the curve when plasma drug concentration is plotted versus time. Drug clearance is equal to the dose administered divided by AUC.

Bioavailability (F)—the fraction of a given drug dose that reaches the systemic circulation.

Biopharmaceutics—the study of the relationship between the nature and intensity of a drug's biologic effects and various drug formulation or administration factors, such as the drug's chemical nature, inert formulation substances, pharmaceutical processes used to manufacture the dosage form, and routes of administration.

Clearance—the process of removing a drug from plasma (expressed as volume of plasma per a given unit of time).

Clinical pharmacokinetics—the application of pharmacokinetic principles to the safe and effective therapeutic management of drugs in an individual patient.

Compartmental model—a basic type of model used in pharmacokinetics. Compartmental models are categorized by the number of compartments needed to describe the drug's behavior in the body. There are one-compartment, two-compartment, and multi-compartment models. The compartments do not represent a specific tissue or fluid but may represent a group of similar tissues or fluids.

Drug distribution—transport processes that deliver drug to body tissues and fluids after absorption.

50% effective concentration (EC_{50})—the concentration at which 50% of the maximum drug effect is achieved.

Elimination rate constant (K)—a constant representing the fraction of drug removed per unit of time (in units of reciprocal time, usually hr^{-1}).

Extraction ratio (E)—the fraction of drug removed from plasma by one pass through an organ. This ratio is a number between 1 and 0. Organs that are very efficient at eliminating a drug will have an extraction ratio approaching 1 (i.e., 100% extraction).

First-order elimination—when the amount of drug eliminated from the body in a specific time is dependent on the amount of drug in the body at that time. A straight line is obtained from the natural log of plasma drug concentration versus time plot only for drugs that follow first-order elimination.

First-pass effect—drug metabolism by the liver that occurs after absorption but before the drug reaches the systemic circulation.

Formation clearance ($CL_{P \to mX}$)—a model-independent parameter that provides a meaningful estimate of a drug's fractional metabolic clearance.

Half-life ($T\frac{1}{2}$)—the amount of time necessary for a plasma drug concentration to decrease by half.

Kinetic homogeneity—the predictable relationship between plasma drug concentration and concentration at the receptor site.

Mean residence time (MRT)—the average time for intact drug molecules to transit or reside in the body.

Minimum inhibitory concentration—the lowest concentration of an antibacterial agent that will inhibit the visible growth of a microorganism after overnight incubation.

Model—a simplified mathematical simulation of physiologic processes used to predict the time course of drug concentrations or effect in the body.

Model-independent parameter—a pharmacokinetic parameter, such as clearance, that can be calculated without the use of a specific model.

Model-independent pharmacokinetics—pharmacokinetic calculations using parameters that do not require the use of specific compartmental models (e.g., one-compartment, two-compartment, etc.).

Pharmacodynamics—the relationship between drug concentrations at the site of action and the resulting effect, including the time course and intensity of therapeutic and adverse effects.

Pharmacokinetics—the relationship of drug dose to the time course of drug absorption, distribution, metabolism, and excretion.

Plasma—the fluid portion of blood (including soluble proteins but not formed elements).

Receptor—a structure on the surface of a cell to which a drug binds and causes an effect within the cell.

Serum—the fluid portion of blood that remains when the soluble protein fibrinogen is removed from plasma.

Steady state—the point at which, after multiple doses, the amount of drug administered over a dosing interval equals the amount of drug being eliminated over that same period.

Therapeutic drug monitoring—determination of plasma drug concentrations and clinical data to optimize a patient's drug therapy.

Therapeutic range—the plasma concentration range that is effective and safe in treating specific diseases.

Tolerance—decreased drug effectiveness with continued use.

Volume of distribution (V)—an important indicator of the extent of drug distribution into body fluids and tissues, V relates the amount of drug in the body to the measured concentration in the plasma. Thus, V is the volume required to account for all of the drug in the body if the concentration in all tissues is the same as the plasma concentration.

Volume of distribution at steady state (V_{ss})—a parameter that relates total amount of drug in the body to a particular plasma concentration under steady-state conditions.

Zero-order elimination—when the amount of drug eliminated for each time interval is constant, regardless of the amount of drug in the body.

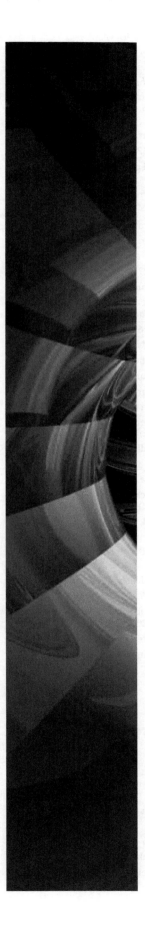

Page numbers followed by an *f* refer to figures; those followed by a *t* refer to tables.